T0325068

UNEQUAL COVERAGE

ANTHROPOLOGIES OF AMERICAN MEDICINE:
CULTURE, POWER, AND PRACTICE
General Editors: Paul Brodwin, Michele Rivkin-Fish, and Susan Shaw

Transnational Reproduction: Race, Kinship, and Commercial Surrogacy in India
Daisy Deomampo

Unequal Coverage: The Experience of Health Care Reform in the United States
Edited by Jessica M. Mulligan and Heide Castañeda

Unequal Coverage

The Experience of Health Care Reform in the United States

Edited by

Jessica M. Mulligan *and* Heide Castañeda

NEW YORK UNIVERSITY PRESS

New York

NEW YORK UNIVERSITY PRESS
New York
www.nyupress.org

References to Internet websites (URLs) were accurate at the time of writing. Neither the author nor New York University Press is responsible for URLs that may have expired or changed since the manuscript was prepared.

Library of Congress Cataloging-in-Publication Data
Names: Mulligan, Jessica M., editor. | Castañeda, Heide, editor.
Title: Unequal coverage : the experience of health care reform in the United States / edited by Jessica M. Mulligan and Heide Castañeda.
Description: New York : New York University Press, [2017] | Includes bibliographical references and index.
Identifiers: LCCN 2017012923 | ISBN 9781479897001 (cl : alk. paper) | ISBN 9781479848737 (pb : alk. paper)
Subjects: LCSH: Health care reform—United States. | Medical policy—United States. | Medical care—United States.
Classification: LCC RA395.A3 U48 2017 | DDC 362.1/0425—dc23
LC record available at https://lccn.loc.gov/2017012923

New York University Press books are printed on acid-free paper, and their binding materials are chosen for strength and durability. We strive to use environmentally responsible suppliers and materials to the greatest extent possible in publishing our books.

Manufactured in the United States of America

10 9 8 7 6 5 4 3 2 1

Also available as an ebook

CONTENTS

ILLUSTRATIONS

ACKNOWLEDGMENTS

This book developed over five years and has enjoyed the help and support of many collaborators along the way. The project initially emerged from a "SMA Takes a Stand" initiative by the Critical Anthropology of Global Health Special Interest Group of the Society for Medical Anthropology (SMA), a section of the American Anthropological Association (AAA). In 2012, a statement was developed to address the issue of health insurance reform and was made publicly available for comment on the SMA website. The statement analyzed the pending Affordable Care Act (ACA) insurance reform in the United States through the lessons learned from transformations of health care systems worldwide, and situated the ACA within the context of broader theoretical questions about recent neoliberal changes in health care, the state, and the social contract. The statement was then revised and published in *Medical Anthropology Quarterly*. Sarah Horton and Fayana Richards organized an invited panel on insurance as part of the 2011 AAA meeting in Montreal, Quebec, which resulted in a special issue of *Medical Anthropology Quarterly* (issue 30[1]) on insurance in 2016.

Continuing the conversation, the editors of this volume, with contributor Emily Brunson, assembled a double, invited session on the ACA at the 2014 AAA annual meetings in Washington, DC. We would like to thank the discussants, Lauren E. Gulbas (University of Texas at Austin) and Sarah B. Horton (University of Colorado-Denver), for their thoughtful feedback on all the papers and for setting us on a path that would eventually develop into a book manuscript.

Many of the presenters from this session then participated in a seminar at the School for Advanced Research (SAR) in Santa Fe, New Mexico in October 2015. Thank you to SAR for funding our seminar, "Transformations in Social Citizenship: Stratification, Risk and Responsibility in Health Care Reform," and for providing the incredible luxury of time, space, and sustenance that allowed us to workshop the chapters and discuss the ideas from which this book developed. We would especially like to acknowledge Michael F. Brown, Nicole Taylor and the staff at Scholar Programs, and Leslie Shipman, Carla Tozcano, and the rest of the Guest Services staff for making us feel at home.

The editors would also like to thank the book's contributors, who all graciously participated in a several-years-long conversation about the Affordable Care Act and responded to countless requests for information, editing, and revision. The themes that run throughout this book are the product of our collective conversations, and we are grateful to have had such engaged and knowledgeable interlocutors.

Other colleagues provided critical feedback and constructive suggestions along the way, including Amy Dao, Tuba Agartan, Janet Bronstein, Karin Friederic, Kyle Kusz, Sarah Horton, Deborah Levine, Laura López-Sanders, Helen Marrow, Mark Nichter, Harris Solomon, and Rebecca Warne Peters. We would also like to acknowledge the contribution of various students who helped with finalizing the book—Paola Gonzalez (USF) assisted with references and Samantha Santos (PC) helped with permissions.

We would like to thank our institutions for support in procuring the images that appear throughout the volume. The images were funded by the Health Policy and Management Program, Providence College; the School of Professional Studies, Providence College; and the University of South Florida's Women in Leadership and Philanthropy (WLP) organization.

Thank you to the anonymous reviewers, who supported the project and whose comments helped to refine and sharpen the final product. Thanks also to the editors of the Anthropologies of American Medicine series—Paul Brodwin, Michele Rivkin-Fish, and Susan Shaw. Finally, we are grateful to NYU Press, and to Jennifer Hammer, Amy Klopfenstein, and other staff for their support of the project and their expertise in transforming our work from a hazy idea to its finished book form.

Jessica M. Mulligan would like to thank her family for hosting many extended research trips to Florida and for the uncompensated child care dispensed in the name of research. The whole family has participated in and supported this project in one way or another. When Norah (who is 5) sees someone talk about health insurance on television, she now says, "Mom, you should interview them." Thank you, Norah and Kyle, for being willing to be enlisted into the research endeavor. And thank you Kyle for shaping my ideas about Trump, whiteness, and resentment (in a good way).

Heide Castañeda would like to thank her family and friends for endless discussions on health care reform and U.S. politics, as well as colleagues and students at the University for South Florida for their encouragement and support of this project.

We hope this book celebrates what worked in the ACA and inspires us to do better in the future, in the name of those who could not afford to use their insurance and those who remain uncovered.

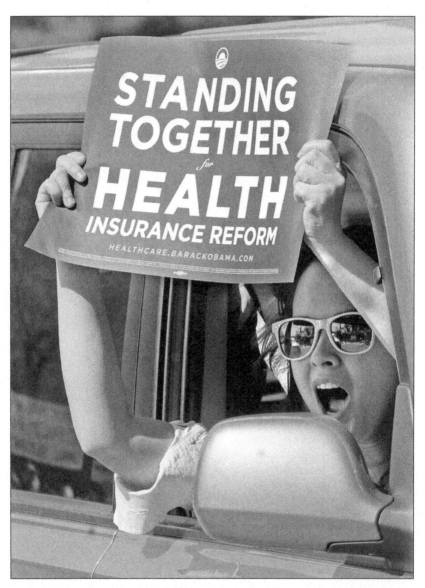

Figure I.1. Standing Together for Health Insurance Reform. A passerby yells in support of health care during a Tea Party protest against the proposed health care plan outside Congresswoman Melissa Bean's office in Schaumburg, Illinois, Tuesday, March 16, 2010. (AP photo/Paul Beaty)

Introduction

JESSICA M. MULLIGAN AND HEIDE CASTAÑEDA

Daniel visited the customer service center at the Rhode Island health insurance exchange close to the last day of open enrollment. He had heard about health reform, but could not figure out how to sign up. Daniel joked with the enrollment specialist about how difficult the application was: "I'm even a computer guy!" he said. The specialist was not chatty; she efficiently took his information and entered it, her screen facing away from Daniel. The waiting room was overflowing with people—some waited in their cars because the building was at capacity. The enrollment specialist would be there late into the evening.

After a few more keyboard clicks and consenting to all the required government legalese, Daniel was happy to find out that he qualified for Medicaid. As a person with Type 1 diabetes who had gone a decade without insurance coverage, Daniel was visibly relieved. He had to pick a Medicaid plan and wanted to make sure that the endocrinologist he had been paying out of pocket to see for years participated in the plan's network. He was upbeat and asked twice about the co-pays. "It's all free?" he asked. "All free," the enrollment specialist assured him.

Three months after Daniel's enrollment, he was interviewed about his experience while seated at the dining room table in his apartment in Pawtucket, a New England mill town whose industries have mostly relocated elsewhere. Daniel lived on the third floor of a triple-decker with angled walls and sloped ceilings. Daniel was single, white, and lived alone with his cat. He was 28 years old and had a high school education. He started technical schools a couple of times because he really wanted to be a computer programmer, but he was never able to finish. He accrued more than $10,000 in student loans from these attempts and was struggling to make the payments. In March, he worked part-time making deliveries for an auto parts store; in May he had a new job with additional hours at a warehouse.

Daniel said he was trying to unlearn some of the habits he developed when he was uninsured: He had stopped checking his glucose regularly because he couldn't afford the test strips; he didn't always have enough medication, so he skipped doses or just ate less; he didn't have enough needles, so he reused them five times or more.

Gaining access to Medicaid greatly reduced Daniel's chances of being hospitalized again in diabetic shock. He was still receiving bills from before he was covered. One thing he didn't miss, he said, was having to complete paperwork for charity care when he was slipping in and out of consciousness. Now that his supplies and medication were covered, he was back on a regular testing and insulin regimen. He was also getting help from his health plan to quit smoking.

Daniel's case shows a best-case scenario for the Affordable Care Act (ACA), a sweeping overhaul of the U.S. health insurance system signed into law in 2010. This legislation was the most dramatic reform to the U.S. health care system since the passage of Medicare and Medicaid in 1965. For some, like Daniel, the ACA represented a huge improvement in their life chances. They were incorporated into new and expanded programs that offered health coverage, including expanded Medicaid for adults in many states, which in Daniel's case gave him a real opportunity to manage his chronic health condition. As a person with diabetes, he would have been uninsurable on the individual market prior to the ACA, since insurance companies could discriminate against those with preexisting health conditions. In 2011, there were 48 million nonelderly uninsured people in the United States, roughly 18% of the nonelderly population (Kaiser Commission on Medicaid and the Uninsured 2012). By 2016, the number of nonelderly uninsured had fallen to 27 million, or 10% of the nonelderly population (Kaiser Commission on Medicaid and the Uninsured 2016). Because of the law's reforms, the U.S. uninsured rate declined by 43% between 2010 and 2015, with improvements in affordability, financial security related to health care debt, and a reduction in the amount of nonelderly adults reporting fair or poor health (Obama 2016).

Yet for others, the ACA did little to address their exclusion from health care. As the chapters in this book detail, some people, such as undocumented and recent immigrants, were intentionally excluded from coverage under the law to establish boundaries around national belonging; others were excluded by affordability, by bureaucratic hurdles, and by choice; and still others were excluded by virtue of state policies in the wake of a Supreme Court decision, *National Federation of Independent Business v. Sebelius*, Secretary of Health and Human Services, in 2012 that made a key provision, the expansion of Medicaid, optional.[1] Thus, while the law represented an extension of social protections to some groups previously excluded from health insurance, in other ways, it created new forms of exclusion as access to affordable coverage options were highly segmented by state of residence, income, and citizenship status. This book documents the everyday experiences of individuals and families across nine states as they attempted to access coverage and care in the wake of the passage of the ACA between 2012 and 2017. It shows that people in the United States desperately wanted and needed affordable health insurance coverage; however, stratified approaches to expanding access generated resentment. Difficult enrollment processes, opaque eligibility rules, expensive premiums, and high deductibles provoked criticism from across the political spectrum. But it was conservative politicians and nativist social movements that most vehemently tapped into and fueled discontent with the law. This book illustrates lessons learned from the ambitious rise of the ACA—a law that aspired to bring affordable health care to most Americans—to its subsequent vulnerability as the political tides changed. We hope future health reforms will build on these lessons, rather than pursue health policies that increase inequality and stratification. We also hope that reformers and students of health policy will see the value in listening to on-the-ground human experience, rather than attending to statistics alone.

The ACA: An Abbreviated Overview

Unlike all other high-income and most middle-income countries, the United States has never made universal health coverage a social right. Instead, health care is delivered through a complex mix of public and private coverage with about half of financing coming from the public sector and half from private sources, which includes employer-based coverage and out-of-pocket spending. This market-based, for-profit health system has resulted in the highest health spending per capita in the world in return for mediocre health outcomes (OECD 2014). The United States has below-average life expectancy among countries of similar economic output and scores poorly on measures of managing chronic disease and access to primary care (OECD 2015). In addition to its unrivaled expense and lagging outcomes, the major shortcoming of the U.S. health care system is its lack of universal coverage.

It is hard to overstate the degree to which the lack of health insurance in the United States was, and for many people continues to be, a humanitarian crisis that exacerbates illness and shortens lives (Kaiser Commission on Medicaid and the Uninsured 2012). For the uninsured, medical needs can quickly lead to financial catastrophe, with medical bills leading the list of reasons for declared bankruptcies (Himmelstein et al. 2009). But industry support for reform only came about because having so many uninsured and underinsured persons in the United States was exerting a drag on the entire health sector. Hospitals and other safety-net institutions strained financially to treat the uninsured because they were obligated by federal law to do so.[2] Insurance premiums showed double-digit increases year after year. Reeling from a deep recession with unemployment swelling, the moment had come for change.

From its passage by the Obama administration with no Republican support to its many days in court, this law was no stranger to controversy. Though the ACA resembled past Republican health proposals, opposition hardened into a scorched-earth approach galvanized by the Tea Party movement, conservative think tanks, and organizations like the American Legislative Council (ALEC) and the Koch Foundation (Haeder and Weimer 2015; Jones et al. 2014). In addition to calling President Obama a "liar" and a "socialist," Republican opposition framed the ACA as government overreach. Anti-ACA advocates voiced wide-ranging objections to specific provisions of the law, including claims that the individual mandate was unconstitutional, accusations that the law would drive up costs, opposition to new taxes, concerns about paying for Medicaid expansion at the state level, and charges that "illegal" immigrants would benefit from the law.

The politics of reform framed the ACA as a much more radical and progressive policy than it actually was. Ultimately, the ACA was a middle-of-the-road policy that built on a legacy of public/private solutions to social problems. It sought to expand access to coverage through two major provisions: first, by expanding Medicaid to adults making less than 138% of the federal poverty level (FPL), and second, by creating insurance exchanges (i.e., online marketplaces) to sell more affordable coverage to individuals, families, and small businesses.

Prior to the ACA, Medicaid programs varied markedly by state and only covered certain categories of low-income individuals: people older than age 65, some disabled individuals, parents, children, and pregnant women. In most states, non-disabled, childless adults were ineligible for the program regardless of their income. Before the ACA, the median eligibility level for working parents was 61% of FPL, meaning that many poor and near-poor parents also went without coverage (Paradise 2015). Medicaid programs were (and continued to be for the populations that were eligible through pre-ACA criteria or in non-expanding states) financed through a Federal Medical Assistance Percentage (FMAP), in which states and the federal government shared the financing for the program. Poorer states enjoy higher FMAPs than wealthier ones; assistance from the federal government ranged from 50% to 73.6% (Paradise 2015). In contrast, the federal government financed the vast majority of costs for the ACA Medicaid expansion; starting at 100%, this was to be gradually phased down to 90%. In other words, the ACA sought to uniformly provide low-income individuals with affordable and comprehensive health coverage through Medicaid, mostly with federal dollars.

The insurance exchanges created through the Affordable Care Act vastly expanded the non–group insurance market by removing some barriers that kept it small: It was no longer legal to bar people, like Daniel, from coverage or to charge them more because of preexisting conditions. Gender rating—which meant that women were charged more for insurance than men—became expressly prohibited. Insurance companies could no longer cancel policies after they were issued (called "excision"). And all insurance products offered on the exchanges were required to comply with the standardized minimum benefit package, meaning that they had to include a comprehensive package of basic services (Cassidy 2013). Risk-pooling strategies known as risk corridors, risk adjustment, and reinsurance were applied to the non-group market and helped to better distribute risk, thereby shielding insurance companies from high losses as well as inordinate profits (Goodell 2014).

Perhaps most important, the ACA addressed the issue of affordability on the non-group market by providing subsidies in the form of tax credits and cost-sharing reductions for households below 400% and 250% of poverty levels, respectively.[3]

The ACA survived multiple legal challenges, but the 2012 U.S. Supreme Court decision that states could opt out of the Medicaid expansion created new and unanticipated problems. Since subsidies were designed to help those who were ineligible for Medicaid, the law was written in such a way that those living below 100% of the federal poverty level were ineligible for help purchasing coverage. And so, in states that decided not to expand Medicaid, millions of people fell into what came to be called "the coverage gap"—they were too poor for subsidies on the exchange, and largely remained uninsured. Chapters in this volume by Mulligan, Sered, and Brunson in particular describe how people experienced falling into this gap, where they often blamed "Obamacare" for their lack of coverage rather than the state governments that opted to turn down federal Medicaid funding that in the first two years would have paid for 100% of the cost of expansion.[4] Because some local and state governments, especially in the South, expressed hostility toward the ACA, in many places the law was only partially implemented.

Its very rocky rollout did not bolster the popularity of the law. The web-based technology platform that hosted www.healthcare.gov, the federally run exchange, encountered debilitating problems. This led to the resignation of the Secretary of Health and Human Services and the appointment of a new Chief Technology Officer (Shear 2014). The law also gave states the option to run their own exchange, default to a federally run exchange, or pursue a hybrid arrangement whereby some responsibility for exchange functions would be split between state and federal actors. Some state-based exchanges were so dysfunctional that they stopped operating and called on the federal exchange to take over. Despite these considerable challenges, millions of people managed to enroll in coverage and many of the exchange's technical difficulties were eventually resolved. Subsequent enrollment seasons were much less controversial than the first year, but enrollment was still lower than initially predicted (Levitt et al. 2016).

In the years following its passage, the law underwent dozens of recall attempts by the U.S. House of Representatives in addition to two challenges brought before the U.S. Supreme Court. It was shielded largely by President Obama's veto power and the threat of a filibuster in the Senate. A politically divisive issue during the 2016 presidential election campaign, the ACA's vulnerability became evident with the transition in executive power. Donald Trump's rise to power was propelled by anti-ACA sentiment. In the Conclusion chapter, we reflect on how his administration radically disrupted the political landscape of the United States and what this might mean for the future of health care access and coverage. Unlike other major health reforms, such as the creation of Medicare and Medicaid in 1965 or the addition of prescription drug coverage to Medicare in 2003, the ACA never transformed into a taken-for-granted and depoliticized health care entitlement program. It remained politically contentious years after its passage. This book helps to explain why by illuminating actual people's experience with health care reform.

Why Study the ACA Ethnographically?

This book presents the stories of communities and individuals located within specific moments of time and contextualized within particular places. The themes that these stories touch upon are not limited to the ACA, but speak as well to the experiences associated with economic restructuring, multiple and overlapping forms of inequality, and the struggle of trying to care for one's self and family in a context of shifting public policy priorities that emphasized personal responsibility and the privatization of public services. This is an anthropological study of policy, and especially the "messy" work of policy implementation. It explores processes and theoretical concepts that have been at the center of social scientific studies of policy—namely, issues of power and governance (e.g., Horton and Lamphere 2006; Okongwu and Mencher 2000; Shore and Wright 1997)—and thus speaks to a wider audience than simply those interested in the recent U.S. health care reform. This book is for scholars, students, and practitioners interested in power, governance, and processes that produce inequality. Using the ACA as a lens on these issues, this book examines how social welfare policies in a multiracial and multiethnic democracy purported to be inclusive while they simultaneously embraced certain kinds of exclusions.

The contributors to this book use ethnographic methods, especially observation and qualitative interviewing, to understand how people made sense of the opportunities and responsibilities that the ACA created for gaining coverage. As researchers, we spent time with people who were providing enrollment assistance and those who were seeking health coverage. When possible, we tried to get to know people in multiple settings, including during formal interviews, at home among family, and even by accompanying them to medical appointments. The ethnographic approach that guides this book differs markedly from most academic accounts of the Affordable Care Act, where there is a strong bias toward quantitative and statistical methods. Ethnographic methods are open-ended, intersubjective, and contingent. Anthropologists follow hunches about what is important, track down as many people who will talk to them as they can, and often spend time during fieldwork simply waiting for something to happen. We do this because we understand that policy is experienced amid other everyday concerns that shape our lives and that health coverage intersects with a wide range of social responsibilities, including caring for one's self and family, seeking financial security, obtaining work, and enhancing well-being.

For those who think that generalizability should be the ultimate goal of research, ethnographic findings can appear maddeningly specific. Some anthropologists argue that we should address our lack of generalizability by reinforcing our methodological rigor, answering practical policy questions that are of interest to health researchers, and better triangulating our data (Closser and Finley 2016). We approach these recommendations with caution, because while relevance is something we strive for, we do not want to lose sight of the unique strengths of ethnographic methods. Specifically, if our methods are always already attuned to producing a list of policy recommendations, using this approach may weaken our ability to broadly contextualize our findings in social and political structures, our ability to embrace the unexpected (Taylor 2014), and our attentiveness to contradictory and subjective understandings that no amount of triangulating can resolve. An important message from this book is that differently situated individuals can have radically different assessments of whether or not a particular health policy benefits them, and these assessments *are* true from their perspective.

In critically examining the call to be useful, which health practitioners sometimes demand of anthropologists, Stacy Leigh Pigg argues that we must remain committed to a methodology that involves sitting and listening: "Whereas global public-health policy looks to ethnography solely as a source of information, pertinent to its goals, ethnographers see their task quite differently, holding that the purpose of patient ethnography is to listen and to be in situ, a practice that opens up a space for the questioning of received certainties through a responsiveness to multiple viewpoints and contested perspectives" (2013, 127). A very similar point could be made about medical anthropologists working in the United States, where there is an increasing desire for "patient-centered" research. Anthropologists have found homes on multidisciplinary research teams, but the methods that are ultimately valued are those of evidenced-based medicine and comparative effectiveness research, in which the purpose is to discover what procedure or intervention is most effective so that it can be widely implemented. Anthropologists have also been caught up in the demands of medical research infrastructures and their "fast" ways of publishing results, scaling up, and churning out programs that should be implemented uniformly in diverse settings (Adams et al. 2014). As anthropologists, we are attentive to particularities and the specificity of places. There is much to be gained by sitting and listening to the people who are involved in health policy projects, both as agents and as targets. Sometimes this listening yields policy insights (for instance, if we really want people to maintain coverage, then the enrollment process shouldn't be so difficult). But other times, what we gain is a richer understanding of the complexities of struggling to care for each other, of political and other forms of belonging, of the reverberations of exclusion, and of the other parts of life that shape and are shaped by health policies. When we are open to the messy contradictions of health policy implementation as it is actually experienced, we see that choosing whether a policy is "good" or "bad" is an impossible task. Instead, we trace the effects of this policy, which continue to shape people's well-being, sense of belonging, and life chances.

This volume is multi-tonal—the authors and the people interviewed are at times strident, outraged, neutral, technocratic, sarcastic, hopeful, and devastated. This is because the stakes were so high. The ACA engendered hope for improved access to care, healing, and financial security.

It also struck fear and worry in those who had coverage or made their living in the health care industry. Instead of aiming for evenhandedness, we have assembled a mix of viewpoints (though not an exhaustive or "representative" list). The chapters do not all take the same approach— some are more overtly critical, some more hopeful, some forlorn. This seems appropriate for a policy that had such diverse and differential effects depending on state of residence, income, immigration status, age, health status, type of insurance coverage, and so on.

Health care advocates have pushed us to refrain from being too critical—they have even said we should avoid emphasizing the negative, especially as the gains the law made in expanding access to coverage seem so fragile and likely to be undone. This criticism has given us pause. We do not want this work to become ammunition for dismantling the law. We would much rather provide evidence and new perspectives for those advocating for a more universal and inclusive coverage expansion policy. But we also acknowledge that our work is likely to have other impacts that we have not anticipated. Ultimately, we feel a responsibility to be honest with the material—and that means not hiding that, for many uninsured people, the law did not improve their circumstances. It means not obscuring the ways in which the law was cynically used to fan racial animus, but also structured in such a way that it created new resentments. It means remembering who the law left out. And finally, it means not shying away from critiquing the misuses of accountability talk and the commitment to market principles over an ethic of care that are enshrined in the law (Horton et al. 2014; Mol 2008). Twenty million people gained access to coverage under the ACA. For many, that access was life-altering. But our job in this volume is a more modest accounting. We seek to illuminate the contradictory effects of this policy in the world, on well-being, on belonging and exclusion, and on felt risks and responsibilities in the everyday contexts and for the ordinary people whose lives it was supposed to make better.

The ACA and Governance: Stratified Citizenship, Risk, and Responsibility

Answering calls to forge a more publicly relevant research practice (Horton et al. 2014), this book brings together ethnographic engagements with the Affordable Care Act and explores three interrelated themes that reflect upon central theoretical concerns: stratified citizenship, risk, and responsibility. Structured under these broad themes, which are woven throughout the book and appear, to some extent, in all the chapters, this book documents how the law produced new social relations, modes of government, and experiences of care.

Stratified Citizenship

While the ACA intended to expand social rights and protections, it did not include everyone. Nor did those who received the law's benefits view it in a uniformly positive light. This book draws attention to the uneven ways in which people experienced the law on-the-ground, based on the insights provided through careful ethnographic research in communities. By talking with the people the ACA brought into coverage and those who were left out, we learned that the responsibilities and benefits of the law were distributed unequally, but in highly patterned ways. We use the term *stratified citizenship* to describe how certain social identities and demographic characteristics—such as immigration status, income, gender, race, and state of residence—mediated how people were included or excluded from health insurance coverage through the ACA.

Citizenship, at its most fundamental, refers to a complex set of practices that constitute political belonging. In this book, the concept of "citizenship" is understood not simply as legal membership in a state, but rather as practices of claims-making in various sites and scales that create political subjectivity. This broader relational definition of citizenship emphasizes that it is a dynamic institution of both domination and empowerment, governing who is citizen, subject, and abject, and how these actors relate to one another in the body politic (Isin 2009). Thus, stratified citizenship refers to the differential gradation of rights and opportunities to different groups residing within the same state. Here, we extend the concept of citizenship beyond legal belonging to a nation-state (as in holding a passport of a particular country) to also include the political, social, and affective experiences of belonging as forms of citizenship for many types of social groups, regardless of nationality. The chapters that do examine juridical statuses for immigrant groups (legal permanent residents, deferred action, undocumented, etc.) show that stratified citizenship is experienced in complex gradations of partial inclusion that tap into feelings of aspiration, hope, and disappointment, while enacting exclusions that can range from ambiguous and incomplete to cruel and life-threatening.

The concept of *health citizenship* recognizes that social inclusion and marginalization are often produced through unequal access to health care, structural barriers to health, and provider attitudes. This concept helps us to understand how stratification can result in some groups experiencing higher levels of access or receiving better quality health care than others, even when all groups are purportedly included in the same system. In particular, ideologies of health-related "deservingness" (Willen 2012) can help to explain the disjuncture between formal entitlement and actual access. This book argues that, in many instances, the ACA reinforced preexisting patterns of exclusion, often by reinforcing longstanding distinctions between the "deserving" and the "undeserving." Means testing is one way in which this occurs; long controversial in the design of poverty relief programs that are stigmatized, it is often used to sort the "deserving" from the "non-deserving" poor (Katz 2008). While addressing some existing inequalities in the U.S. health care system, the ACA also exacerbated or produced others through the differential opportunities afforded various groups, such as legal permanent resident immigrants or LGBTQ communities. In other words, "[t]he ACA aims to redress systemic inequalities in access to care, but not all populations will benefit equally" (Horton et al. 2014).

The Affordable Care Act's impact on racial inequalities in health and health coverage has been complex. Many provisions of the law aimed to reduce health disparities, such as improving data collection on race and ethnicity, diversifying the health care workforce, and funding research on disparities and health equity (RWJ 2011). And importantly, blacks and Latinos experienced some of the biggest gains in coverage under the law (McMorrow et al. 2015). Nonetheless, these groups continued to be disproportionately uninsured: At the end of 2015, 21% of Hispanics, 11% of blacks, and 7% of whites were uninsured nationally (KFF 2016a). Because undocumented and some lawfully present immigrants were explicitly excluded from coverage, those populations remained uninsured at much higher rates than citizens (see chapters by Castañeda, Joseph, and Melo in this volume). Furthermore, the partial implementation of the ACA through non-Medicaid expansion and insufficient in-person assistance in states with governments hostile to the ACA disproportionately impacted blacks and Hispanics. One study estimated that 1.4 million more blacks would have been covered if Medicaid expansion had not been optional (Clemans-Cope et al. 2014; McMorrow et al. 2015).

As we argue in this volume, it is no accident that people of color were disproportionately impacted by the decision to exclude some immigrants from coverage and to opt out of Medicaid expansion. Repeated attempts to repeal and disrupt the implementation of the law are part of a long history in the United States of opposing programs that are perceived as benefiting communities of color, especially, though not exclusively, in the South (Haney López 2014). As of 2016, 90% of people in the coverage gap lived in the South (Garfield and Damico 2016). Voting to repeal the ACA and blocking implementation join a long list of practices (such as onerous application procedures, frequent eligibility re-verification, work requirements, and literacy tests) designed to disenfranchise people of color and thwart policies that might result in greater financial, educational, and racial equality.

The ACA both built upon but also remedied existing stratification by gender, sex, and sexuality. The law ended gender rating—the practice of charging men and women different rates for identical health plans—and protected women from higher premiums, in addition to lifetime and preexisting condition limits. Prior to the ACA, women paid up to $1 billion more than men each year for identical insurance plans on the individual market (the practice was already banned in the case of employer-based plans) (NWLC 2012). The law also expanded access to basic women's health services and mandated the inclusion of maternity care and coverage without cost-sharing for preventive services such as contraceptives. However, contraceptive coverage applied only to women; men using vasectomy or condoms were left with out-of-pocket costs, despite a long history of inclusion in other public and private programs. These gendered exclusions generated resentments and led to a backlash, with conservative lawmakers and media outlets objecting to and fanning outrage over the inclusion of maternity care in the individual market, since men must contribute to covering the cost for this particular service that, by definition, they do not use (Franke-Ruta 2013).

The law also remedied some heteronormative exclusions, requiring insurance plans to offer coverage to same-sex married spouses; it also extended nondiscrimination protections (KFF 2016b). For people living with HIV/AIDS, the removal of the preexisting condition bar was an important victory and allowed this segment of the population to access comprehensive insurance policies. The Ryan White HIV/AIDS Program began to transition its role to assist people in obtaining coverage through the ACA marketplaces and Medicaid expansion (HRSA 2016). However, health plans have used other means to discourage enrollment of HIV-positive people, such as discriminatory formularies that make HIV medications inordinately expensive (NHeLP 2014). The removal of the preexisting condition clause, along with the fact that the ACA prohibits discrimination based on sexual identity, also greatly benefited transgender persons. Major advocacy organizations for transgender people interpreted the law to mean that transition-related health services should be covered by ACA plans (NCTE 2016).

We link stratified citizenship to a longer history of allocating access to medical care based on notions of deservingness that were articulated in their contemporary form in the Personal Responsibility and Work Opportunity Reconciliation Act (PRWORA), which essentially repealed prior social safety net programs. Passed in 1996 by the U.S. Congress and signed into law by President Clinton, PRWORA transformed the welfare system by replacing it with state-run, block-grant programs using new criteria that included time limits for benefits, tying receipt of benefits to employment, and providing incentives for reduced caseloads. As the name suggests, it increased the emphasis on "personal responsibility" of the poor, adding a work requirement and a lifetime benefits limitation of five years. PRWORA also set the precedent of tightly intertwining eligibility for federal benefits with immigration status, denying eligibility to most legal immigrants during their first five years of U.S. residence. Through the ACA, these practices of conferring eligibility to "deserving" versus "non-deserving" immigrants and requiring that recipients of public benefits demonstrate and enact responsibility were intensified and became even more commonplace. Thus, the ACA was layered upon an existing patchwork of policies that already created exclusionary effects for some populations. This volume is attentive to the landscape of health care access already in place when the ACA was implemented, and highlights the ways in which it emerged under already highly stratified conditions of eligibility.

A key concern that this book raises is whether—and to what extent—the ACA succeeded in including the large segment of the U.S. population that was previously uninsured or underinsured. More broadly, the chapters by Castañeda, Melo, Joseph, and Andaya each unveil the processes associated with projects of stratified citizenship by exploring who gained access and who was excluded. Because the ACA maintained many prior exclusions—such as the exclusion of "nonqualified" immigrants from Medicaid—while simultaneously creating new exclusions (such as that of DACA recipients), the law created a complex landscape of eligibility for immigrants in mixed-status families (Castañeda, this volume). Moreover, as the federal government has devolved to states the decision about whether to restore inclusion in Medicaid for certain unqualified immigrants (such as legal permanent residents who have been in the United States for less than five years) (Joseph)—as well as what services Emergency Medicaid should provide undocumented immigrants (Melo), this landscape of exclusion varied dramatically across states. Furthermore, as Andaya suggests, there is a difference between health inclusion and health equality, arguing that we must move beyond studying coverage as an either/or scenario and instead illustrate how different *forms* of health coverage can also contribute to experiences of stratification. As people were unequally included in the rights and responsibilities engendered by this law, how did that create new and further entrench earlier affective feelings of belonging and external evaluations of deservingness? Of course, ideas of deservingness are also connected with notions of risk and responsibility, as we illustrate in the following sections.

Risk

The ways people assess and experience risks are deeply connected to their class positions, sense of vulnerability, and social resources. Therefore, we treat risk as an embodied, relational concept rather than an abstract property. Our focus in this volume is on how people experienced multiple forms of risk and found ways to navigate them in the new health care landscape created by the ACA. Measuring and predicting risk is a core part of the concept of "insurance": Insurers profit when the actual health costs of their risk pools are lower than the premiums they collect. Insurance can serve as a way to socialize risk, but it can also segment risk into smaller and more profitable pools that take precedence over broad social protection (Dao and Mulligan 2016; Ericson et al. 2003). In financial terms, more risk is not always a bad thing, since it can mean higher rates of return when risk refers to the probability that an investment will make or lose money. But risk isn't just the product of prediction and formulas; it can be affective, too. Talking about health insurance coverage often brings up feelings of being "at risk" or in danger; people we spoke with described the sense that they were "risking" something important, such as their health or security. And risk can also refer to behavior: Risk is something we do, like drink alcohol or use drugs. And sometimes it becomes something we are. Risk is used as a label to describe a person—for example, poor pregnant women are often deemed "high risk" and subject to intense surveillance because of it (see Andaya, this volume).

Many of the chapters here show how individuals and families calculated their health and financial risks when they enrolled in coverage and attempted to access health care services. Perceived health risks, both for oneself and for family members, play a big role in shaping whether coverage is considered necessary and desirable. People who lived with a chronic condition or who experienced serious injury were more likely to view insurance as a necessity. This may be why those who signed up for coverage in the first few years of the ACA turned out to be sicker than initially predicted (Pear 2015a). Those with unmet medical needs were among the first to enroll, in part because preexisting condition clauses had prevented those with medical needs from signing up for coverage on the individual market.

Obtaining insurance to mitigate risk was a common strategy employed by the people we collectively studied, but other approaches were also noted. In a neoliberal era when many risks have been transferred from state programs onto individuals (such as indexed retirement accounts in the form of 401(k)s replacing guaranteed pensions), some individuals and families "embraced risk" (Baker and Simon 2002). They shopped extensively, calculated the cost of various disaster scenarios such as a car accident that might injure the entire family, and negotiated with providers to obtain the maximum return on their health care investment (see Brunson, this volume). These individuals understood their decisions within a framework of being responsible risk-takers and were often ideologically hostile to government insurance or "Obamacare." However, this risk-embracing strategy was a response to highly circumscribed conditions, where the deck was stacked against middle-income individuals and families, who chose between spending tens of thousands of dollars on insurance premiums and deductibles or risking their family's health and financial security by gambling on remaining uninsured.

As these "risk embracers" illustrate, health insurance can both protect families from financial risks as well as generate new risks as families strain to keep up with the costs of high premiums and deductibles. As noted earlier, medical bills are the leading cause of bankruptcy in the United States (Himmelstein et al. 2009), so remaining uncovered can be financially risky for those in the middle class, who have assets to lose. But increasingly, having coverage does not provide complete protection against catastrophic medical bills. Most plans on the exchanges had substantial cost-sharing in the form of deductibles that made it difficult for people to access health services even when they were able to pay their premiums. A *New York Times* analysis found that more than half of the plans offered on exchanges had a deductible of $3,000 or more in 2015 (Pear 2015b).

In the wider medical anthropology and sociology literature, risk has also been interpreted as a form of medicalization or diagnostic creep. Pre-disease states (pre-diabetes, obesity, or pre-hypertension, for example) signal an elevated probability of developing an illness and can come to be experienced as disease states themselves. In *Drugs for Life* (2012), Joseph Dumit argues that pharmaceutical marketing strategies explicitly seek to inculcate the idea that we are always at risk of impending illness. Risks are perceived in society in a way that naturalizes a need to always be treated, even if a person shows no actual sign of disease.

This calculable and medicalized understanding of risk as described by Dumit did not resonate with many of the people we studied who remained uncovered. They did not know their specific risk factors and biomarkers, as pharmaceutical marketers might wish, because they were cut off from consistent care and lab work is often not covered by safety net institutions. Instead, many intrinsically felt the risks of managing their chronic conditions without insurance, of worsening health when insulin, asthma inhalers, and addiction treatment were out of reach, of sliding into disability and unemployment when their unmet medical needs made it impossible to maintain their previous levels of functioning. They weren't always already at-risk so much as experiencing the kinds of subprime risks that make being poor so dangerous to one's health.

Similar to the subprime financial instruments that made the poor profitable for payday, auto, and high-risk mortgage lenders, the health risks that poor and uninsured populations experience in the United States both worsen their health status and undermine their financial stability, all the while generating revenue for outpatient clinics, insurance carriers, hospitals, and debt collection agencies. In the financial meltdown that preceded the passage of the ACA, subprime financial instruments (like payday loans and high-interest and balloon mortgages) were aggressively marketed to low-income people. These expensive and often misleading loans undermined the ability of the working poor to achieve financial security through home ownership and exacerbated unemployment-related insecurity (Dwyer and Lassus 2015). Just as poor Americans are cut off from traditional financial instruments like 30-year fixed-rate mortgages, so too are many cut off from integrated health care and comprehensive, low-cost health insurance. The ACA attempted to address this intermingling of health and financial risks—and for those who were able to enroll in expanded Medicaid, their financial status and access to care improved (Antonisse et al. 2016; Christopher et al. 2016). Nonetheless, the ACA's exchanges provided coverage that was beyond the financial means of many. We argue that the health system itself generates new subprime risks, where health is precarious and always in danger of unraveling. And so, the chapters in this volume ask: How did individuals and families navigate the new financial and health risks created by the ACA? And how does the segmented and disjointed health system in the United States create risks for the covered and the uncovered alike?

Responsibility

The ACA created new responsibilities for individuals and families and new opportunities for providers and contractors to transform the health care of the poor and underserved into a revenue-generating enterprise. The law's responsibilities were unequally distributed—individuals and families came under increased scrutiny and surveillance while technology and other service contractors entered into lucrative agreements and benefited from a lack of oversight at the highest levels of government. The ACA's individual mandate transformed health coverage from an employment perk and a protection into a *responsibility*. Before the ACA, health coverage in the United States was a middle-class benefit that some workers received from their employers.[5] Coverage was also available through a mix of public programs for some protected groups: poor pregnant women, some poor children, some people with disabilities, those over 65, and some veterans. The ACA required that individuals and families obtain coverage or pay a fine. But the new responsibilities engendered by the law did not stop at coverage; they fanned out into state governments and the private sector and involved a wide range of actors and organizations in the work of implementation.

The ACA must be seen as part of a longer history of welfare reform that has devolved responsibility for public services onto community organizations, businesses, and individuals over the last three decades (Clarke 2004; Goode and Maskovsky 2001; Kingfisher 2002; and Horton et al. 2014). For example, following the PRWORA welfare reform in 1996, recipients of TANF (Temporary Aid to Needy Families) had to prove they were actively looking for work or enrolled in job training, and they were subject to drug testing and other forms of invasive monitoring (Soss et al. 2011). The job training programs funded through the TANF program were contracted out to private firms and community organizations. Likewise, the ACA focused on personal responsibility by requiring that individuals obtain health insurance, and famously relied on private subcontractors and partners to carry out many of its key provisions (Jain et al. 2015).

Like other government-funded social service programs in the United States, the ACA is an example of "delegated governance" (Morgan and Campbell 2011). Responsibility for carrying out the key purpose of the law—expanding insurance coverage—was placed on individuals, families, and employers with government agencies and their contractors serving as middlemen. More specifically, the ACA expanded access to health insurance by extending and adding on to existing programs, which were largely administered at the state level (Medicaid) or by private entities like employers and insurance companies. The federal government's ascribed role was actually quite limited; it included writing regulations, enforcing the tax provisions of the law, running insurance exchanges if states opted not to, and paying for the Medicaid expansion and insurance subsidies. State governments had to decide whether to expand their Medicaid programs to poor adults or to operate an insurance exchange, and oversee and regulate insurers (Morgan and Campbell 2011).

Though this well-established model of delegated governance was employed in the ACA, it is important to point out that the law reversed a long-standing trend to cut benefits received by working-aged, non-disabled adults. Instead, the ACA established that insurance was important and necessary and provided new avenues for childless adults to access coverage through the expanded Medicaid program and insurance exchanges. Likewise, the responsibilities the law created were not always burdensome or oppressive for marginalized groups; in emphasizing collective responsibility, the ACA also provided more funding for community health centers and mandated a focus on the recording and alleviation of health disparities. For all of its flaws, the law contained a fundamental conception that the state was responsible for making health care available and affordable. Nonetheless, access to health coverage was still not considered a right, since the law obligated people to purchase insurance and did not guarantee universal coverage.

Together, federal and many state governments expanded public insurance eligibility and created new insurance marketplaces, but the actual responsibility for obtaining, maintaining, and paying for coverage fell to employers, individuals, and families, thanks to the employer and individual mandates. The mandates were one of the most controversial aspects of the law, since they required that most people get covered. Exceptions existed for religious objectors, people who were incarcerated, ineligible immigrants, those who still did not have an affordable insurance option (including millions who fell into Medicaid gaps in non-expanding states), those experiencing certain kinds of hardships, and members of certain groups including federally recognized tribes (CMS 2016). Though 26 states sued the federal government on the grounds that the mandates were unconstitutional, the Supreme Court decided in

2012 that the government does have the authority to require U.S. residents to purchase health insurance coverage as part of Congress's power to levy taxes (KFF 2012b). Penalties for not having coverage thus fell on individuals and were assessed as part of their tax filing in what the law terms a "shared responsibility payment."

While the ACA did expand government's responsibility for providing health coverage to U.S. residents, it fell short of universal coverage and asked much of individuals and families in the process. This downstreaming of responsibility meant that those with the least amount of power to affect the system had new obligations to get covered and pay for their insurance and health care costs in a health care landscape with increasingly stingy insurance plans and exorbitant cost sharing for consumers (Collins et al. 2015). Chapters by Brunson, Mulligan, and Sered explore how people made sense of their new responsibilities to get covered. Other chapters examine how coverage also promoted a responsibility to maintain health. In Susan Shaw's example of medication adherence programs for patients with chronic conditions in Massachusetts and Mary Alice Scott and Richard Wright's case study of a formerly free clinic in New Mexico, patients who gained access to coverage through health reform also experienced new pressures to maintain and improve their health status. As earlier studies of managed care have pointed out, providers commonly fill the gaps left when care is not coordinated or covered. Given their social commitment to serving the poor, many community health centers and charity providers try to buffer the impacts of disruptive policy changes, inadequate patient education, and technological snafus by simply doing more (Boehm 2005; Horton et al. 2001). Cathleen Willging and Elise M. Trott show how policymakers in New Mexico, in an example of "organized irresponsibility," used antifraud provisions of the ACA to dismantle the non-profit, community-based safety net for mental health services, thus undermining the ability of the safety net to serve poor clients.

As ethnographers of health reform, we have sought to show how people reacted to and assumed the new responsibilities created by the ACA. How were these new responsibilities socially distributed? As individuals, families, and employers were charged with the responsibility to obtain coverage, did governments and institutions face similar levels of accountability?

Overview of Book Organization and Chapters

Section I: Inclusions and Exclusions

The first section of the book explores how the ACA emerged as an extension of social protections to some groups but also created new forms of exclusion, as access to affordable coverage options were highly segmented by state of residence, income, and citizenship status. In doing so, it built upon a legacy of existing stratification that had long excluded people by class, occupation, race, ethnicity, immigration status, gender, and sexuality.

The chapter by Heide Castañeda argues that the ACA (re)produced and stratified juridical categories of immigrants with sometimes contradictory results. It highlights the fact that immigrant groups in the United States are not monolithic, but instead are stratified by many chaotic bureaucratic categories. The ACA intensified immigrants' exclusion from the health care system, exacerbating a costly spiral of disability and death. Using three case studies derived from longitudinal research in Texas, this chapter illustrates the unanticipated and contradictory effects of the law by examining how immigration categories influenced eligibility and participation. The ACA not only explicitly excluded more than 11 million undocumented immigrants from coverage, it even distinguished between "qualified" and "non-qualified" immigrants among those who were considered "lawfully present." Through three cases, this chapter illustrates the impacts of these exclusions and inclusions. We see how these distinctions produced ripple effects on U.S. citizen children in mixed-status families. In addition, the exclusion of youth holding deferred action for childhood arrival (DACA) status—produced through an unusual case of administrative rollback—created a new pattern of formal disenfranchisement, while a loophole allowed some immigrants to qualify for insurance subsidies that U.S. citizens living in the same state could not.

In "Stratified Access: Seeking Dialysis Care in the Borderlands," Milena Andrea Melo ethnographically explores a marginalized population who must negotiate exclusionary practices to access treatment to prolong their lives as they struggled with renal failure. This chapter examines the impact of the lack of health insurance coverage for low-income, undocumented immigrants who required regular dialysis to stay alive. Undocumented immigrants were deemed undeserving of most publicly funded health care services by virtue of their "illegal" status. Those with chronic, debilitating illness struggled to navigate public and private health care institutions as indigent patients in order to locate lifesaving but substandard treatment. Since they were uninsured, receiving irregular and costly dialysis treatments in hospital emergency rooms, paid by Emergency Medicaid, was their only option. Melo demonstrates that the health system itself exacerbated health risks for dialysis patients by requiring that they come close to death before they were offered emergency services. This chapter raises questions concerning belonging, deservingness of care, and American notions of human rights in cases where those with nothing more than "bare life" are excluded.

In "Stratification and 'Universality': Immigrants and Barriers to Coverage in Massachusetts," Tiffany D. Joseph examines how stratification of access by immigration status effectively undermined a "universal" health policy. While the ACA only extended coverage to U.S. citizens and eligible documented immigrants, Massachusetts pursued a universal health care system at the state level and offered coverage to all residents regardless of documentation status. Despite this policy that aimed for inclusion, immigrants in Massachusetts were still more likely than non-immigrants to remain uninsured. Joseph interviewed Brazilian and Dominican immigrants, health care professionals, and immigrant/health organization employees to find out why immigrants remained uninsured. She identified immigration-related, health care system, and bureaucratic barriers that prevented individuals from effectively accessing care. She found that bureaucratic disentitlement processes tied to applying for coverage and re-enrollment created major difficulties for immigrants who were unfamiliar with the U.S. health care system and who had limited English proficiency. As Joseph argues, Massachusetts served as both a model and a cautionary tale for ACA implementation, with barriers exacerbated for immigrant, low-income, and minority populations.

"Stratification through Medicaid: Public Prenatal Care in New York City" by Elise Andaya focuses on Medicaid-covered prenatal care in New York State to illustrate how health care for low-income people after the passage of the ACA has reconstituted preexisting patterns of exclusion and reinforced long-standing moral divisions between the "righteous" and the "undeserving" poor. Given that Medicaid expansion accounted for more than half of the population newly insured under the ACA, this chapter investigates how the long-standing division between "consumers" of private health insurance and Medicaid "recipients" had effectively been maintained. Those covered under Medicaid faced a cultural landscape in which public aid was inextricably entangled with judgments about "proper" citizenship and moral worth. Stratification was especially evident in pervasive beliefs about the disposability of poor people's time and the disciplinary power of waiting for services that were viewed as "free" or "charity." In addition, poor women were singled out as medically and socially high-risk patients, justifying increased state-medical oversight in the name of risk that sharply underscored the interplay between discipline and nurturance by the state. Finally, their inclusion in the body politic was only temporary; shortly after pregnancy ended, women and their infants were reincorporated into society through new or existing categories of stratified health citizenship, including noncitizenship. Andaya suggests that the experiences of Medicaid-covered pregnant women reveal the difference between health inclusion and health equality, and the consequences of this distinction for the ACA. This chapter suggests we must go beyond understanding lack of coverage to also take account of how different *forms* of health coverage can also contribute to experiences of health inequality. The failure to dismantle the public/private division places into question the degree to which health reform has transformed ideologies of health citizenship in the contemporary United States.

Section II: Implementation along the Red/Blue Divide

This section examines how the larger politics of the "red/blue divide"— that is, partisan political divisions that led to profound geographic differences in the law's implementation—shaped both understandings of the ACA and how those affected negotiated the risks of being or not being covered. The chapters in this section show that people made sense of the divisions created by the ACA by using the language of deservingness, individualism, dependence, and responsibility.

Drawing on the concepts of "dog whistle politics" and white resentment, Jessica M. Mulligan illustrates how repeated attempts to repeal and disrupt the implementation of the ACA must be understood as part of a long history of strategic opposition to programs that are perceived as benefiting communities of color. This chapter examines the different meanings and impacts of the law for differently situated individuals and families, which derive from three overlapping sources. First, they emerge from the contradictions of using means-tested, actuarially rated programs to increase insurance access rather than universal access. They are also the result of the move by some states to reject the expansion of Medicaid and therefore deprive millions of access to medical insurance. Finally, they derive from racial politics that structure how many people make sense of the law. She concludes that there is no shared sense of the social created through the law, which has impacted its success. Instead, people's experience of health care reform, and potentially enhanced health care access, is mediated by a politics of resentment, eligibility and actuarial categories, past experiences with insurance and illness, and attempts to care for loved ones.

Susan Sered, author of the seminal work *Uninsured in America: Life and Death in the Land of Opportunity* (2005), revisits the American health care landscape following the implementation of the ACA and in her chapter returns to the same communities to learn how the people she originally interviewed are faring now. The ACA, she argues, was never designed to overhaul the U.S. health care landscape; rather, it was a political compromise in a health care "system" made up of a chaotic multitude of financing and delivery mechanisms. Of the people she met on her return trips, not a single person had remained in the same coverage status and situation for more than a few years at a time. Even with insurance, she notes, health care is hardly affordable for most Americans. The return visits made it clear that health and access to health care greatly depend upon where one lives. Geographically driven health disparities have been exacerbated by the 2012 Supreme Court ruling, leaving large numbers of people to fall into the "coverage gap." The existence of these gaps, together with the inconsistent nature of coverage and the absence of a human rights ethos, created barriers and hostilities, with many people feeling that other categories of people received greater benefits.

In "'Texans Don't Want Health Insurance': Social Class and the ACA in a Red State," Emily K. Brunson examines how the ACA has unfolded in Texas, a state with significant popular and political sentiment against the law despite being home to the highest percentage of uninsured persons in the nation. State leaders introduced numerous road blocks to coverage, including the decision to not expand Medicaid coverage as well as other less successful efforts to undermine ACA implementation. This has increased the number of *under*insured persons, who cannot afford health care because of the high costs associated with their expensive and inadequate insurance plans. Providing a deep analysis of longitudinal case studies of three previously uninsured women—some of whom were able to access insurance coverage following the ACA—Brunson shows how each person struggled with issues of choice, responsibility, and risk in relation to their health care. The chapter also considers how social class and gender affected these women's experiences and their understandings of health, health care, and the ACA. Brunson concludes that while the ACA improved health care access and health outcomes for some Texans, it also deepened inequalities by increasing stratification based on social class. Those who were better off economically could use their social capital to navigate the decision to buy coverage or remain uninsured, while the working poor remained without options and continued to live uncovered.

Section III: The ACA's Accountability Contradictions

The final section of the book examines the social distribution of new responsibilities under the ACA and how people responded to the call to get enrolled, improve their health, and pay for coverage. Collectively, these chapters demonstrate that the accountability, responsibility, and transparency that were demanded of patients, clients, and providers were not equally expected from lawmakers, administrators, and insurance companies.

Susan J. Shaw examines the management and regulation of low-income residents' access to and coverage for medications in Massachusetts, the "canary in the coalmine of U.S. health care reform." In this chapter, she shows how Medicaid patients experienced accountability in health care as they struggled to pay out-of-pocket costs for their medications and endured frequent eligibility re-certifications for insurance coverage. Their physicians were subject to insurers' cost-savings measures that included changing lists of covered medications. Finally, patients received monthly statements from their insurance companies detailing the patients' share compared to the actual costs of their medications. Shifts in medication benefits intersect with complex pharmaceutical beliefs that shaped low-income patients' adherence to biomedical care for chronic disease. Utilizing insights about the importance of "audit culture" to regimes of accountability, she argues that the Massachusetts experience of health care reform serves as a cautionary tale of the diverse costs of health care reform in neoliberal moral economies of care.

In "Outsourcing Responsibility: State Stewardship of Behavioral Health Care Services," Cathleen E. Willging and Elise M. Trott argue that politically driven processes of the past have shaped the current context of mental health care delivery in New Mexico. New Mexico is an economically challenged, mostly rural state, where mental health care disparities, a product of structural violence and of contemporary efforts to privatize, corporatize, and outsource public sector services, disproportionately impact Hispanic, Latino, and Native American citizens. Provisions of the ACA, including the expansion of Medicaid and outreach to underserved populations, offered the possibility of improving access and services for New Mexicans struggling with unmet treatment needs. However, as the authors argue, public stewards manipulated key ACA provisions to propagate unsubstantiated allegations of waste, fraud, and corruption against safety-net service providers. This chapter shows how public-private partnerships in the Medicaid arena, discourses of transparency, and technologies of accountability can engender truthiness claims, obscure vital information, destabilize a behavioral health care safety net, and deny low-income citizens care. They argue that scholars have the responsibility to attend to the "total bureaucratization" of government-funded health care systems that also allows such abuse of authority.

The chapter by Mary Alice Scott and Richard Wright explores the intersections of seemingly opposing understandings of health—as a "right" or a "responsibility"—in health care professionals' commentaries on ACA implementation in a formerly free clinic in southern New Mexico. In doing so, it challenges an often-unexamined moral framework that obscures structural barriers to achieving health. The concepts of co-responsibility and of patient engagement—increasingly central to health care and other social programs globally—were reflected in staff framing of health care problems, clinic activities, and conceptualizations of patients. Patient engagement relies on "shared responsibility" among patients, providers, health care administrators, and communities; it requires motivating patients to increase participation in their own health care, empowering patients to develop self-efficacy, and improving health literacy so that patients can be more fully informed in making health care decisions, along with other processes to increase patient accountability. As this chapter shows, there is often a mismatch between provider expectations of shared responsibility and the highly constrained actions of patients, who in this study confronted structural barriers including being unhoused, lack of regular transportation, undocumented immigration status, competing priorities including work, and missing important identification documents that were necessary for obtaining coverage.

* * *

This book guides readers through the tumultuous U.S. health care system through the lens of the Affordable Care Act. Using ethnographic methods, the contributors provide up-close, intimate portraits of individuals who gained coverage and remained uninsured as well as the providers tasked with delivering health care to the newly insured. We see the moral, financial, and health stakes of a sweeping social policy as it touched down in people's lives. The volume answers the question of whether or not the Affordable Care Act worked, arguing that it unevenly expanded access to care and in so doing, the ACA addressed some inequalities and stratification, sustained or exacerbated others, and created new ones.

NOTES

1 *NFIB v. Sebelius* considered the constitutionality of the individual mandate and the Medicaid expansion. The Supreme Court maintained the constitutionality of the individual mandate under Congress's power to tax. The individual mandate is the provision of the Affordable Care Act that requires most residents of the United States to obtain health insurance coverage or pay a fine. However, the Court found that the Medicaid expansion was "unconstitutionally coercive" because states could be penalized for not expanding Medicaid by losing all of their Medicaid funding (which also covers long-term care, coverage for children,

pregnant women, parents, poor seniors, and people with certain disabilities) Instead, states had to affirmatively opt in to expand their Medicaid programs to adults at 138% or below the federal poverty level (KFF 2012). This decision created "the coverage gap" wherein many adults in non-expanding states were ineligible for both Medicaid and ACA subsidies that made coverage more affordable.

2 The Emergency Medical Treatment and Labor Act (EMTALA) of 1986 requires that people with emergency conditions be treated and stabilized in emergency rooms regardless of ability to pay (CMS 2012). While some politicians have construed this law to mean that nobody goes without coverage in the United States, in fact, the law is quite limited since it only covers emergency care and patients are still billed for services used (Carroll 2012). See Melo (this volume) for an account of the deadly consequences of relying on emergency care to manage chronic illness.

3 The ACA is a long and complicated law that includes many other provisions, such as requirements for improved data collection on health disparities, funding for more primary care graduate training, and rules for employers offering coverage. These provisions are not discussed at length in this book. Instead, we focus on the coverage expansions that were at the heart of the law.

4 Throughout the book, we employ the term Affordable Care Act or ACA to refer to the health reform legislation. Sometimes we also use "Obamacare," as this was the nomenclature often used in the press and was also the name that many of the people who we interviewed responded to and recognized. As discussed in the chapter by Mulligan, the term Obamacare was initially used derisively and was part of efforts to racialize the law. However, the Obama administration then tried to reclaim the term by putting a positive spin on it: Obama cares. When referring to the legislation, we use the term ACA. When appropriate to the context of the discussion, we also occasionally use Obamacare throughout the text.

5 Employer-based health insurance expanded rapidly in the United States after World War II in part because employer contributions to insurance were tax-exempt. Employer sponsored insurance coverage has been declining since its peak in the 1980s (Enthoven and Fuchs 2006).

REFERENCES

Adams, Vincanne, Nancy J. Burke, and Ian Whitmarsh. 2014. Slow Research: Thoughts for a Movement in Global Health. *Medical Anthropology* 33 (3): 179–197.

Antonisse, Larisa, Rachel Garfield, Robin Rudowitz, and Samantha Artiga. 2016. The Effects of Medicaid Expansion under the ACA: Findings from a Literature Review. *Kaiser Commission on Medicaid and the Uninsured* (November 30). kff.org.

Baker, Tom, and Jonathan Simon. 2002. *Embracing Risk: The Changing Culture of Insurance and Responsibility*. Chicago: University of Chicago Press.

Boehm, Deborah A. 2005. The Safety Net of the Safety Net: How Federally Qualified Health Centers "Subsidize" Medicaid Managed Care. *Medical Anthropology Quarterly* 19(1): 47–63.

Carroll, Aaron. 2012. Why emergency rooms don't close the health care gap. www.cnn.com.

Cassidy, Amanda. 2013. Essential Health Benefits. *Health Affairs.* Health Policy Briefs. www.healthaffairs.org.

Christopher, Andrea S., Danny McCormick, Steffie Woolhandler, David U. Himmelstein, David H. Bor, and Andrew P. Wilper. 2016. Access to Care and Chronic Disease Outcomes Among Medicaid-Insured Persons versus the Uninsured. *American Journal of Public Health* 106(1): 63–69.

Clarke, John. 2004. *Changing Welfare, Changing States: New Directions in Social Policy.* Thousand Oaks, CA: Sage.

Clemans-Cope, Lisa, Matthew Buettgens, and Hannah Recht. 2014. Racial/ethnic differences in uninsurance under the ACA: Are differences in uninsurance rates projected to narrow? *Urban Institute.* www.urban.org.

Closser, Svea, and Erin Finley. 2016. A New Reflexivity: Why Anthropology Matters in Contemporary Health Research and Practice, and How to Make It Matter More. *American Anthropologist* 1118(2): 385–390.

CMS (Centers for Medicare and Medicaid Services). 2012. Emergency Medical Treatment & Labor Act (EMTALA). www.cms.gov.

———. 2016. Exemptions from the requirement to have health insurance. www.health care.gov.

Cohen, Robin A., and Michael E. Martinez. 2015. Health Insurance Coverage: Early Release of Estimates from the National Health Interview Survey January–March 2015. *Centers for Disease Control and Prevention/National Center for Health Statistics.* www.cdc.gov.

Collins, Sara. R., Petra W. Rasmussen, Sophie Beutel, and Michelle M. Doty. 2015. The problem of underinsurance and how rising deductibles will make it worse—findings from the Commonwealth Fund Biennial Health Insurance Survey. *Commonwealth Fund.* www.commonwealthfund.org.

Dao, Amy, and Jessica Mulligan. 2016. Toward an Anthropology of Insurance and Health Reform: An Introduction to the Special Issue. *Medical Anthropology Quarterly*, 30(1): 5–17.

Dumit, Joseph. 2012. *Drugs for Life.* Durham, NC: Duke University Press.

Dwyer, Rachel E., and Lora A. Phillips Lassus. 2015. The Great Risk Shift and Precarity in the U.S. Housing Market. *ANNALS of the American Academy of Political and Social Science* 660(1): 199–216.

Enthoven, Alain C., and Victor R. Fuchs. 2006. Employment-Based Health Insurance: Past, Present, and Future. *Health Affairs* 25(6): 1538–1547.

Ericson, Richard V., Aaron Doyle, and Dean Barry. 2003. *Insurance as Governance.* Toronto: University of Toronto Press.

Franke-Ruta, Garance. 2013. Why Is Maternity Care Such an Issue for Obamacare Opponents? *The Atlantic*, November 22.

Garfield, Rachel, and Anthony Damico. 2016. Issue Brief: The Coverage Gap: Uninsured Poor Adults in States that Do Not Expand Medicaid. *Kaiser Family Foundation.* kff.org.

Goode, Judith G., and Jeff Maskovky. 2001. *The New Poverty Studies: The Ethnography of Power, Politics and Impoverished People in the United States*. New York: New York University Press.

Goodell, Sarah. 2014. Health Policy Brief: Risk Corridors. *Health Affairs*. healthaffairs .org.

Haeder, Simon F., and David L. Weimer. 2015. You Can't Make Me Do It, but I Could Be Persuaded: A Federalism Perspective on the Affordable Care Act. *Journal of Health Politics, Policy and Law* 40(2): 281–323.

Haney López, Ian. 2014. *Dog Whistle Politics: How Coded Racial Appeals Have Reinvented Racism and Wrecked the Middle Class*. New York: Oxford University Press.

Health Resources & Services Administration (HRSA). 2016. About the Ryan White HIV/AIDS Program. hab.hrsa.gov.

Himmelstein, David U., Deborah Thorne, Elizabeth Warren, and Steffie Woolhandler. 2009. Medical Bankruptcy in the United States, 2007: Results of a National Study. *American Journal of Medicine* 122(8): 741–746.

Horton, Sarah, and Louise Lamphere. 2006. A Call to an Anthropology of Health Policy. *Anthropology News* 47(1): 333–336.

Horton, Sarah, Cesar Abadía, Jessica Mulligan, and Jennifer Jo Thompson. 2014. A Critical Medical Anthropological Approach to the U.S.'s Affordable Care Act. *Medical Anthropology Quarterly* 28(1): 1–22.

Horton, Sarah, Joanne McCloskey, Caroline Todd, and Marta Henriksen. 2001. Transforming the Safety Net: Responses to Medicaid Managed Care in Rural and Urban New Mexico. *American Anthropologist* 103(3): 733–746.

Isin, Engin F. 2009. Citizenship in Flux: The Figure of the Activist Citizen. *Subjectivity* 29: 367–388.

Jain, Sachin H., Brian W. Powers, and Darshak Sanghavi. 2015. Big Plans, Poor Execution: The Importance of Governmental Managerial Innovation to Health Care Reform. *Journal of General Internal Medicine* 30(4): 395–397.

Jones, David K., Katharine W. V. Bradley, and Jonathan Oberlander. 2014. Pascal's Wager: Health Insurance Exchanges, Obamacare, and the Republican Dilemma. *Journal of Health Politics, Policy and Law* 39(1): 97–137.

Kaiser Commission on Medicaid and the Uninsured. 2012. *The Uninsured: A Primer, October 2012*. Kaiser Family Foundation, Menlo Park, CA.

———. 2016. *The Uninsured: A Primer, November 2016*. Kaiser Family Foundation, Menlo Park, CA.

Kaiser Family Foundation (KFF). 2012. A Guide to the Supreme Court's Affordable Care Act Decision. kff.org.

———. 2016a. Disparities in Health and Health Care: Five Key Questions and Answers, kff.org.

———. 2016b. Health and Access to Care and Coverage for Lesbian, Gay, Bisexual, and Transgender (LGBT) Individuals in the U.S., kff.org.

Katz, Michael B. 2008 (2001). *The Price of Citizenship: Redefining the American Welfare State*. Philadelphia: University of Pennsylvania Press.

Kingfisher, Catherine. 2002. *Western Welfare in Decline: Globalization and Women's Poverty*. Philadelphia: University of Pennsylvania Press.

Levitt, Larry, Gary Claxton, Anthony Damico, and Cynthia Cox. 2016. Assessing ACA Marketplace Enrollment. *Kaiser Family Foundation*. kff.org.

McMorrow, Stacey, Sharon K. Long, Genevieve M. Kenney, and Nathaniel Anderson. 2015. Uninsurance Disparities Have Narrowed for Black and Hispanic Adults under the Affordable Care Act. *Health Affairs* 34(10): 1774–1778.

Mol, Anne Marie. 2008. *The Logic of Care: Health and the Problem of Patient Choice*. New York: Routledge.

Morgan, Kimberly J., and Andrea Louise Campbell. 2011. Delegated Governance in the Affordable Care Act. *Journal of Health Politics, Policy and Law* 36(3): 387–391.

National Center for Transgender Equality (NCTE). 2016. HHS issues regulations banning trans health care discrimination. www.transequality.org.

National Health Law Program (NHeLP). 2014. NHeLP and the AIDS Institute file hiv/aids discrimination complaint against Florida health insurers. www.healthlaw.org.

National Women's Law Center (NWLC). 2012. *Turning to Fairness: Insurance Discrimination again Women Today and the Affordable Care Act*. www.nwlc.org.

Obama, Barack. 2016. United States Health Care Reform: Progress to Date and Next Steps. *Journal of American Medical Association* 316(5): 525–532.

Okongwu, Anne Francis, and Joan P. Mencher. 2000. The Anthropology of Public Policy: Shifting Terrains. *Annual Review of Anthropology* 29: 107–124.

Organization of Economic Cooperation and Development (OECD). 2014. OECD Health Statistics 2014. How does the United States compare? www.oecd.org.

———. 2015. Health at a Glance 2015: OECD Indicators. www.oecd.org.

Paradise, Julia. 2015. "Medicaid Moving Forward." Kaiser Commission on Medicaid and the Uninsured. kff.org.

Pear, Robert. 2015a. Health Insurance Companies Seek Big Rate Increases for 2016. *New York Times*, July 3.

———. 2015b. Many Say High Deductibles Make Their Health Law Insurance All but Useless. *New York Times*, November 14.

Pigg, Stacy Leigh. 2013. On Sitting and Doing: Ethnography as Action in Global Health. *Social Science & Medicine* 99: 127–134.

Robert Wood Johnson Foundation (RWJ). 2011. Issue Brief: How does the Affordable Care Act address racial and ethnic disparities in health care? www.rwjf.org.

Sered, Susan S., and Rushika Fernandopulle. 2005. *Uninsured in America: Life and Death in the Land of Opportunity*. Berkeley: University of California Press.

Shear, Michael D. 2014. Sebelius Resigns After Troubles Over Health Site. *New York Times*, April 10.

Shore, Chris, and Susan Wright. 1997. Policy: A New Field of Anthropology. In *Anthropology of Policy: Critical Perspectives on Governance and Power*, ed. Chris Shore and Susan Wright, Pp. 3–39. Oxford: Routledge.

Soss, Joe, Richard C. Fording, and Sanford F. Schram. 2011. *Disciplining the Poor: Neoliberal Paternalism and the Persistent Power of Race*. Chicago: University of Chicago Press.

Taylor, Janelle S. 2014. The Demise of the Bumbler and the Crock: From Experience to Accountability in Medical Education and Ethnography. *American Anthropologist*, 116: 523–534.

Willen, Sarah S. 2012. Migration, "Illegality," and Health: Mapping Embodied Vulnerability and Debating Health-Related Deservingness. *Social Science & Medicine* 74(6): 805–811.

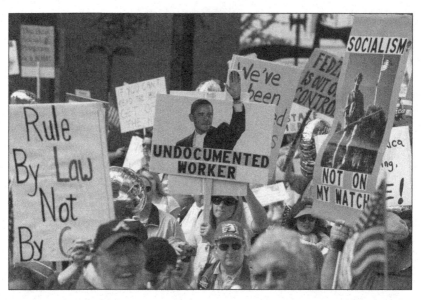

Figure S1.1. Undocumented Worker. The Taxpayer March on DC proceeds down Pennsylvania Avenue toward the Capitol on Saturday, September 12, 2009. (CQ Roll Call via AP Images)

Inclusions and Exclusions

When the Affordable Care Act (ACA) was enacted, it represented a sweeping transformation of the U.S. health care system designed to make access to health insurance more equitable and affordable. However, it built upon a legacy of existing stratification that had long excluded people by class, occupation, race, ethnicity, gender, and sexuality. This foundation was coupled with a series of political and legal compromises and concessions, including the U.S. Supreme Court ruling that permitted states to decide whether or not to expand Medicaid (in those that didn't, the "coverage gap" was created). As a result, while many people found themselves newly included, others experienced no change to their health insurance status or were purposely shut out. While the law represented an extension of social protections to some groups, it also created new forms of exclusion as access to affordable coverage options were highly segmented by state of residence, income, and citizenship status.

Many immigrants were explicitly excluded from the ACA, including undocumented persons and those with less than five years of residency in the United States. The ACA is layered on an existing patchwork of policies that already created segregated effects, especially the Personal Responsibility and Work Opportunity Reconciliation Act (PRWORA). However, as the following chapters show, immigrant groups in the United States are not monolithic but instead are stratified by many chaotic bureaucratic categories. Because the ACA maintained most of these prior exclusions—such as the exclusion of "nonqualified" immigrants from Medicaid—while simultaneously creating new exclusions (such as that of DACA recipients, who arrived as children and were granted a temporary reprieve under President Obama), this lead to quite a checkered landscape of eligibility for immigrants in mixed-status families (Castañeda). Moreover, as the federal government has devolved to states the decision about whether to restore inclusion in Medicaid for certain unqualified immigrants (such as legal permanent residents, who have

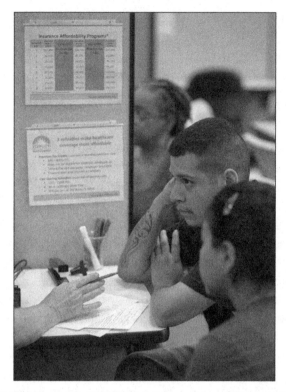

Figure S1.2. Texas Insurance Sign-Up. Eric Sosa, center, and Nancy Maldonado, right, listen to a volunteer counselor with Insure Central Texas explain health insurance options, Tuesday, October 1, 2013, in Austin, Texas. Texas hospitals, clinics, and charities are gearing up to help uninsured Texans enroll in health care exchanges after Governor Rick Perry declared the state government would do as little as possible to help implement the Affordable Care Act. (AP photo/Eric Gay)

been in the United States for less than five years) (Joseph)—as well as what services Emergency Medicaid should provide undocumented immigrants (Melo), this landscape of exclusion varies dramatically across states. In addition, some states that had inclusive practices before the ACA and that included these immigrants (e.g., Massachusetts) continued to do so, while others later used the state option to expand eligibility to these groups (e.g., California). Finally, the chapter by Andaya shows that some groups experienced exclusions and inequality not because they were left out of the ACA, but because of the kind of coverage they were afforded.

1

Stratification by Immigration Status

Contradictory Exclusion and Inclusion after Health Care Reform

HEIDE CASTAÑEDA

While the Patient Protection and Affordable Care Act of 2010 (ACA) extended public and private insurance to some 20 million individuals (Garrett and Gangopadhyaya 2016), this chapter argues that it stratified immigrants with harsh and sometimes contradictory results. The ACA squarely addressed the problem of uneven access, though it stopped well short of universal health care. However, the sheer size of the excluded immigrant population in the United States stands in the way of the goal of expanding coverage (Panday et al. 2014). Immigrant communities cannot be viewed as monolithic as they are stratified by a multitude of chaotic bureaucratic categories that are created by the state and set specific parameters for inclusion and exclusion.

This chapter provides evidence that juridico-legal categories of immigration status mattered just as much as means-tested categories for the ACA. Experiences of inclusion were complex, and especially evident in the unexpected grey areas I present here, where particular categories of immigrants were included or excluded from the benefits associated with the ACA in often-contradictory ways. Less unexpected, perhaps, is the explicit exclusion of an estimated 11.2 million undocumented immigrants. Marrow and Joseph (2015) have argued that the health care reform intentionally increased the "brightness" of immigrants' symbolic and social exclusion within the U.S. health care system, creating a massive boundary shift that resulted in a stronger and clearer separation of undocumented immigrants from the rest of the morally "deserving" U.S. body politic. This shift occurred, first, through a *boundary expansion* for U.S. citizens and long-term legal immigrants, and second, through a *boundary contraction* for undocumented immigrants.

This chapter furthers this analysis by arguing that the boundary contraction worked alongside other policies and within household structures to complicate the issue not only for some *authorized* immigrants, but also for *U.S. citizens*. It illustrates these unanticipated and contradictory effects by examining eligibility categories delineating between "qualified" and "non-qualified" immigrants. Both of these designations applied only to those considered "lawfully present immigrants"; as the law already explicitly excluded undocumented immigrants, they are not the subjects of the current chapter. Instead, I focus on three cases in which the inclusion of lawfully present persons became muddled and resulted in unexpected and contradictory situations: first, U.S. citizen children in mixed-status families; second, the exclusion of young adults holding deferred action for childhood arrival (DACA) status; and third, a loophole that allowed some immigrants to qualify for insurance subsidies while U.S. citizens living in the same state did not. Although not focused on undocumented persons, this chapter does speak to the extended, indirect effects of excluding them from health care access through the resulting impacts on lawfully present immigrants and U.S. citizens.

Following the passage of the ACA, different state governments took quite diverse approaches to implementing the law, with some creating state-based exchanges, expanding Medicaid, and supporting the application process. Texas, however, remained in adamant opposition to the law; its position is best described as "absolute non-collaboration" (Jones et al. 2014). A large portion of the population remained ineligible for Marketplace insurance and subsidies, either because they were undocumented or were among the working poor who made less than 100% of the federal poverty level. Texas rejected the expansion of adult Medicaid, which would have insured 1.5 million low-income working adults and brought in billions in federal funding to remedy this gap. Thus, the benefits associated with the ACA remained uncertain for a large percentage of those living in the region, and the burden of filling gaps in health care continued to fall on the severely underfunded local levels.

While certain contradictions are best highlighted through a specific research site such as the one presented here, this chapter also steps back to examine processes and implications on a much wider scale, arguing that the policy convergence of immigration and health care reform is a useful lens with which to understand the reinforcement of categories of deservingness and stratified citizenship, even within a diverse migrant population.

Methods

This chapter draws from data gathered from ethnographic fieldwork along the Texas/Mexico border, where through a series of projects we have been talking with immigrants of various statuses along with community stakeholders in order to understand how the state and its agents demarcate the contours of inclusion (Castañeda and Melo 2014). This region remains home to the highest rate of uninsured persons in the nation, having garnered first place in a list of "Counties that Need the Affordable Care Act the Most" (Chu and Posner 2013). While Texas has the highest uninsurance rate in the nation, this county has the highest rate in the state.

This research was informed by semi-structured interviews with 167 individuals living in mixed-status families in Hidalgo County, Texas. Of these, 75 individuals completed a follow-up interview one year later, providing a longitudinal picture of their lives, while ten participants completed two additional interviews and were followed for more than four years. Participants were recruited using purposive referral (snowball) sampling after initial individuals who met the inclusion criteria were identified with the assistance of local community-based organizations. A $20 gift card to a local retailer was provided as an incentive. Interviews lasted from 35 minutes to two hours and took place at a location of the participant's choice, typically in their homes. The author or research assistant Melo (see chapter 2) conducted all initial and follow-up interviews. Interviews were conducted in Spanish (n=94), English (n=61), or both languages (n=12) and audio-recorded with the participant's consent.

Another source of data was informal interviews with health care providers, caseworkers, navigators, social workers, organizational staff, public health officials, researchers, and other key stakeholders (n=62). Five of these interviews were conducted in Spanish, while the rest were in English. Because they were the result of different project phases, only 21 were audio-recorded and the rest relied on extensive note taking. These interviews provided background information about county characteristics, historic efforts at improving health care, availability of services, and major challenges and successes experienced.

All interviews were transcribed verbatim and then analyzed with the aid of MAXQDA (Version 12) software. The coding process utilized both deductively derived codes identified from an initial pilot study, as well as inductively derived codes emerging from the data and reflecting the particular concepts and concerns of participants. Descriptive coding was utilized to draw out major phrases and concepts and to compare and contrast data points across interviews. Systematic analysis identified categories and concepts that emerged from the text, which were linked to the theoretical constructs in an iterative process. The preliminary analyses were brought back to organizational partners in August 2016 for critique and validation through summaries and small group discussions.

The results sections that follow describe major themes that emerged relating to the ACA and health care access. All Spanish quotes have been translated into English by the author, and all names are pseudonyms.

Immigration Status and Health Care Reform

The ACA utilized several distinct categories of juridico-legal status to determine individuals' eligibility for programs. These categories were first constructed by Congress in 1996 as part of the Personal Responsibility and Work Opportunity Reconciliation Act (PRWORA) and distinguish between "qualified" and "non-qualified" immigrants for federal benefits purposes. Eligibility for marketplace coverage through the ACA utilized a similar framework, although it *first* distinguished between "lawfully present immigrants" (which includes both "qualified" and some "non-qualified" categories from the PRWORA framework) and "not lawfully present immigrants."

"Lawfully Present" Immigrants under the ACA

Under the ACA, lawfully present immigrants included lawful permanent residents (i.e., green card holders), refugees, asylees, Cuban and Haitian entrants, certain victims of domestic violence and trafficking survivors and their derivatives (his/her spouse, child, sibling, or parent), persons granted withholding of deportation/removal, temporary protected status, lawful temporary residents, individuals with nonimmigrant status (including holders of worker visas and student visas), those with deferred enforced departure, and deferred action status (with the exception of Deferred Action for Childhood Arrivals), as well as applicants for any of these statuses. However, not all lawfully present persons were "qualified" persons. For example, nonimmigrants—the official term for students, visitors, and temporary guest workers, who are not legal permanent residents—are categorized as "lawfully present" but were ineligible for benefits under the ACA, including purchasing coverage on the exchanges. Only those who were both "lawfully present" and "qualified" were eligible for exchange subsidies, as well as premium tax credits and cost-sharing tax credits toward plans that met the essential benefits package outlined in the ACA, regardless of how long they have been in the United States.

Furthermore, lawfully present immigrants' eligibility for Medicaid—a public program—remained restricted under the ACA, with "qualified" immigrants barred for the first five years and those with "non-qualified" statuses (e.g., non-immigrants) barred indefinitely unless their status changed. Lawfully residing immigrant adults who have been in the country five years or less are not eligible for Medicaid coverage (in states that have opted to expand adult Medicaid). However, some lawfully residing immigrant children who have been in the country less than five years were eligible for Medicaid coverage at state option.[1] In other words, opportunities for Medicaid coverage for both children and adults varied depending on the state in which they live.

"Not Lawfully Present" Immigrants under the ACA

The Affordable Care Act expressly excluded undocumented immigrants from participating in the federally subsidized state health exchanges and the Medicaid expansion. They were also exempt from the individual mandate requiring insurance coverage or payment of a penalty. The only program for which they qualified—as before—was prenatal care under Medicaid and emergency room care (see chapter by Melo in this volume). They may also receive health care from Federally Qualified Health Centers (FQHCs) and some state and local programs regardless of immigration status. FQHCs are a major source of primary care for populations that remained uninsured through the ACA; however, despite increased funding and bipartisan political support, they struggle with financial self-sufficiency, health professional shortages, inadequate networks of specialists, and low-quality outcomes. FQHCs are only located in one-quarter of the areas designated as medically underserved and provide only limited primary and preventive services. In the past, local for-profit hospitals claimed 10–20% of their annual budgets as uncompensated care and recuperated costs from Medicaid Disproportionate Share Hospital (DSH) funds, Emergency Medicaid, and county indigent programs. However, DSH funds were greatly reduced under the ACA, based on the assumption that there would be an increase in insured patients.

Efforts to limit health care have remained a standard and predictable tool for enforcing immigration control in the United States. In September 2009, when President Obama addressed a joint session of Congress to outline his plans for health care reform that would ultimately lead to the passage of the ACA, it was his assurance that the proposal would *not* cover undocumented immigrants that drew the most attention. During Obama's speech, Representative Joe Wilson of South Carolina shouted, "You lie!" and in the following weeks, this prompted another round of debate over immigration policy. It was but one of many examples of Americans' continuing public confusion and unease regarding undocumented immigrants' access to the health care system, but also one of the few moments where anxieties over "rationing" health care has been discussed explicitly and openly. Even after the passage of the ACA, health care in the United States remained conceptualized as a scarce and limited good, with no acknowledgment that it is a right, and that it is explicitly withheld from those who are viewed as undeserving.

Thus, the undocumented had already been symbolically and socially excluded, even relative to previously uninsured individuals who became insured. Under the ACA, the U.S. government explicitly reserved and allocated most resources for insurance coverage and care to U.S. citizens and long-term legal immigrants, illustrating how juridical mechanisms such as labeling now more strongly classify and stereotype undocumented immigrants as illegal, immoral, and undeserving outsiders (Marrow and Joseph 2015; Light 2012).

Contradictions of Inclusion and Exclusion: Three Cases

While the exclusion of those not lawfully present was clearly defined in the ACA and has been explored elsewhere, this chapter examines the ambiguity, "messiness," and spillover effects for other categories of immigrants, permanent residents, and U.S. citizens. I argue that efforts to exclude some groups viewed as "undeserving" led to unintended consequences for others. In other words, the intimate linking of immigration and health care resulted in curious and contradictory situations.

Case 1: Mixed-Status Families

> When my parents came here, they really weren't looking for anything, being supported by the government, feed off the government. They were just looking for a better life. I went to a doctor when I was six and a social worker came up to my mom and told her that she could get Medicaid for us kids. But we have talked in my family that we're going to have to pay back all that money that the government provided to us to go to the doctor, or that there was going to be a penalty for having Medicaid for us who were born here in the United States.

In this quote, Lisa, a 23-year-old U.S. citizen who grew up in a mixed-status family, describes her family's decision-making process regarding enrolling eligible children into the Medicaid program. As she recalls, because her parents were undocumented, they hesitated to enroll their children, believing that they would ultimately have to "pay back all that money," even though the federal program is designed to provide benefits to low-income children with no or inadequate medical insurance (and is not a loan to be paid back). Their fear stemmed from the belief that accepting any form of government assistance would jeopardize the entire family's future, since being perceived as a "public charge"—that is, dependent on the government—impacts chances of future regularization of legal status. However, the U.S. Citizenship and Immigration Services has a policy clearly stating that the use of non-cash public benefits—including Medicaid—will not be used to determine if someone is a public charge when applying for residency or citizenship. Enrolling eligible family members in these programs does not put other members at risk for being a public charge, and parents should not have to fear repercussions for accessing them on behalf of their children. Nonetheless, in mixed-status families across the nation, people described a desire to avoiding "being on the list" or having any "debts" to the government, including through the provisions of the ACA, such as subsidies or tax credits. In the end, Lisa's parents decided to enroll her and her brother in Medicaid, which covered regular doctor and dentist visits until they turned 18. As she says, "In times of need, for our parents our health is more important than having to pay a fee afterwards."

Lisa's story highlights the dilemma faced by mixed-status families in the United States. There are 2.3 million families with varied constellations of citizens, permanent legal residents, undocumented immigrants, those holding visitor visas, and individuals in legal limbo, e.g., temporary protected status or deferred action. The majority of children in such families—about 4.5 million—are U.S. citizens by birth. Their composition is not static, as members may move in and out of households and between statuses over time. In recent years, the number of migrant families with complex legal status configurations has sharply increased; indeed, mixed-status families must be considered a primary feature of the contemporary immigration experience (Castañeda and Melo 2014).

Mixed-status families are analytically significant as social units in which the relationship to the state differs among individual members, who are sharply separated on the basis of rights and opportunities. The ways individuals are categorized by the state—which has the power to demarcate boundaries and define inclusion—in fact establishes the very contours of the family. Family and immigration law in the United States has failed to keep pace with the fluid and complex configurations of migrant families; rather than preserving, law has become a mechanism for dividing families. This has implications that ripple through kin networks and permeate daily life via the threat of deportation, restrictions on mobility, and lack of access to education and health care. Thus, experiences in mixed-status families are repeatedly mediated by the discursive formation of "illegality" (de Genova 2002), the impact of which can be examined in everyday, embodied experiences, even for those who are lawfully present. Lisa's case illustrates that, because individuals are always members of larger family units, the production of "illegality" for some shapes experiences and opportunities for all.

In the case of mixed-status families, exclusionary effects can be read as unintended consequences of policy or as a deliberate effect of state power. Abrego and Menjívar (2011) describe the "legal violence" that occurs when laws protect the rights of some while simultaneously marginalizing other groups and leaving them more vulnerable. This is especially devastating when it restricts practices at the core of family dynamics via ideas of "good parenting," such as the ability to access resources for children in times of illness. Furthermore, policies restricting or mystifying access have broad spillover effects on others living in the same household. The structure of public health insurance entails the potential for variable eligibility to occur within families, which is associated with decreased access to care for all (Hudson 2009). This creates dilemmas for parents, who may worry about favoritism and thus not enroll any children in programs (Pereira et al. 2012), resulting in reduced overall household resources (Hagan et al. 2003).

Citizen children like Lisa are directly impacted by the "illegality" of family members. Despite their eligibility for benefits such as Medicaid and Children's Health Insurance Program (CHIP), they access these at a lower rate than those with citizen parents (Fix and Passel 2002; Hagan et al. 2003; Huang et al. 2006; Pereira et al. 2012). Complex eligibility rules produce a "chilling effect" on participation by mixed-status families (Sommers et al. 2012). Fear of deportation leads some families to limit or delay services for children (Abrego and Menjívar 2011; Capps et al. 2004), or withdraw from programs altogether (Hagan et al. 2003; Xu and Brabeck 2012). Moreover, as described earlier in Lisa's family's case, some undocumented parents fear that enrolling children will affect future chances at regularization, because of variability in and misunderstanding of public charge assessment (Castañeda and Melo 2014; Mendoza 2009; Park 2011). When immigration and health care access policies are combined, an environment is created "in which immigrants are often ineligible, discouraged or frightened from obtaining public health insurance coverage and health care services" (Hagan et al. 2003, 459).

Under the ACA, some mixed-status families had taxpaying members who could not purchase health insurance through the Marketplace, alongside other family members who were eligible to use the Marketplace as citizens or lawfully present immigrants. Similarly, some members were eligible for Medicaid or CHIP while others—for example, undocumented siblings—were not. For undocumented family members, the result was an exacerbation of existing health disparities, since access to services was reduced for undocumented immigrants under the ACA (Arredondo et al. 2012; ASPE 2014; Barnes 2013; Bustamante et al. 2012; Hinojosa-Ojeda et al. 2010; Warner 2012; Zuckerman et al. 2011). They became more isolated from the general, formerly uninsured population, and were ineligible for coverage through the purchase of subsidized insurance from health insurance exchanges, even out of their own pocket. Public support and funding for programs that treat uninsured persons also diminished (Sommers 2013). New identification requirements meant that some eligible mixed-status family members were likely to avoid preventative care (Hinojosa-Ojeda et al. 2010). Finally, the ACA provided specific rules for calculating subsidies that reduced the amounts for mixed-status families (Siskin 2011). At the same time, however, those ineligible for subsidized coverage (such as undocumented persons) may have benefited indirectly from the ACA because other family members did qualify for Medicaid or subsidized coverage, thus reducing the financial burden on the entire family (ASPE 2014). A focus on individuals might reveal little impact regarding eligibility or affordability of health care; however, there is a cumulative effect on families.

In our work, we have heard many stories like Lisa's, in which parents, social workers, and eligibility specialists described families' hesitancy to enroll citizen children in programs such as Medicaid due to fear of deportation or to avoid jeopardizing chances of future regularization. Another example is Juliana, who is 33 years old and has lived in the United States for 11 years. She has four children, all U.S. citizens. She said, "Well, at first I was hesitant to enroll them [in Medicaid] because they told me that if I ask for assistance, it will affect me later when there is immigration reform." Benefits specialists with whom we spoke were well aware of these policies and encouraged parents to enroll children, but still faced skepticism. This may be because some other programs do fall under the public charge assessment, namely cash assistance programs such as Supplemental Security Income and Temporary Assistance for Needy Families. Furthermore, various reports of information—not entirely incorrect—circulate within the community and are weighed alongside enrollment specialists' attempts to persuade parents. The broader implication was that some refused to accept *any* services to avoid the perception of being a public charge. In addition, undocumented parents sometimes hesitated to enroll their children because eligibility was based on household income; this required them to enter all of their personal information (address, employer, etc.) in the system, which they may have been unwilling to do because of their precarious legal status.

Of particular significance here is the self-exclusion that accompanies this process. Some parents opted to not enroll eligible children in programs with an eye toward the greater good of the family because they did not want to be viewed as a public charge. This, along with the desire to "pay back" services—despite clear contributions to the federal tax base and to local economies—is a means to demonstrate one's contribution and is practiced as a marker of citizenship and worthiness of membership. These are not simply difficult decisions made by parents who hesitate or refuse to enroll eligible children. Rather, these possibilities are constructed by the state and its disciplinary practices through juridical categorization. The production of categories of semi-membership, as well as the persistent hope for an imminent comprehensive immigration reform, repeatedly promise the prospect of change and add significantly to the insecurity experienced by these households.

Case 2: DACA Recipients

A second incongruity presented by the stipulations of the ACA was that recipients of Deferred Action for Childhood Arrivals (DACA) fell into the category of "non-qualified" immigrants, despite the fact that they were considered lawfully present. In other words, they were an exception to the rule: lawfully present, but not qualified. How did this come to be, and how did people experience this contradiction?

In an effort to address some of the challenges that undocumented youth face in the midst of ongoing debates and political stagnation over the proposed DREAM Act[2] and comprehensive immigration reform, President Obama exercised administrative discretion to announce the DACA program on June 15, 2012. However, unlike the DREAM Act,

DACA did not give undocumented youth lawful permanent resident status or a path to legal permanent residency or citizenship; it simply provided temporary relief from deportation and a work authorization that could be renewed every two years. DACA had a massive effect on the lives of almost 800,000 young adults in a relatively short amount of time.

However, the program also produced patterns of formal and informal disenfranchisement. DACA recipients, like undocumented immigrants, were explicitly exempted from all provisions of the ACA and remained ineligible for regular Medicaid, Medicaid expansion, and the ability to purchase private insurance through the state-based health exchanges. On July 30, 2012, the Department of Health and Human Services' Centers for Medicare and Medicaid Services published an interim final rule that excluded DACA recipients from all key components of ACA program eligibility. Unlike other recipients of deferred action programs or persons granted a withholding of removal, they were deemed "non-qualified" immigrants. The treatment of DACA recipients presents a special case of *administrative rollback* among the eligibility categories for the Affordable Care Act. For those recipients, deservingness stopped short of insurance coverage and access to care (Marrow and Joseph 2015).

On the other hand, DACA recipients had access to employer-based insurance, since they were provided with a work permit. Many of the young adults in our study were thus able to acquire health insurance coverage for the first time in their lives (as undocumented children, they would not have been eligible for Medicaid growing up). At the time of our interviews, however, most had not yet used the insurance, since they were healthy overall and unaccustomed to regular primary and preventive care. The insurance, in these cases, served as a form of security should an accident occur. For example, Josue, a 24-year-old DACA recipient who worked at a large supermarket chain earning $1,200 a month, was able to obtain insurance from his employer.

> JOSUE: Everyone was hoping that there would be some sort of way that we could achieve a medical insurance. But there's nothing that ties DACA with medical insurance, so for the most part that was some-

thing that people had to seek out on their own and we can't apply
for Obamacare. We're excluded. But thankfully at my current job I'm
employed full-time and they have offered me insurance and I've been
able to take it.

HC: Have you used it yet?

JOSUE: I actually haven't. But it's nice to know that it's there if I need it.
And if something, god forbid, something really bad happens, I know
that I won't be up to my eyeballs in debt.

However, some young adults had difficulties utilizing the insurance
when they needed to because of their unfamiliarity with co-pays, deductibles, and the referral process after a lifetime of being uninsured. In
other cases, the deductibles in their plans were too high and made necessary care unaffordable. Several months after our interview, Josue was
involved in a car accident. After his emergency room care, he required
several follow-up surgeries with an orthopedic specialist to fully repair
a shattered bone. No longer considered an emergency, he now faced a
$5,000 deductible for the surgery that he could not afford. In addition,
because of his injury (not to mention a totaled vehicle), his supervisors
no longer scheduled him to work any shifts. There was simply no alternative work task for him while temporarily disabled. While he was able
to keep his job, over the course of those two months he earned no wages,
putting him even further into debt and leaving him unable to pay for
the necessary surgeries. In this case, the experience resulted in the same
outcome as if he had still been undocumented. He was indeed "up to his
eyeballs" in debt, as he had feared.

There is yet another contradiction. While DACA recipients were
sometimes able to acquire health insurance through their employers,
they were not *required* to do so under the individual mandate provisions of the ACA. In other words, because they were explicitly excluded,
they faced no penalty for being uninsured when they filed their income
taxes, as others do. In our work, we encountered numerous mispercep-
tions and instances of confusion among DACA recipients regarding the
individual mandate resulting in high levels of anxiety and a desire to
"do the right thing." For instance, 27-year-old Luis stated: "From my understanding, everyone is supposed to have insurance or they will get

fined. . . . We still don't have access. What are the consequences going to be for not having insurances if it is going to be mandatory? What category are we falling into?"

In many cases, the confusion was heighted because different individuals within the same family had different obligations to maintain coverage. In Luis's case, his two U.S.-born younger siblings fell under the individual mandate, while his undocumented parents did not. He himself, like others in our study with DACA, fell into a "grey zone" in which he was lawfully present but ineligible for the reform's benefits. However, it is also noteworthy that, rather than expressing relief that they were exempt from the mandate, most participants were instead very interested in opportunities to purchase affordable health insurance (Castañeda and Melo 2014).

Other DACA recipients viewed their exclusion from obtaining affordable coverage as "understandable" or even stated that that would be "asking too much." Many called DACA "just the first step." For instance, 26-year-old Martin, a college junior also working full-time with his new permit, stated that

> The focus right now is to give a social security [number] to the people who are already here. I think that is already asking enough, don't you? Like us, deferred action, they just gave us a social security number, but we can't have access to other things. And in my opinion if we could have both things it would be awesome, but if not, we will compromise simply with a social security number because like that you can work and if something costs money, medicines cost money, the money you would have there.

As Andaya (this volume) has pointed out, marginalized populations often face "the doxa of waiting"; this is the penalty for non-deservingness and socializes people into their place in the hierarchy of health citizenship. This leads some individuals like Martin to rationalize that it is simply a "compromise"—even though he lacks the social and political positioning to negotiate one—and that they have perhaps not "earned" full citizenship rights.

However, others felt that this was unfair since they did pay federal income and Medicare taxes in accordance with the work permit they were provided. In the words of 21-year-old Servando: "When it comes to fairness, we're paying the taxes like everyone else, and they're benefitting from it? How is that fair?" Sebastian, a 19-year-old DACA recipient who worked full-time at a lumber yard as he completed his college degree, continued:

> We're paying taxes, I'm paying Medicare taxes, aren't I? So why should I be giving the government money if I already paid my application, I work, paying taxes, I'm doing everything like every other citizen is doing, but yet I can't get the benefit. Sometimes I'm paying more than what they're paying. Yeah! I'm a real nerd, I was doing my math, and since January, I've paid like more than $400 to the government, and I could have helped my parents with $400. When I'm sick, I could use those $400. So if they're not giving me benefits, why should I pay? Shouldn't I use that money to pay for my own health care? A lot of us, thousands of us, don't have a choice.

Here we see the irony of having all the responsibilities of citizenship—working and paying taxes "like every other citizen"—without any of the benefits, including affordable health insurance options through the ACA Marketplace and no possibility to ever receive the Medicare benefits to which they are contributing.

Case 3: Immigrants Receive Subsidies Where Citizens Do Not

While the exclusion of DACA recipients is an example of a *boundary contraction* for some lawfully present immigrants, other situations resulted in unanticipated forms of inclusion for immigrants. A little-noticed provision of the ACA allowed some low-income lawfully present immigrants to qualify for subsidies to buy private insurance through online marketplaces. This "loophole" existed only in states that rejected Medicaid expansion.

Here is the background: the law's framers created a special option for lawfully present legal immigrants, who were barred from enrolling in Medicaid for five years. If those immigrants in the five-year waiting period earned less than the federal poverty level, they could qualify for a subsidy to help them buy private insurance. In addition, those earning between 100% and 400% of the poverty level were eligible for the same subsidies as U.S. citizens.

Thus, states that rejected the Medicaid expansion unintentionally created a disparity between citizens and immigrants, providing immigrants with a subsidy not available for U.S. citizens. In the initial version of the ACA, Medicaid coverage was to be extended to adults at 138% or below of the federal poverty level, until the 2012 U.S. Supreme Court ruling made this provision voluntary at state option. As a result, U.S. citizens caught in that gap were no longer eligible for subsidies if they lived in a state that opted to not expand Medicaid. But eligible immigrants did, because of the aforementioned provision at the federal level. Ironically, the original intent was exactly the opposite—namely, to disadvantage immigrants in the receipt of federal benefits—but the state option for Medicaid provision turned the situation around. As the director of Health and Civil Rights at the National Council of La Raza, an Hispanic advocacy group, noted: "It makes it look like legal immigrants are getting better treatment than U.S. citizens, but this was born out of Congress being punitive to immigrants . . . [wanting] to maintain the restrictions that prevent low-income immigrants from Medicaid" (Kaiser Health News 2014).

This situation had some remarkable political effects in states with large populations of immigrants, including Texas, where conservative policymakers generally opposed to the ACA used this loophole to advocate for expansion of their state's Medicaid program. They argued (correctly) that a failure to extend the program would deprive low-income U.S. citizens of access to insurance that is currently available to some legal immigrants. In Florida, for instance, a state with a large foreign-born population, this argument worked well by drawing on ideological debates around immigration, since an estimated 760,000 citizens remain ineligible for either subsidies or Medicaid. In Arizona, concerns about the political fallout of this issue helped persuade Republican governor Jan Brewer, initially an ardent foe of the health law, to expand Medicaid eligibility in 2013. Brewer's budget advisers said that without expanding the program, "only legal immigrants, but not citizens [below the federal poverty line], would be eligible for subsidies." In Texas, however, hundreds of thousands of working, low-income U.S. citizens remained locked out of subsidized insurance as the governor and other state leaders refused a federally paid expansion of Medicaid.

There was uneven knowledge about this provision among navigators and enrollment specialists. In many parts of Florida, for instance, enrollment specialists generally claimed a lack of awareness about this provision, which would have helped many low-income Haitian and Hispanic immigrants to qualify for subsidies. In the first two enrollment periods, technical issues with the healthcare.gov website contributed to this confusion; the site would automatically indicate that a person was ineligible for Medicaid or the subsidies if they were located in a non-expansion state. By contrast, in our work in Texas, the option was known by navigators and enrollment specialists and openly discussed at a regional Marketplace Assistance Working Group meeting we attended.

Conclusion

More than 20 years ago, the Personal Responsibility and Work Opportunity Reconciliation Act (PRWORA) set the precedent of tightly intertwining immigration status and eligibility for federal benefits purposes. This set the stage for immigrant exclusion that, with the ACA, intensified and became commonplace. However, we also saw grey areas, apertures, and unexpected contradictions. Using three case studies derived from longitudinal research in Texas, this chapter has illustrated the unanticipated and contradictory effects of the ACA by examining how legal categories influenced eligibility and participation. In each of the cases described here, the inclusion of lawfully present persons became muddled and resulted in unexpected situations: first, the ripple effects of exclusion on U.S. citizen children in mixed-status families; second, the exclusion of young adults holding deferred action for childhood arrival status (DACA); and third, a loophole that allowed some immigrants to qualify for insurance subsidies while U.S. citizens living in the same state could not, due to politicians' refusal to expand Medicaid.

Unlike some of the other chapters in this book (see those by Brunson, Mulligan, and Sered), the people described here were very eager to be included in health care reform, even though many of them were "excluded and frozen out" (Marrow and Joseph 2015) and, as I have shown, even described their own situation as unworthy. This chapter also shows that there was an ongoing balance between responsibilities and benefits: inclusion was complex, and in some cases people contributed to the overall system without receiving anything in return. This was especially poignant for the estimated 11.2 million undocumented immigrants, who remained without coverage despite contributing to the overall tax base. Some analysts have pointed out that covering the relatively healthy population of undocumented migrants would lower health premiums for everyone else. In other words, health care reform "could be motivated by enlightened self-interest for the insured as well as by an interest in social justice" (Brown et al. 2015, 991).

In the first case presented in this chapter, we saw that in mixed-status families, the effects of "illegality" extended to those who were lawfully present, including U.S. citizens. This challenges assumptions that anti-immigrant policies only affect the undocumented. In the second case, that of DACA recipients, we saw a special case of administrative rollback. Recipients of other forms of deferred action did, in fact, have access to the health care system. Notably, these gradations of inclusion are created only because they arrive in the form of an executive order, which may be reversed at any time. Thus, we see the formation of new and complex political subjectivities, as the constant vacillation between hope and fear engendered by the possibility of immigration reform acts as a major disciplinary practice (Chavez 2014; Gonzales and Chavez 2012). Finally, in the third case, states that rejected the Medicaid expansion unintentionally created a disparity between low-income citizens and legal immigrants. This is unique in its use of nationalist rhetoric on the political right to actually argue *for* Medicaid expansion, since not extending the program would have deprived low-income U.S. citizens of access to insurance available to some legal immigrants.

The ACA intentionally increased and intensified immigrants' exclusion from the health care system. It illustrated how symbolic boundaries have become more institutionalized into national health legislation and practice, yielding escalating symbolic and social exclusion for some—and especially undocumented—immigrants. Prior to 2010, these boundaries were at least blurred by the fact that 32 million other Americans also lacked insurance. As this chapter has argued, the effects and con tradictions of the ACA expanded beyond the exclusion of 11 million un- documented immigrants to affect authorized immigrants and even U.S. citizens. The political logic of utilizing access to affordable health care as a tool of immigration policy is faulty, and the negative effects ultimately affect groups that are otherwise designated as "lawfully present" (e.g., DACA recipients) and, perhaps even more poignantly, citizens—as in the case of U.S.-born children in mixed-status families and low-income, working-class Americans shut out of the opportunity to receive subsi- dies in states that refused to expand Medicaid.

ACKNOWLEDGMENTS

Funding for this project was provided by the National Science Foun- dation (Award #1535664) and the Wenner-Gren Foundation for Anthropological Research. I am profoundly grateful to families who shared their experiences with me. I appreciate the thoughtful feedback on this material from the participants in the 2015 School for Advanced Research Seminar on health care reform. I would like to thank Milena A. Melo for her invaluable assistance with data collection, and Nora Brick- house Arriola, Carla Castillo, Ryan Logan, and Aria Walsh-Felz for their assistance with transcription.

NOTES

1 The state option was made available since PRWORA, allowing states to decide to affirmatively include legal permanent residents who had been in the United States for fewer than five years with their own state Medicaid funds. This option is still available to states under the ACA.

2 The DREAM (Development, Relief, and Education for Alien Minors) Act was a legislative proposal introduced to the U.S. Senate in 2001 to grant conditional res- idency for undocumented immigrant youth who arrived before the age of 16 and who met strict eligibility requirements. Upon meeting further requirements, these youth would have qualified for permanent residency. The bill was re-introduced several times following its initial rejection, but has failed to pass.

REFERENCES

Abrego, Leisy, and Cecilia Menjívar. 2011. Immigrant Latina Mothers as Targets of Legal Violence. *International Journal of Sociology of the Family* 37(1): 9–26.

Arredondo, Armando, Emanuel Orozco, Steven P. Wallace, and Michael Rodriguez. 2012. Health Insurance for Undocumented Immigrants: Opportunities and Barriers on the Mexican Side of the U.S. Border. *International Journal of Health Planning and Management* 27(1): 50–62.

ASPE (Office of the Assistant Secretary for Planning and Evaluation, U.S. Department of Health and Human Services). 2014. The Affordable Care Act Coverage Implications and Issues for Immigrant Families. aspe.hhs.gov.

Barnes, Nielan. 2013. What Does the 2010 Affordable Care Act Mean for Securing Immigrant Health in North America? In *North American Integration: An Institutional Void in Migration, Security and Development.* Edited by Gaspare M. Genna and David A. Mayer-Foulkes, 152–176. New York: Routledge.

Brown, Henry S., Kimberly J. Wilson, and Jacqueline L. Angel. 2015. Mexican Immigrant Health: Health Insurance Coverage Implications. *Journal of Health Care for the Poor and Underserved* 26(3): 990–1004.

Bustamante, Arturo V., Hai Fang, Jeremiah Garza, Olivia Carter-Pokras, Steven P. Wallace, John A. Rizzo, and Alexander N. Ortega. 2012. Variations in Healthcare Access and Utilization among Mexican Immigrants: The Role of Documentation Status. *Journal of Immigrant and Minority Health* 14(1): 146–155.

Capps, Randolph, Michael E. Fix, Jason Ost, Jane Reardon-Anderson, and Jeffrey S. Passel. 2004. *The Health and Well-Being of Young Children of Immigrants.* Washington, DC: Urban Institute.

Castañeda, Heide, and Milena A. Melo. 2014. Health Care Access for Latino Mixed-Status Families: Barriers, Strategies, and Implications for Reform. *American Behavioral Scientist* 58(14): 1891–1909.

Chavez, Leo R. 2014. Illegality across Generations: Public Discourse and the Children of Undocumented Immigrants. In *Constructing Immigrant "Illegality": Critiques, Experiences, and Responses.* Edited by Cecilia Menjívar and Daniel Kanstroom, 84–110. Cambridge, MA: Cambridge University Press.

Chu, Anna, and Charles Posner. 2013. The Counties that Need the Affordable Care Act the Most. *Center for American Progress Action Fund.* www.americanprogressaction.org.

De Genova, Nicholas P. 2002. Migrant "Illegality" and Deportability in Everyday Life. *Annual Review of Anthropology* 31: 419–447.

Fix, Michael E., and Jeffrey S. Passel. 2002. Lessons of Welfare Reform for Immigrant Integration. *Urban Institute.* www.urban.org.

Garrett, Bowen, and Anuj Gangopadhyaya. 2016. Who Gained Health Insurance Coverage Under the ACA, and Where Do They Live? *Urban Institute.* www.urban.org.

Gonzales, Roberto G., and Leo R. Chavez. 2012. "Awakening to a Nightmare": Abjectivity and Illegality in the Lives of Undocumented 1.5-Generation Latino Immigrants in the United States. *Current Anthropology* 53(3): 255–281.

Hagan, Jacqueline, Nestor Rodriguez, Randy Capps, and Nika Kabiri. 2003. The Effects of Recent Welfare and Immigration Reforms on Immigrants' Access to Health Care. *International Migration Review* 37(2): 444–463.

Hinojosa-Ojeda, Raul, Max Hadler, and Paule Cruz Takash. 2010. *What Health Care Reform Means for Immigrants.* Los Angeles: Council of Mexican Federations, UCLA.

Huang, Zhihuan Jennifer, Stella M. Yu, and Rebecca Ledsky. 2006. Health Status and Health Service Access and Use among Children in U.S. Immigrant Families. *American Journal of Public Health* 96(4): 634–640.

Hudson, Julie L. 2009. Families with Mixed Eligibility for Public Coverage: Navigating Medicaid, CHIP, and Uninsurance. *Health Affairs* 28(4): w697–w709.

Jones, David K., Katharine W. V. Bradley, and Jonathan Oberlander. 2014. Notes on Pascal's Wager: Health Insurance Exchanges, Obamacare, and the Republican Dilemma. *Journal of Health Politics, Policy and Law* 39(1): 97–137.

Kaiser Health News. 2014. States that Reject Medicaid Expansion Could Create Disparity Between Legal Immigrants and Citizens. www.kff.org.

Light, Donald W. 2012. Categorical Inequality, Institutional Ambivalence, and Permanently Failing Institutions: The Case of Immigrants and Barriers to Health Care in America. *Ethnic & Racial Studies* 35(1): 23–39.

Marrow, Helen B., and Tiffany D. Joseph. 2015. Excluded and Frozen Out: Unauthorised Immigrants' (Non)Access to Care after U.S. Health Care Reform. *Journal of Ethnic and Migration Studies* 41(4): 2253–2273.

Mendoza, Fernando S. 2009. Health Disparities and Children in Immigrant Families: A Research Agenda. *Pediatrics* 124(Suppl 3): S187–195.

Pandey, Sanjay K., Joel C. Cantor, and Kristen Lloyd. 2014. Immigrant Health Care Access and the Affordable Care Act. *Public Administration Review* 74(6): 746–759.

Park, Lisa Sun-Hee. 2011. Criminalizing Immigrant Mothers: Public Charge, Health Care, and Welfare Reform. *International Journal of Sociology of the Family* 37(1): 27–47.

Pereira, Krista M., Robert Crosnoe, Karina Fortuny, Juan Pedroza, Kjersti Ulvestad, Christina Weiland, Hirokazu Yoshikawa, and Ajay Chaudry. 2012. Barriers to Immigrants' Access to Health and Human Services Programs. *Urban Institute* (May). aspe.hhs.gov.

Siskin, Alison. 2011. Treatment of Noncitizens Under the Patient Protection and Affordable Care Act. *Report to Congress.* Washington, DC: Congressional Research Service. www.nafsa.org.

Sommers, Benjamin D. 2013. Stuck between Health and Immigration Reform—Care for Undocumented Immigrants. *New England Journal of Medicine* 369(7): 593–595.

Sommers, Benjamin D., Meredith Roberts Tomasi, Katherine Swartz, and Arnold M. Epstein. 2012. Reasons for the Wide Variation in Medicaid Participation Rates among States Hold Lessons for Coverage Expansion in 2014. *Health Affairs* 31(5): 909–919.

Suárez-Orozco, Carola, Hirokazu Yoshikawa, Robert Teranishi, and Marcelo M. Suárez-Orozco. 2011. Growing Up in the Shadows: The Developmental Implications of Unauthorized Status. *Harvard Educational Review* 81(3): 438–473.

Warner, David C. 2012. Access to Health Services for Immigrants in the U.S.A.: From the Great Society to the 2010 Health Reform Act and After. *Ethnic and Racial Studies* 35(1): 40–55.

Xu, Qingwen, and Kalina Brabeck. 2012. Service Utilization for Latino Children in Mixed-Status Families. *Social Work Research* 36(3): 209–221.

Zuckerman, Stephen, Timothy A. Waidmann, and Emily Lawton. 2011. Undocumented Immigrants, Left Out of Health Reform, Likely to Continue to Grow as Share of the Uninsured. *Health Affairs* 30(10): 1997–2004.

2

Stratified Access

Seeking Dialysis Care in the Borderlands

MILENA ANDREA MELO

As the doctor leads me into the dialysis ward of the hospital, I spot Reynaldo lying in the last corner bed. Although his hands look rough from the construction work he has done all of his life in the United States, I notice how skinny and sickly his body looks, especially compared to his feet. His feet are so swollen that his shoes do not fit him. Although he is only wearing socks, it looks like he is hiding big bulky shoes, like skateboarder shoes, underneath them. "That is what happens when there is too much fluid built up," the doctor says. Reynaldo is a 48-year-old, undocumented Mexican immigrant receiving emergency dialysis for end-stage renal disease caused by his Type II diabetes. If he is lucky, he gets dialysis twice a week, although that almost never happens. Alternatively, he must survive with the bare minimum to keep him alive: treatment about once a week depending upon his potassium levels. He has been awake since 4 a.m., when his brother dropped him off at the hospital on his way to work. He has waited in the ER for over seven hours; it is now almost 3 p.m. and Reynaldo will finally be done with his dialysis treatment within the hour. However, his brother cannot pick him up until after work. Therefore, Reynaldo will return to the ER lobby and continue to wait until 6 p.m. Today the entire process took over 14 hours, but the effects of this treatment will soon wear off. When that happens, Reynaldo will have to once again return to the ER and hope to qualify for the treatment that will save his life.

Introduction

Undocumented immigrants in the United States are deemed undeserving of most publicly funded health care by virtue of their "illegal" status. Though they pay taxes, they are not afforded the same benefits that citizens and some legally present immigrants receive, such as federal aid. This population does not fit within the normal boundaries of substantive citizenship claims. Therefore, those excluded members with chronic, debilitating illness must struggle to navigate public and private health care institutions to locate lifesaving treatment, such as dialysis.

As argued in the introduction to this volume, exclusions in the ACA built upon and combined with national and state health care and immigration policies to shape the illness experiences of uninsured and undocumented low-income immigrants. This chapter features case studies of Mexican immigrant dialysis patients and explores the substandard treatment available to the uninsured and undocumented. The exclusion of certain populations from the ACA reveals the limits of belonging, discourses of deservingness, and American notions of human rights. What were the lived effects and risks of these exclusions on the lives of the low-income undocumented and uninsured? I argue that Giorgio Agamben's (1998) concept of "bare life" can be applied to dialysis patients excluded by biopolitical institutions (Foucault 1978) and the ACA. I will also detail and question the effects of the ACA failing to address this particular population of excluded patients who risk their lives to stay alive.

The U.S.-Mexico Borderlands of South Texas

Data for this chapter are derived from research focused on immigrants who receive dialysis treatment for end-stage renal disease (ESRD) in the U.S.-Mexico borderlands of South Texas, better known as the Rio Grande Valley (RGV). The South Texas borderlands have some of the highest rates of poverty and undocumented immigrants in the country. The study site, Hidalgo County, had a population estimated at 815,996 in 2013, of which 91% were Latino. According to the 2010 U.S. Census, 29.5% of Hidalgo County residents were foreign born, of which 97% were from Mexico. Hidalgo County's per capita income in 2012 was $14,126, compared to Texas at $25,809. Hidalgo's poverty rate of 35% was approximately double the state average (17.4%) (U.S. Census Bureau 2013).

Furthermore, Hidalgo County is one of the most medically underserved areas of the United States, characterized by gaps in public health services, poor access to care, significant environmental health concerns, elevated rates of chronic disease, one of the highest rates of obesity in the country (Bryner 2012), and the highest uninsured rate in the country at almost 40% (Hidalgo County Health and Human Services 2012). With the prevalence of ESRD risk factors such as obesity, hypertension, and diabetes (Montoya 2011), the RGV is a "hot spot" for dialysis treatment. As one dialysis patient told me, "Here in the Valley, *estamos en la raíz.* We are at the root of dialysis."

The RGV is effectively sealed off from both Mexico and the rest of the United States for undocumented immigrants. To the east lies the Gulf of Mexico, and to the south and west, Mexico. The northern edge of the RGV is lined with Border Patrol interior checkpoints. While undocumented immigrants who live north of the checkpoints may travel throughout the United States to find treatment for their medical needs, undocumented immigrants who live in the RGV cannot go north or south without facing inspection, surveillance, and probable deportation. Furthermore, increasing militarization of this geopolitical border has made crossing into Mexico for health care a virtual impossibility for undocumented immigrants. Thus, the RGV borderlands are a particularly resonant ethnographic site from which to understand the lived effects of health care policy on undocumented immigrants (Castañeda and Melo 2014).

Methods

Ethnographic data informing this chapter were derived from participant observation, semi-structured interviews, and case studies with 100 low-income Mexican immigrant dialysis patients (50 "documented," naturalized U.S. citizens or lawful permanent residents and 50 undocumented persons) and 42 health care professionals (social workers, dieticians, hospital administrators, nurses, dialysis technicians, financial directors, primary doctors, nephrologists, radiologists, biotechnicians, and dialysis facility administrators) conducted across 14 months of fieldwork. Health care professionals were recruited based on their occupation through dialysis centers, hospitals, and clinics. Of the 100 patients interviewed, eight (four documented and four undocumented) served as case studies; I met with these patients at least twice a month over a period of six months. Case study visits included everyday life activities, such as driving and accompanying patients to dialysis, doctor's appointments, errands, cooking together, attending family events such as birthday parties, barbeques, and *quinceañeras*, and simply talking around the kitchen table over a meal or cup of coffee. Interviews were conducted in English and Spanish, depending on interviewee preference. Recruitment of dialysis patients was facilitated through a local federally qualified health center and snowball sampling. I utilize pseudonyms to protect the identities of interviewees.

End-Stage Renal Disease and Dialysis

End-stage renal disease (ESRD) is complete, permanent kidney failure requiring regular, maintenance dialysis treatment three times a week to remove toxins and excess fluid while cleaning the blood. Without dialysis, people with ESRD suffer and die from associated complications. Dialysis involves several restrictions that impact patients for the rest of their lives (Hamdy 2008). Patients must spend three to four hours being dialyzed at each treatment. They may suffer from side effects such as nausea, vomiting, dizziness, cramping, fatigue, and many other symptoms before, during, and after treatment. Dialysis patients are on extremely strict diets that involve avoiding potassium and phosphorus-rich foods and drinking as little fluid as possible. Their ability to work is limited according to how they feel, as well as a variety of factors such as available dialysis schedules, transportation, Medicare and Medicaid income restrictions, and ability to freely travel. Furthermore, dialysis can cause severe strains on family relationships as well as emotional and psychological well-being.

Standard Maintenance Dialysis

To fully appreciate the differences in dialysis treatment between those who are covered and those who are excluded, it is important to first explore the basics of who receives the standard line of treatment in the United States as well as where, when, and how. Upon diagnosis of ESRD, almost all U.S. citizens and lawful permanent residents (LPRs) qualify to receive the standard of care consisting of thrice weekly maintenance dialysis treatments for ESRD through Medicare, Medicaid, and/or commercial insurance at private, for-profit outpatient dialysis centers.

Coverage also pays for surgery to prepare vascular access through an arteriovenous (AV) fistula or graft several months to a year before it becomes necessary to start dialysis. AV fistulas allow the entry vein to grow stronger and larger for increased blood flow at the site, which will be utilized for dialysis. Patients who do not have veins that can withstand constant use are implanted with a graft to serve the same purpose (Hamdy 2008). AV fistulas are considered the best long-term vascular access for dialysis because of their low rates of complications, adequate blood flow, and longevity, with grafts being a close second (NIDDKD 2006). Once the AV fistula or graft has had the proper amount of time to heal (usually about three months), strengthen, and grow, ESRD patients are able to easily transition into dialysis when determined necessary according to the nephrologist. Therefore, ideal dialysis treatment involves an appropriate, permanent vascular access, which will be utilized three times a week on set days and times in an outpatient dialysis clinic. Hortencia told me:

> I had been seeing Dr. John for several years—maybe like 4 or 5—when he told me that we were getting close, that my kidneys were at 18% and that I would need to start dialysis soon. He told me that I needed to get ready for this transition and asked to schedule my fistula surgery. I had my fistula for four months before I landed in the hospital and had to start dialysis.

Hortencia's experience provides a glimpse of the ideal transition into maintenance dialysis care. She had continuous treatment with a nephrologist for years who was able to slowly prepare her for the likelihood of dialysis. Hortencia also prepared herself by opting to have her fistula surgery before starting dialysis in order to be physically ready when the time came. Furthermore, because of her legal status as a U.S. citizen, she had access to health insurance, which covered the great majority of her medical costs. Before she was even released from the hospital, Hortencia was admitted to an outpatient facility where she goes three times a week for her dialysis treatments. She qualified for Medicare based on her kidney disease, working quarters, and legal status, and was therefore able to easily transition into the regular dialysis routine without ever having to ask about the price of dialysis.

Substandard, Emergency Care for the Excluded

In 1972, U.S. Public Law 92–603 granted access to dialysis for patients with ESRD with no requirement of citizenship or legal status for eligibility of treatment (Campbell et al. 2010). This, however, changed in 1986 when two revisions were passed as the Consolidated Omnibus Budget Reconciliation Act. The first revision prohibited federal Medicaid payments from applying to undocumented immigrants, unless it was an emergency and the patient would have otherwise qualified for Medicaid based on income (i.e., Emergency Medicaid). The second revision was the inclusion of the Emergency Medical Treatment and Active Labor Act (EMTALA). EMTALA requires all hospitals receiving Medicare funds to triage and treat/stabilize patients who request services at emergency departments regardless of their ability to pay or legal status. In 1996, the PRWORA placed the responsibility on individual states to determine what coverage they would provide for their undocumented immigrant population. Texas provides no other coverage. This act, along with the Illegal Immigration Reform and Immigrant Responsibility Act passed in 1996, has created serious barriers to accessing health care, since it requires patients to provide a social security number in order to qualify for publicly funded health care.

As a result of these changes in health care and immigration policy, the treatment protocol is drastically different for those who are excluded from insurance coverage through the patchwork of programs that include Medicare, Medicaid, and coverage bought on insurance exchanges. In order to qualify for Medicare, which covers 80% of dialysis treatment costs for the majority of patients, U.S. citizens and LPRs must have earned at least 40 working quarters (approximately 10 years) throughout their lifetime. For patients who are too young to have worked that long, they must rely on their parents or spouses to "transfer" quarters to them. U.S. citizens and LPRs who do not fulfill these criteria fall into very similar gaps of care as undocumented immigrants. As a result of their "unproductive" work history—as determined by these standards insinuating that they have not contributed enough tax dollars to the government—undocumented immigrants and non-qualifying U.S. citizens and LPRs are excluded from the standard of care. This chapter presents case studies of patients who fall into both of these treatment gaps.

Laws of exception and other forms of neoliberal governance that regulate and manage bodies restrict access to adequate ESRD dialysis treatment to U.S. citizens and LPRs, but only if they qualify. Individuals must have accrued sufficient annual quarters in their work history to be eligible for Medicare; otherwise, they can only access treatment if they self-pay the full cost of dialysis. Since undocumented immigrants with ESRD are not only non-citizens but also in the United States under an undocumented immigration status, government policies make irregular dialysis treatments in hospital emergency rooms the most common and often only option for undocumented immigrants in Texas (Hurley et al. 2009).

As I sat with Andres, an undocumented 49-year-old patient, in the hospital dialysis wing during his treatment, I listened attentively to the conversation he had with his Hispanic dialysis nurse in Spanish.

NURSE DIEGO: Dialysis patients are supposed to go to outpatient centers for their regular treatments. They are all over the place, you know, those big companies you see all over: Fresenius, DaVita, U.S. Renal. And they go three times a week but on a schedule.
ANDRES: So why haven't they sent me there to get dialysis?
NURSE DIEGO: Well you don't qualify. . . . you know . . . because you're not from here [the U.S.].
[Long pause as I saw Andres think about what he had just heard and digest it.]
ANDRES: Oh . . . right.

Diego nodded and looked solemnly at the floor before turning the swivel chair back to his laptop. In this conversation, Diego did not directly state that Andres did not have access to standard care because of his legal status, but he alluded to it, as is a common way of implying issues of legal status in this region on an everyday basis. Furthermore, Andres not only learned that there is a standard of care for dialysis outside of hospitals, but that he had been excluded from this option since he's not "from here." However, it is not an entirely correct portrayal. The problem is not that Andres was born and raised in Mexico, i.e., "not here," but that he does not have the validation provided by legal status to deem him deserving of U.S. benefits such as Medicare and Medicaid.

This scenario not only demonstrates why he is excluded, but also brings into question his belonging (Coutin 2003; Chavez 1992; Rosaldo 1997) and deservingness of care (Willen 2012a, 2012b) in the United States as a non-citizen. In this case, both Andres and Diego accepted emergency dialysis as the only option for Andres because of his legal status. In addition, simply saying he was not from the United States was enough of an answer for Andres to understand and accept it as fact. There was no awkward tension, just a long pause, and only a couple of minutes passed before the two started up another conversation, this time about cars.

This liminal and uncertain state of treatment produces additional harm to the already fragile social, economic, and political worlds of this marginalized population. The result is a cycle of increased suffering and reduced treatment, demonstrated by higher morbidity and mortality rates, and significantly higher economic costs (Campbell et al. 2010; Hurley et al. 2009). Ironically, undocumented immigrants are excluded from standard treatment partially based on economic justifications—since many believe (erroneously) that undocumented immigrants do not pay taxes, it follows that they should not receive publicly subsidized medical care. However, a study conducted in Texas (Sheikh-Hamad et al. 2007) compared costs associated between maintenance and emergency dialysis. They discovered that emergency dialysis costs 3.7 times more than maintenance dialysis, averaging $284,655 versus $76,906 per year. In this case, undocumented immigrants' "illegality" invokes a discourse about their lack of "deservingness" for any treatment that goes beyond the bare emergency minimum as dictated by government regulation.

When examining legal immigration status as a category of exclusion in health care policy, the concepts of illegality and deservingness are key to understanding the experiences of undocumented individuals who were almost completely excluded and documented immigrants who were partially included in the ACA (Castañeda 2009; De Genova 2002, 2005; Gomberg-Muñoz 2010, 2011; Willen 2012a, 2012b; Sargent 2012). Federal and state policies that deny undocumented immigrants regular health care, health-promoting resources, and workplace protection place them at greater risk for injury and illness (Fassin 2001, 2009, 2011; Horton 2004, 2006; Chavez 1986, 1991, 2008, 2012; Castañeda 2009; Willen 2012a, 2012b; Sargent 2012; Holmes 2013). Lives in illegality are compounded by poverty, conscripting immigrant bodies and well-being to be largely determined by state exclusionary practices (Becker 2004; Castañeda 2009; Willen 2012a, 2012b; Fassin 2001, 2009, 2011; Viladrich 2012; Marrow 2012). Abrego and Menjívar (2011) describe this as "legal violence," referring to laws that protect the rights of some while at the same time marginalizing certain groups, leaving them unprotected and ultimately more vulnerable. This legal violence can be experienced as stratified citizenship, impacting the experiences of individuals based on a variety of factors, including familial support, income, gender roles, and disability.

Although the great majority of undocumented immigrants have paid social security and Medicare taxes throughout their lives working in the United States, they have no legal record or status documenting the required working quarters to qualify them for Medicare. Therefore, undocumented dialysis patients not only do not qualify for Medicare to cover their dialysis, but they also cannot receive treatment in outpatient facilities because of their inability to self-pay the out-of-pocket costs associated with dialysis, which average approximately $6,000 per treatment.[1] They were also unable to purchase health care coverage from an insurance agency or through the ACA marketplace in the United States because of their legal status. Therefore, undocumented immigrants must rely on Emergency Medicaid as the last and only resource to cover their unscheduled and irregular intermittent care in hospital emergency rooms if deemed necessary by the attending physician (Sheik-Hamad et al. 2007; Hurley et al. 2009; Campbell et al. 2010). According to health care professionals interviewed, this is usually based on potassium levels, but can also be determined according to physical signs of distress such as shortness of breath or critically low heart rate.

Emergency Medicaid is available to anyone, regardless of legal status, who has been residing in the United States for at least six months and whose income falls below a given threshold (usually below 200% of the federal poverty level). However, in order to qualify for Emergency Medicaid, the emergency room visit must be deemed a "true emergency," defined by federal legislation as "a medical condition (including emergency labor and delivery) manifesting itself by acute symptoms of sufficient severity (including severe pain) such that the absence of immediate medical attention could reasonably be expected to result in—(a) placing the patient's health in serious jeopardy, (b) serious impairment to bodily functions, or (c) serious dysfunction of any bodily organ or part" (Campbell et al. 2010: 185).

Although it varies based on hospital policy and severity at presentation, most undocumented immigrants receive dialysis only once or twice a week. This occurs when the emergency room physician and lab results determine that they are "sick enough" to need dialysis according to physical state and potassium levels. In this condition, elevated potassium levels place patients at risk of cardiac arrest. Therefore, they literally risk death in order to extend their lives through dialysis. By setting this criterion, the health care system is not letting them die, but only allowing patients to maintain a "bare life" (Agamben 1998). Agamben's concept of bare life is drawn from the Roman *Homo sacer*, an individual who could be exiled from society, stripped of their political and social rights awarded to them by citizenship, and reduced to solely biological life, i.e., "bare life." Since undocumented immigrants are not awarded the political rights of citizenship due to their lack of legal status, their bodies are only treated based on a critical physical state, reduced to qualifying criteria determined by lab results and bodily symptoms. Their bodies must always register a near-death state, while qualifying U.S. citizens and LPRs are granted access based on their political rights as lawful and deserving members of society.

Qualifying U.S. citizens and LPRs are served by outpatient facilities when scheduled for dialysis, but undocumented and uninsured immigrants can spend several days in emergency room lobbies, waiting for their chance to obtain treatment, since they are often turned away if they do not meet hospital criteria (i.e., potassium levels) and therefore have to continue returning until the criteria are met. If a patient arrives in a more critical state than those waiting, they are given priority and less critical patients may have to continue to wait due to limited dialysis machines and staff to run them. Furthermore, unlike most U.S. citizens and LPRs, uninsured and undocumented immigrants are ineligible for an AV fistula surgery before and often even after beginning dialysis treatment. While some hospitals eventually provide AV fistulas to undocumented patients after several months of dialysis, the great majority of undocumented ESRD patients receive dialysis through a temporary venous catheter. This catheter must be inserted and removed at every dialysis session. However, temporary catheters are associated with higher rates of infection and death compared to the permanent AV fistulas. The catheters can clog, become infected, and result in narrowing of the veins in which they are placed (NIDDKD 2006). While it is possible to live a long and normal life on dialysis after being diagnosed with ESRD, physicians I interviewed stated that undocumented immigrants on irregular dialysis typically have a life expectancy of less than 4 to 5 years after reaching ESRD.

Dr. Smith, an internal medicine doctor working at one of the clinics that serves the uninsured and undocumented, has been treating dialysis patients like Andres for more than 15 years in the RGV. During my interview with him, he expressed his opinion on the topic by describing the inhumanity and toll that dialysis takes on patients who are only able to receive emergency care. He said,

> Receiving dialysis treatment only when you are on the verge of death is like a bizarre form of hospice. The health care system provides just enough treatment to keep them barely alive. Most of these patients' appearances change dramatically as ESRD affects their bodies. As horrible as it sounds, most of them look like something out of [TV show] *The Walking Dead*.

I propose that the suffering of these undocumented and uninsured ESRD patients should be understood as a peculiar form of bare life that is partially managed by biopolitical institutions. These patients' lives become "accursed" and "excluded" (Agamben 1998) through the institutional and government policies that limit access to care (Foucault 1978). Exclusion from regular dialysis care places patients constantly at risk, since they must weekly appear near death in order to be granted life-saving treatment. Immigrants are placed in a complicated position, in which they are constantly aware of the standard of treatment from which they are excluded due to their precarious legal status. In this case, the severity of their condition is known but the patients are not properly assigned treatment as it would be if they had legal status. As a result, their limited access extends to increased suffering, enhanced by greater morbidity and mortality rates. Furthermore, substandard treatment results in vastly higher costs than regular care (Melo and Fleuriet 2016; Hurley et al. 2009; Campbell et al. 2010).

Between the Cracks

Carlos is a 58-year-old Type II diabetic LPR who receives dialysis on an emergency basis at one of the RGV hospitals. Carlos moved to the United States from a Mexican border town two years ago once the cartel violence escalated. Luckily for Carlos, his son was a U.S. citizen who had just turned 21 and was therefore able to petition for his residency. While he waited for his residency, Carlos received dialysis treatment in the hospital ER every 8 to 10 days. The first hospital he went to told him to go back to Mexico and that he "did not belong" there, but upon talking to neighbors about hospitals in the area, he went to another one that received him with more courtesy. In the meantime, he qualified for the county health care indigent program that covered his regular doctors' visits and a few medications. Carlos expected that gaining his residency would allow him more access to health care and regularly scheduled dialysis treatment. However, when Carlos received it, he still was unable to qualify for Medicare because he did not have any working quarters in the United States.

Carlos told me:

> I started dialysis about 2 years ago. I have two U.S. citizen children. When my son turned 21 he processed the paperwork for my residency. I used to receive help from the county health program, but as soon as I was given my residency, they took away that help and because I haven't lived here long, I do not qualify for more help. Now, I only qualify for Emergency Medicaid and I struggle to pay for medications, doctor bills, and even food.

While the great majority of documented immigrants and U.S. citizens qualify for dialysis in outpatient facilities, there are exceptions besides the undocumented, such as Carlos, who fall in between the cracks. While the Medicare system allows for U.S. citizen parents to transfer working quarters to their children, it does not allow for U.S. citizen children to transfer them to their aging parents. In this instance, U.S. citizen children experience stratified citizenship by being unable to fulfill common caretaking roles as it is part of Mexican culture and tradition to look after and help elderly family members. Once again, this gives the impression that some patients are more deserving of care than others, and therefore have restricted opportunities to qualify for health care based on not only legal immigration status and income, but also age and familial relationships. Just as is the case for age restrictions on kidney transplantation (Kaufman 2013), limiting transfer of quarters only to children shows that younger patients are seen as more deserving of a longer life. For those who migrated "legally" later in life, whose spouses are also immigrants, and who may have briefly or never entered the U.S. workforce, the only option is to purchase Medicare and pay a high monthly premium, which at $400–$750 a month is usually not an option for low-income families. Because of the toll his disease is taking on him, Carlos cannot work and is therefore supported financially by his daughter on a limited income.

A common theme regardless of immigration status is that dialysis patients often experience stratified citizenship through their inability to work and the attendant financial limitations. Constrained by their disease, they must rely on other family members not only for financial support, but for general support in daily tasks, thereby blurring the traditional roles of family caretaker and often making dialysis patients feel inept or straining family relationships. This has been further exacerbated as a result of Carlos not being able to obtain any ACA plans, afford the Medicare premium, nor qualify for disability.

These exclusionary loopholes not only demonstrate the cracks in the U.S. health care system, but also complicated notions of deservingness and belonging for immigrants. In these cases, legal status alone does not qualify or disqualify an ESRD patient for dialysis. Immigrant ESRD patients must also have contributed to the workforce and economy through taxes for a substantial portion of their lives. By doing so, they are fulfilling the ideals of the "good" or "right" type of immigrant in order to be deemed deserving of the benefits reserved for productive citizens, such as federal assistance with health care. Coutin further demonstrates this by stating, "Migrants are desired as laborers but are excluded from certain public benefits" (2003: 508). For those individuals, like Carlos, who do not fulfill these ideals, adequate treatment is unattainable and equivalent to that of those formally excluded from the system due to legal status or citizenship. Therefore, because he does not qualify for coverage, Carlos is still excluded from standard dialysis treatment, just as he was when he was undocumented. He must continue attempting to qualify for dialysis through the emergency room.

Policy Implications

> FINANCIAL COORDINATOR: Don't even get me started on
> Obamacare!
> M: No, I really want to know. How has it changed dialysis for your
> patients?
> FINANCIAL COORDINATOR: Well that's the thing, it really hasn't. Out
> of the hundreds of patients I see, I think I have seen only one person
> qualify for coverage under Obamacare. It has been much more of
> a big headache for us because it is a lot of paperwork and it doesn't
> provide a better option or solution. At least maybe not here in the
> Valley or Texas.

While the reality may be different for states that expanded Medicaid under the ACA (Horton 2016), in Texas, dialysis care seemed to be largely unchanged for undocumented patients. Most of the health care professionals I interviewed about the ACA simply answered with a "no" or "it hasn't" when I asked them how the ACA had affected or changed the dialysis access. As one of the directors of the federally qualified health center said, "The ACA really will not affect the majority of our patients because they do not qualify and therefore will continue to have to seek treatment in our clinics or emergency rooms."

While this may be true in most cases, by excluding these populations from the potential benefits of the ACA, many states' failure to expand Medicaid resulted in fewer Disproportionate Share Hospital (DSH) funds for hospitals serving patients who fell into the coverage gap. An expansion of Medicaid and greater inclusion in the ACA would have also meant more money flowing into the region, allowing uncompensated care and charity funds to serve more patients. For states like Texas, where so many of the uninsured did not qualify for the ACA or Medicaid due to income or legal immigration status, the results could be detrimental, especially for an area like the RGV, which lacks a county hospital.

The exclusion of undocumented immigrants from the ACA and the absence of Medicaid expansion in states like Texas revealed the limits of

American notions of human rights and deservingness. When is health care a human right according to U.S. health care laws? National health care policies clearly view health care as a commodity the majority of the time and in most circumstances. This case study also demonstrates the ACA's failure to challenge American discourses of deservingness by failing to incorporate and offer social protection to the most vulnerable populations in the United States. While discourses of deservingness may vary in the case of undocumented immigrants' access to health care, the existence of EMTALA suggests that there is at least an American ideological frame for administering emergency and life-saving care under the argument that medical treatment in this dying state is a human right, regardless of political, social, or economic factors (Goodale 2006, 2009; Farmer 1999; Willen 2012c; Biwas et al. 2013). However, it also raises many questions. Why is health care considered a human right only in emergency situations? Why are undocumented immigrant bodies recognized as human and considered deserving of health care only in the case of emergencies? Why is preventing an immediate death more acceptable than providing regular, long-term treatment that can avoid and postpone death altogether?

In order to address these questions, health care professionals, medical anthropologists, and policymakers must challenge the exclusionary policies of limited health care access and humanitarian aid. The dire health consequences that result from insufficient aid suggest that changes such as closing the Medicaid gap, expanding the right to health care access beyond emergency care to regular standards of care, and removing exclusionary criteria such as sufficient working quarters and legal status would result in better quality of life and health outcomes overall.

Some states and counties have taken matters into their own hands to address the flaws in the federal health care system. In Houston, county funds were utilized to open a dialysis center that specifically serves patients who have been excluded from regular dialysis due to documentation or uninsured status. This has allowed the county to avoid the extremely high financial costs associated with emergency dialysis while allowing patients to receive the same standard of care as their qualifying counterparts (Raghavan 2012). Some states such as California, Arizona, Massachusetts, New York, and North Carolina have reinterpreted Emergency Medicaid standards to cover maintenance dialysis treatment in outpatient facilities, eliminating the requirement for patients to reach a critical state before granting them access to life-saving treatment (Linden et al. 2012). However, undocumented and uninsured dialysis patients remain barred from a more permanent solution—receiving kidney transplants—as a result of the high costs of surgery and the inability to prove they will be able to continue to afford their anti-rejection medications. Transplant policies must change this stipulation not only to provide a better quality of life for patients, but to avoid a lifetime of dialysis costs (Linden et al. 2012). These models demonstrate a glimpse of what could possibly alleviate, if not solve, the complex issues related to ESRD and dialysis for uninsured and undocumented patients.

Conclusion

The harsh reality is that those who were excluded from qualifying for the ACA or Medicare receive insufficient dialysis when emergency rooms are their only option for treatment of ESRD. Emergency dialysis as the only available care for undocumented immigrants allows for survival (Agamben 1998), but not well-being (Campbell et al. 2010). The case of dialysis for undocumented immigrants shows how health care access is related to social evaluations of belonging, deservingness, and human rights. Categorical exclusion from program eligibility together with incomplete and inadequate inclusion in emergency care has the effect of producing and prolonging social and physical suffering for immigrant kidney failure patients. As can be seen in this examination of different legal statuses on availability and quality of care, exclusionary political and economic practices directly impacted subjective experiences of well-being. Undocumented immigrants who lack financial resources are denied almost all forms of primary and specialty care in Texas, except for emergency care. In that instance, immigrants are treated under American moral and humanitarian reasoning that the most basic, life-saving health care may and should be a human right (Goodale 2006, 2009; Farmer 1999; Willen 2011, 2012c; Willen et al. 2011; Biwas et al. 2013). Furthermore, by examining case studies of undocumented immigrants and other populations excluded by the ACA, medical anthropologists can explore how individuals work against and within this restricted construction of health care as a human right in emergency situations. Last, when examining the ACA and those who it excluded, it is important for medical anthropologists and social scientists to examine how health care providers and state policymakers accommodated and contested exclusive definitions of health citizenship.

This chapter has analyzed the tensions and creative actions of a hidden, marginalized population that negotiates exclusionary practices of health care institutions and immigration policies to access treatment that will prolong life, albeit a life of relatively increased morbidity and mortality. It also contributes to policy dialogues by using ethnography to highlight the drastic health implications and costs resulting from an intentional lack of formal policy addressing resources and care for those who were excluded from the health care system and the ACA. It demonstrates that, in spite of the benefits that the ACA provided for some, the U.S. health care system remains broken for many of those whom it has continually excluded.

ACKNOWLEDGMENTS

I would like to acknowledge all of the dialysis patients, their families, and the health care professionals without whom this project could not have been possible. I would also like to thank the National Science Foundation, Ford Foundation, American Anthropological Association, and the University of Texas at San Antonio's Mexico Center for their generous funding during data collection and writing.

NOTE

1 These costs can vary greatly. While the average emergency dialysis bill was $4,000–$6,000 per treatment, outpatient facilities claimed to charge an average of $500–$1,000 per treatment. However, one uninsured patient showed me a bill that had various dialysis charges for a two-month period, ranging from $4,000 to $15,000 per treatment.

REFERENCES

Abrego, Leisy J., and Cecilia Menjívar. 2011. Immigrant Latina Mothers as Targets of Legal Violence. *International Journal of Sociology of the Family* 37(1): 9–26.

Agamben, Giorgio. 1998. *Homo Sacer: Sovereign Power and Bare Life*. Redwood City, CA: Stanford University Press.

Becker, Gay. 2004. Deadly Inequality in the Health Care "Safety Net": Uninsured Ethnic Minorities' Struggle to Live with Life-Threatening Illnesses. *Medical Anthropology Quarterly* 18(2): 258–275.

Biwas, Dan, Brigit Toebes, Anders Hjern, Henry Ascher, and Marie Norredam. 2013. Access to Health Care for Undocumented Migrants from a Human Rights Perspective: A Comparative Study of Denmark, Sweden, and the Netherlands. *Health and Human Rights Journal* 14(2): 49–60.

Bryner, Jeanna. 2012. The Skinniest and Fattest U.S. Cities Revealed. *Foxnews.com*. www.foxnews.com.

Campbell, G. Adam, Scott Sanoff, and Mitchell H. Rosner. 2010. Care of the Undocumented Immigrant in the United States with ESRD. *American Journal of Kidney Disease* 55(1): 181–191.

Castañeda, Heide. 2009. Illegality as Risk Factor: A Survey of Unauthorized Migrant Patients in a Berlin Clinic. *Social Science & Medicine* 68(8): 1–9.

Castañeda, Heide, and Milena A. Melo. 2014. Health Care Access for Latino Mixed-Status Families: Barriers, Strategies, and Implications for Reform. *American Behavioral Scientist* 58(14): 1891–1909.

Chavez, Leo. 1986. Mexican Immigration and Health Care: A Political Economy Perspective. *Human Organization* 45(4): 344–352.

———. 1991. Outside the Imagined Community: Undocumented Settlers and Experiences of Incorporation. *American Ethnologist* 18(2): 257–278.

———. 1992. *Shadowed Lives: Undocumented Immigrants in American Society*. New York: Harcourt Brace.

———. 2008. *The Latino Threat: Constructing Immigrants, Citizens, and the Nation*. Redwood City, CA: Stanford University Press.

———. 2012. Undocumented Immigrants and Their Use of Medical Services in Orange County, California. *Social Science & Medicine* 749(6): 887–893.

Chu, Anna, and Charles Posner. 2013. *The Counties that Need the Affordable Care Act the Most*. Washington, DC: Center for American Progress Action Fund. www.americanprogressaction.org.

Coutin, Susan Bibler. 2003. Cultural Logics of Belonging and Movement: Transnationalism, Naturalization, and U.S. Immigration Politics. *American Ethnologist* 30(4): 508–526.

De Genova, Nicholas. 2002. Migrant "Illegality" and Deportability in Everyday Life. *Annual Review of Anthropology* 31: 419–447.

———. 2005. *Working the Boundaries: Race, Space, and "Illegality" in Mexican Chicago*. Durham, NC: Duke University Press.

Farmer, Paul. 1999. Pathologies of Power: Rethinking Health and Human Rights. *American Journal of Public Health* 89(10): 1486–1496.

Fassin, Didier. 2001. The Biopolitics of Otherness: Undocumented Foreigners and Racial Discrimination in French Public Debate. *Anthropology Today* 17(1): 3–7.

———. 2009. Another Politics of Life Is Possible. *Theory, Culture & Society* 26(5): 44–60.

———. 2011. Policing Borders, Producing Boundaries: The Governmentality of Immigration in Dark Times. *Annual Review of Anthropology* 40: 213–226.

Foucault, Michel. 1978. *The History of Sexuality. Volume 1*. New York: Random House.

Gomberg-Muñoz, Ruth. 2010. Willing to Work: Agency and Vulnerability in an Undocumented Immigrant Network. *American Anthropologist* 112(2): 295–307.

———. 2011. *Labor and Legality: An Ethnography of a Mexican Immigrant Network.* New York: Oxford University Press.

Goodale, Mark. 2006. Toward a Critical Anthropology of Human Rights. *Current Anthropology* 47(3): 485–511.

———. 2009. *Surrendering to Utopia: An Anthropology of Human Rights.* Stanford: Stanford University Press.

Hamdy, Sherine F. 2008. When the State and Your Kidneys Fail: Political Etiologies in an Egyptian Dialysis Ward. *American Ethnologist* 35(4): 553–569.

Hidalgo County Health and Human Services. 2012. *Diabetes Awareness: November Is Diabetes Awareness Month.* Edinburg: County of Hidalgo, TX. www.co.hidalgo .tx.us.

Holmes, Seth. 2013. *Fresh Fruit, Broken Bodies: Migrant Farmworkers in the United States.* Oakland: University of California Press.

Horton, Sarah. 2004. Different Subjects: The Health Care System's Participation in the Differential Construction of the Cultural Citizenship of Cuban Refugees. *Medical Anthropology Quarterly* 18(4): 472–489.

———. 2006. The Double Burden on Safety Net Providers: Placing Health Disparities in the Context of the Privatization of Health Care in the U.S. *Social Science & Medicine* 63(10): 2702–2714.

———. 2016. *They Leave Their Kidneys in the Fields: Illness, Injury, and Illegality among U.S. Farmworkers.* Oakland: University of California Press.

Hurley, Laura, Allison Kempe, Lori A. Crane, Arthur Davidson, Katherine Pratte, Stuart Linas, L. Miriam Dickinson, and Tomas Berl. 2009. Care of Undocumented Individuals with ESRD: A National Survey of U.S. Nephrologists. *American Journal of Kidney Diseases* 53(6): 940–949.

Kaufman, Sharon R. 2013. Fairness and the Tyranny of Potential in Kidney Transplantation. *Current Anthropology* 54(7): S56–S66.

Linden, Ellena A., Jeannette Cano, and George N. Coritsidis. 2012. Kidney Transplantation in Undocumented Immigrants With ESRD: A Policy Whose Time Has Come? *American Journal of Kidney Diseases* 60 (3): 354–359.

Marrow, Helen. 2012. Deserving to a Point: Unauthorized Immigrants in San Francisco's Universal Access Healthcare Model. *Social Science & Medicine* 74(6): 846–854.

Melo, Milena A., and K. Jill Fleuriet. 2016. Who Has the Right to Access Health Care and Why? Immigration, Incorporation, and Health Care Policy. In *Mexican Migration to the United States: Perspectives from Both Sides of the Border.* Edited by Harriett D. Romo and Olivia Mogollon-Lopez. Austin: University of Texas Press.

Montoya, Michael. 2011. *Making the Mexican Diabetic: Race, Science, and the Genetics of Inequality.* Oakland: University of California Press.

NIDDKD (National Institute of Diabetes and Digestive and Kidney Diseases). 2006. *Treatment Methods for Kidney Failure: Hemodialysis.* Washington, DC: U.S. Department of Health and Human Services. kidney.niddk.nih.gov.

Raghavan, Rajeev. 2012. When Access to Chronic Dialysis Is Limited: One Center's Approach to Emergent Hemodialysis. *Seminars in Dialysis* 25(3): 267–271.

Rosaldo, Renato. 1997. Cultural Citizenship, Inequality, and Multiculturalism. In *Latino Cultural Citizenship: Claiming Identity, Space, and Rights.* Edited by William V. Flores and Rina Benmayor. Boston: Beacon.

Sargent, Carolyn F. 2012. Special Issue Part I: "Deservingness" and the Politics of Health Care. *Social Science & Medicine* 74(6): 855–857.

Sheik-Hamad, David, Elian Paiuk, Andrew J. Wright, Craig Kleinmann, Uday Khosla, and Wayne X. Shandera. 2007. Care for Immigrants with End-Stage Renal Disease in Houston: A Comparison of Two Practices. *Texas Medicine* 103(4): 53–58.

U.S. Census Bureau. 2013. Hidalgo County Quick Facts. Washington, DC: U.S. Census Bureau. quickfacts.census.gov.

Viladrich, Anahi. 2012. Beyond Welfare Reform: Reframing Undocumented Immigrants' Entitlement to Health Care in the United States, a Critical Review. *Social Science & Medicine* 74(6): 822–829.

Willen, Sarah S. 2011. Do "Illegal" Im/migrants Have a Right to Health? Engaging Ethical Theory as Social Practice at a Tel Aviv Open Clinic. *Medical Anthropology Quarterly* 25(3): 303–330.

———. 2012a. How Is Health-Related "Deservingness" Reckoned? Perspectives from Unauthorized Immigrants in Tel Aviv. *Social Science & Medicine* 74(6): 812–821.

———. 2012b. Migration, "Illegality," and Health: Mapping Embodied Vulnerability and Debating Health-Related Deservingness. *Social Science & Medicine* 74(6): 805–811.

———. 2012c. Anthropology and Human Rights: Theoretical Reconsiderations and Phenomenological Explorations. *Journal of Human Rights* 11(1): 150–159.

Willen, Sarah S., Jessica Mulligan, and Heide Castañeda. 2011. Take a Stand Commentary: How Can Medical Anthropologists Contribute to Contemporary Conversations on "Illegal" Im/migration and Health? *Medical Anthropology Quarterly* 25(3): 331–356.

3

Stratification and "Universality"

Immigrants and Barriers to Coverage in Massachusetts

TIFFANY D. JOSEPH

Yolanda is a naturalized U.S. citizen who arrived to Boston from her native Dominican Republic in 1989 after marrying an American whom she met there. She became a U.S. citizen in 1995, which she admits has made her life much easier. Unfortunately, she and her husband divorced in 1999 after ten years of marriage. While married, she was a home-maker and lived in white American neighborhoods, where she and her mixed-race children were the only minorities. But she did not recall experiencing any discrimination. Because she had fair skin and took her husband's American surname, it was not always obvious that she was Latina. After divorcing her husband, she reclaimed her maiden name and moved to Dominican neighborhoods in Boston. It was then that she began to notice how differently Dominicans and other Latinos, includ-ing her, were treated. She noticed that customer service representatives treated her with less respect and patience over the phone after she gave her Spanish surname. Yolanda is now a Spanish freelance interpreter, who is currently enrolled in a local college.

When asked about her experiences with health care reform in Mas-sachusetts (pre-ACA implementation), she responds that she has had dif-ferent types of health coverage and feels fortunate to have good health for the most part. She has been diagnosed with an iron deficiency, but not yet with anemia. So, she must periodically get blood tests to monitor her iron levels. When married, she had what she felt was very good private cover-age through her husband's employer. After her divorce, she was eligible for the state's Medicaid program called MassHealth, which she felt covered all of her medical needs. She had this coverage until she enrolled in col-lege and switched plans to be covered under her college's student health insurance plan, unaware it would cover very few of her medical expenses. As a result, she spoke about how her medical bills, from regular medical appointments and annual physicals, were mounting because her doctors do not accept her plan. She also noted that her plan has high co-pays and deductibles, which she cannot afford. Despite her dissatisfaction with the coverage, Yolanda was unable to switch back to MassHealth from her student plan, as the state's open enrollment deadline had passed.

Yolanda's experience highlights both the benefits and pitfalls of comprehensive health reform in Massachusetts (MA) prior to ACA implementation. Like more than 97% of Massachusetts residents, Yolanda was fortunate that she had health coverage, which was required of all eligible MA residents. However, as her experiences with different types of coverage demonstrate, any coverage is not necessarily good coverage. Her current college insurance plan does not meet her needs and she has difficulty paying her medical bills. But, Yolanda is also fortunate because, even though she is an immigrant, she has more structural access as an English-speaking naturalized (Latina) citizen who can pass as white. This allows her to have a better, albeit not ideal, experience with the health care system compared to her undocumented, non-English-speaking, and darker-skinned immigrant counterparts, who may experience race- and immigrant-based discrimination in their health care encounters.

Unlike many other parts of the country, the state of Massachusetts and the city of Boston in particular are socially progressive locations where immigrants have historically been able to access some state-funded public benefits, one of which was health care. When Massachusetts became the first state to implement comprehensive health reform, known as Chapter 58, in 2006, income-eligible state residents of any documentation status could apply for and receive full or partially subsidized coverage (Joseph 2016). Chapter 58 was considered successful, as it reduced the state's uninsured population to 3% (Long et al. 2013; BCBS 2013). This is one reason why Chapter 58 was used to craft the 2010 Affordable Care Act (ACA), which aimed to improve Americans' access to health insurance and care (Patel and McDonough 2010). Unlike the ACA, which explicitly excluded undocumented and some documented immigrants, Chapter 58 included provisions for *all* MA residents (Joseph 2016). However, preliminary studies of Chapter 58 found that immigrants, especially the undocumented, were likely to remain uninsured despite their inclusion in the policy (BCBS 2013; Pryor and Cohen 2009). This research suggests that immigrants experienced difficulty accessing coverage due to undocumented status, complexity of (re) enrollment, and inability to afford premiums and co-pays (BCBS 2013; Maxwell et al. 2011). Yolanda's experiences with her current college plan illustrate one of the shortcomings of Chapter 58; though it has improved MA residents' likelihood of being insured, the coverage is not always affordable.

Seeking to more clearly understand Boston immigrants' experiences with the health care system post-Chapter 58 and pre-ACA implementation, this chapter identifies and examines how various barriers limit health care access even when individuals have access to health coverage. I use interview data collected from a sample of 70 Latino immigrants, health care professionals, and immigrant and health organization employees in Boston under Chapter 58 to show that these barriers stratify access by citizenship in various ways. This volume looks at stratified citizenship in reference to multiple, overlapping categories that impact access to rights and responsibilities as well as feelings of belonging and exclusion. Though my analysis focuses on how legal immigration statuses, such as undocumented, green card holder, legal permanent resident, and so on, affect the ability to access coverage and care in Massachusetts, I draw attention to how race, income, and gender interact with immigration status to magnify and at times lessen vulnerability. I also discuss how these barriers are created through the politics of health reform, which effectively undermine "universal" health policies. As U.S. and foreign-born Latinos comprise a significant proportion of Massachusetts's population and are highly concentrated in Boston, the importance of exploring the impact of Chapter 58 and its implications for vulnerable populations cannot be overstated. It is vital for policymakers, health care professionals, and researchers to understand and potentially minimize such barriers for immigrants and the general population in the aftermath of ACA implementation.[1]

Chapter 58 and Its Impact on Immigrants

Massachusetts implemented Chapter 58 to make health coverage accessible for all of its residents with: (1) an individual mandate requiring all eligible residents to have coverage; (2) a Medicaid expansion to cover low-income residents; (3) an insurance exchange where private insurance companies could offer coverage to middle- and higher-income residents; and (4) an employer mandate requiring large employers to provide coverage to their employees (Patel and McDonough 2010).[2] The state also maintained its preexisting safety net system primarily funded by state hospitals, renaming it the Health Safety Net (HSN) to provide primary care to those who remained uninsured post-Chapter 58 due to ineligibility for federal or state-funded coverage. Residents of *any* documentation status with an income of less than 400 percent of the federal poverty level (FPL) were HSN eligible and entitled to receive care at 160 designated health care facilities throughout Massachusetts (Joseph 2016). To be eligible for MassHealth, the state's Medicaid program, applicants had to be U.S. citizens or have legal permanent residence (hereafter, LPR) status for five years, and have an income of up to 200 percent FPL (Joseph 2016). But, MA developed a state-funded program called Commonwealth Care to subsidize privately purchased coverage for middle income short-term LPRs with less than five years of residency (ineligible for Medicaid) and citizens (Joseph 2016).

Overall, Chapter 58 reduced the state's uninsured population, and parts of the policy were used to craft the ACA, namely the individual mandate, Medicaid expansion, and health care marketplace exchange (BCBS 2013). Nevertheless, cost containment remains an issue and studies conducted in MA after Chapter 58 but before ACA implementation found that low-income residents, many of them immigrants, reported receiving less care than higher income residents (BCBS 2013). One in five adults reported being denied care because doctors would not accept their public coverage (BCBS 2013).[3] Ethno-racial minorities, low-income individuals, and people with poor health were still more likely to be un(der)insured, utilize health services less, and unable to afford coverage or out-of-pocket spending costs (BCBS 2013). The remaining uninsured generally had unstable employment status, fluctuating income, and undocumented status (BCBS 2013).

The 2008 recession also affected residents' coverage under Chapter 58, as MA reduced reimbursement rates and cut funding to some public health programs and mental health services (Long and Stockley 2010). Documented and undocumented immigrants were significantly affected by these cuts. First, funds for Health Safety Net—the program through which both federally ineligible immigrant and low-income MA residents receive primary care—were reduced as more residents obtained insurance (Long and Stockley 2010). Second, the state reduced coverage for 40,000 short-term LPRs who were eligible for Commonwealth Care by shifting their coverage to a cheaper program that was only accepted at hospitals outside of Boston (Health Law Advocates 2013). This coverage shift created lapses in care for immigrant patients as they could no longer see their Boston-based providers.

In 2012, the Health Law Advocates group successfully sued the state for this action, arguing that it was unconstitutional to discriminate against these immigrants based on their short-term LPR status (Health Law Advocates 2013). The state subsequently reinstated Commonwealth Care coverage to those LPR patients who had lost their coverage. Both of these changes illustrate how Chapter 58 was stratified by legal citizenship and income. When it was necessary for legislators to address the state's fiscal situation, noncitizens' and low-income residents' health care benefits were reduced, which illustrates how their documentation status and income made them expendable and vulnerable for exclusion (Gottleib 2015; Lockwood 1996).

Methods

Data for this chapter come from my larger project examining immigrants' experiences with the Boston health care system after the passage of Chapter 58 and prior to ACA implementation in Massachusetts. I conducted qualitative interviews with 70 individuals that consisted of immigrants, health care professionals, and immigrant and health organization employees. The immigrant sample included 21 Brazilian and 10 Dominican immigrants—two of Boston's largest immigrant groups—to assess how documentation status influenced their health care access. These groups demonstrate the heterogeneity in national origins, migration histories to the United States, documentation status, and language among Latino immigrants. These interviews explored: (1) immigrant profile; (2) self-reported physical/mental health pre-migration and in United States; and (3) insurance coverage/health care access pre-migration and to the United States.

To learn more about the institutional factors that influence immigrants' experiences with the health care system, I interviewed 19 health care professionals at the Boston Health Coalition (BHC),[4] a network of hospitals and clinics with a reputation of providing quality health care to minority populations. The 19 respondents were from six sites and interviews explored their perceptions of: (1) challenges serving immigrant populations; (2) availability of multilingual/ cultural staff; (3) impact of Chapter 58 on serving patients; (4) major health problems of patients; and (5) how being an immigrant affects their patients.

Finally, to assess how local immigration policy influenced immigrants' health care access, I interviewed 20 employees of local immigrant and health organizations. These organizations primarily served Brazilian or Dominican immigrants or were health advocacy organizations that assisted state residents in Chapter 58 enrollment. These interviews examined: (1) social climate for immigrants; (2) local enforcement of state/ federal immigration policy; and (3) challenges immigrants face living and navigating the health care system.

To recruit the sample, I volunteered at and attended relevant community events at immigrant organizations throughout Boston. My Brazilian Portuguese and Spanish proficiency and previous travels to and research in Brazil and the Dominican Republic aided in gaining access to these communities, and I used purposive snowball sampling. For the immigrant sample, I recruited women and men who had been in the United States for at least one year and were ages 25 to 60 years, as these individuals were likely to be oriented in the United States and needed to use the health care system. BHC respondents consisted of physicians, case workers, medical interpreters, and other staff who mostly have Brazilian, Dominican, and/or other immigrant patients. Interviews were audio-recorded, conducted in Brazilian Portuguese, Spanish, or English, lasted from 60 to 90 minutes, and were then professionally transcribed.

Data analysis consisted of importing and closely reading each interview transcript into NVivo software. I then developed an exhaustive list of codes—one- to three-word phrases that describe different types of barriers identified by respondents in the data. I also created subcodes for each barrier that corresponded to each stakeholder group to compare perceptions between immigrants, health care professionals, and organization employees. I then re-read each transcript and organized all words, phrases, and sentences under the associated codes. I continued this process until all transcripts were analyzed. I analyzed each interview in the language in which it was conducted to minimize nuances being lost in translation.

My access to undocumented immigrants allowed me to explore their experiences, which are underrepresented in survey research on Chapter 58 and the ACA. Although the data were collected in Massachusetts, studies of Chapter 58 prior to ACA implementation were used to assess the potential national impact of the ACA. Thus, while these factors limit the generalizability of the findings, the results may have some implications for other populations that have been and may remain uninsured (i.e., minorities, low-income) after ACA implementation.

Immigrants' Barriers to Health Care

My interviews with immigrants, health care professionals, and immigrant/health organization employees revealed that various health care barriers remained for Boston immigrants even though nearly all of the immigrant respondents had health coverage. These barriers fit into three main overlapping categories: (1) immigration-related, (2) bureaucratic, and (3) health care system. Each of the barriers illustrates stratification by citizenship and/or the politics of health reform in that they have a significant impact on local immigrants' health care access, who are typically low-income and also ethno-racial minorities. Cumulatively, these social positions highlight immigrants' marginality in the writing and implementation of health policy in Boston and elsewhere. I incorporate anecdotes from respondents where appropriate to illustrate how each barrier affected immigrants' health care access.

Immigration-Related Barriers

One of the biggest barriers that many respondents across all of the stakeholder groups referenced was related to being an immigrant. Documentation status, difficulty producing eligibility information for coverage (re)enrollment, non-English proficiency, and immigration enforcement negatively affected immigrants' ability to sign up for or use health coverage. Although most of the immigrants I interviewed were documented, a few were undocumented at some point in their lives and discussed how that created a barrier to health care. In our conversations,

I also discovered that some immigrants were unaware of Chapter 58, or that the coverage that many had was because of Chapter 58. Most of the immigrants had coverage through the Health Safety Net Program. As a result, lack of knowledge about coverage or what services could be used with their coverage also affected immigrants' ability to receive care. Yet, the fact that most immigrant respondents had coverage indicated that they were a select group who could access health services.[5] Marilza, a Brazilian immigrant who had been informed enough to apply for and use HSN, told me about her friend who had remained uninsured:

> There are many Brazilians who don't know about the coverage and are liv-
> ing more difficult lives. The friend here who helped me get settled hasn't
> been to the doctor in 10 years because the policy said she only had ER
> coverage. She's also afraid to go because she is undocumented and could
> be arrested. So there's a lack of knowledge, maybe on the part of the gov-
> ernment, that does not share information.

Marilza's quote demonstrates how lack of awareness of HSN, but also fear of being undocumented, leads many eligible immigrants to forgo access to coverage and care.[6] Being willing to seek resources and services and having social ties that could guide respondents to those services influenced whether immigrants would use available resources. But, Marilza also feels that the state government has not done enough to spread the word to immigrant communities about the availability of these programs, which contributes to the lack of awareness that mini-mizes immigrants' health care access. BHC health care professionals and immigrant organization employees echoed these sentiments. Christina, a BHC social worker, shared her frustrations about how immigrants' iso-lation makes it difficult to incorporate them into the health care system. She also feels that the government, in partnering with community orga-nizations, can bridge the gap to better inform immigrant communities and improve immigrants' trust of local health care facilities:

> But everybody [has] access to health care if income eligible. But the peo-
> ple, the population doesn't know that until they talk to somebody like us.
> But we don't know who is out there, who doesn't access health care. And
> then that's a big problem because the whole population [immigrants],

they kind of isolate themselves and are afraid. If they do not have a social security [number] or—if they do not have the immigration documents. So we need the community agency. The only way I think will be the community agency developing a partnership with the government because otherwise there won't be trust.

When it comes to seeking health care, Christina also told me that male immigrant patients are even harder to reach. While they may fear health care facilities, they are also usually working multiple jobs, which makes it difficult for them to find time to come in and apply for and use coverage.

When immigrants do eventually come to Christina to receive assistance applying for coverage, many face another immigration-related obstacle: providing necessary documentation for coverage enrollment. To apply for "subsidized" Chapter 58 coverage, applicants had to submit proof of income, state residency, and in some cases, citizenship status. Immigrants working in the informal economy do not receive paystubs or have irregular work periods, which makes it difficult to provide proof of income and establish income eligibility. Because immigrants working in low-paying jobs have roommates in order to reduce living expenses, they are unable to provide proof of residence if their names are not on apartment leases or bills. This, combined with the inability to obtain government-issued identification, makes it impossible to provide proof of residence. Finally, although no proof of citizenship status is required for enrollment in HSN, it was required for MassHealth and other subsidized coverage under Chapter 58. Sociologist Helen Marrow (2012) has described this predicament of being eligible for health services but unable to produce necessary documentation as a condition of eligibility as "bureaucratic disentitlement."[7]

Beyond this bureaucratic disentitlement in terms of ability to provide proper documentation, having to submit personal identifying information to the government and/or health care facilities to apply for coverage or receive care also incited fear in immigrant communities. Carmen, executive director of a Brazilian immigrant organization, commented:

Going to the doctor means giving your name, your address, disclosing that you're in this country and that is the first big barrier for most people to get treated. And they only go [to doctor] when they have to. So it's real hard to follow up on preventive care. They may go for just Emergency Care and not follow up, given how much is asked of them about their private life. And when they hear that word social security, all bets are off. People will freak out, [at] many places, you have to provide a valid ID to get any kind of care too. And if you don't have that valid ID and you are not dying, they won't even see you.

Carmen's quote illustrates the additional vulnerability that Boston immigrants feel when attempting to use health services and how this fear sometimes prevents them from receiving proper care. Often at doctor's offices, patients of any documentation status are asked to provide identification and insurance cards during check-in. And throughout the doctor's visit, patients are usually repeatedly asked for their birth date, first by front-door staff, next by the nurse practitioner or physicians' assistant, and again by the doctor as a way to verify the patients' medical records. These standard verification methods are harmless for most patients, but create additional concerns for immigrant patients, especially the undocumented, who fear that their use of health services may affect their immigration status. After all, passage of the 1996 immigration and welfare reforms led to a broad misconception that, being considered a public charge, via use of public benefits like subsidized health care, could be cause for deportation or might jeopardize future naturalization attempts (Park 2011). BHC health care providers and immigrant organization employees also mentioned this misconception was prevalent among some of their immigrant patients, which influenced their use of health services.

Some immigrants were able to overcome the initial barriers of providing documentation and fear of using health services by finding a trusted place to go for care that accepted their coverage. But, concerns about being stopped *in transit* also affected their decisions to seek health care. The increase in immigration enforcement alongside policies that prevent immigrants from obtaining driver's licenses have put many immigrants in fear of leaving their homes (Hacker et al. 2012). This has indirectly affected Boston immigrants' health care access, particularly as Massachusetts was a pilot state for the Secure Communities program and does not allow driver's licenses for undocumented immigrants.[8] BHC health care providers like social worker Peggy cited this as a big issue:

We face issues with patients who are facing deportation because they were coming to the clinic and they were pulled over. So, then we have to work with the patients in terms of getting a lawyer or service in terms of that. There was a period of time when the new reform [Chapter 58] came about and the new law [Secure Communities] was put in place [so] that the police were going and stopping people and doing raids and stuff. So a lot of our patients got caught. We had a patient who was coming to the clinic one day, and they called to say, I'm not going to make it to the visit because on my way to the clinic I saw a police car, so I'm turning around. So all that plays in with the patients.

Peggy's anecdote illustrates how federal immigration policy enforced at the local level also deterred immigrants from coming to BHC even though her immigrant patients feel it is a safe space. However, the route to BHC is not always as safe, posing a deportation risk if immigrant patients are pulled over and detained or arrested by local law enforcement.

All of these immigration-related barriers illustrate how immigrants' ability to actually use their Chapter 58 coverage was stratified by citizenship, in terms of formal documentation status, but also in terms of income and types of services they could use. Although they could apply for coverage, being a noncitizen disadvantaged them in the enrollment process due to inability to provide necessary documentation and when attempting to seek care. Despite being legally *included*, immigrants felt and were vulnerable to deportation and informal exclusion. Furthermore, the coverage for which most immigrants were eligible was through the Health Safety Net Program, which could only be used in certain locations. Because HSN is a government-subsidized program, it only allows patients to receive services that are available at HSN-designated locations. But, for some types of specialty care unavailable at those locations, immigrants are unable to receive referrals elsewhere, as their documentation status limits their access (Marrow and Joseph 2015). Finally, because most immigrant respondents were low-income, they used HSN or MassHealth as they were unable to afford more expensive health coverage elsewhere. Being low-income also affected their ability to pay co-pays for doctors' visits or prescription medications when necessary.

Bureaucratic disentitlement processes also tied to applying for coverage and re-enrollment created additional barriers, as applicants did not understand that they needed to reapply each year. Providers and immigrant organization employees reported that immigrants would come for appointments only to discover they were no longer insured. Immigrant patients may have received reenrollment documentation via mail, but disregarded it due to language proficiency or confusing instructions. Annette, a BHC insurance supervisor, explained that after applying for HSN, many immigrants receive:

> A four-page letter that makes no sense. But it starts off saying you have been denied. The first side of the letter says that. So every time a patient comes to us with that denial letter, we say, did you turn [it over]? Did you see your name there? They [Mass Health] only send out letters in English and Spanish and there are other [language-speaking] populations that get it.

Because the letter, enrollment materials, and other correspondence are written in formal bureaucratic English, they are very difficult for applicants, especially those with limited English proficiency and education, to understand. The Massachusetts government prepared documentation for its different health coverage plans in English and Spanish, although non-English- and non-Spanish-speaking immigrants live in the state. The state has a high number of residents who speak Portuguese, Haitian Creole, and a range of Asian languages. But, application procedures and enrollment assistance have yet to accommodate this diversity. Thus, language provides a barrier to coverage enrollment.

Bureaucratic Barriers

After interviewing Annette and employees from some of the immigrant and health advocacy organizations and hearing about the difficult application procedure, I went to the MassHealth website to view and attempt to complete the application. Despite having a doctorate degree and being a health policy researcher, I too found the English application cumbersome to complete. It had 16 pages with tiny font and different instructions about what documentation needed to be submitted if applying for HSN, in which case citizenship status proof was not needed. But, if applying for MassHealth and Commonwealth Care, citizenship status proof was needed. When it came to establishing income eligibility and state residence, various documents could be provided, such as a paycheck stub, or lease/mortgage, or utility bill. If MassHealth employees have difficulty understanding or verifying any of the information provided in the application, this may stall the enrollment process, taking longer for the applicant to receive notification of their coverage. My interview with Diana, a Portuguese-speaking health helpline employee, discussed this complexity:

> The people that call and speak Portuguese, I basically [hear about] language barriers. [The application is] complicated to understand, [callers] requesting information. [It's] complicated for them to understand how it's [application] going to be processed or sending the right information because [of] the language barrier, lack of information. They don't know where to go, who to talk to. When they call the helpline I feel that they could have called a long time ago but sometimes they get referred by a friend or family members. They've been trying to navigate the system but they really don't understand it. I think they don't understand because it's complicated, even [in] English, the language is not so simple.

One of the ways that organizations like Diana's reduce these bureaucratic barriers is by completing the application with individuals over the phone. Without the efforts of Diana's organization to demystify the politics of health reform, more eligible individuals would not be able to apply for coverage or navigate the system. Local immigrant organizations have also attempted to address these gaps by providing assistance in their respective constituents' languages. These organizations' efforts underscore the importance of official or informal navigators in helping patients enroll in and understand their health coverage.

Barriers within the Health Care System

Beyond immigration-related and bureaucratic barriers, navigating the complex U.S. health care system also posed a significant challenge. Respondents across all groups mentioned that immigrant patients typically do not understand how the U.S. health care system works. For example, the difficulty immigrants had using the Boston health care system was tied to their inability to go directly to a specialty doctor rather than having to get a PCP referral, which is typically required in the United States. Navigating the financial aspects of the system was challenging, as immigrants did not understand differences between co-pays and deductibles or costs associated with physician-provided or ER services. Even under coverage programs that had low premiums, co-pays, and deductibles, patients still experienced difficulty paying for care or prescription co-pays because they were considered low-income. This represented another form of bureaucratic disentitlement, and a BHC social worker named Margaret commented on this barrier:

> We still have patients struggle [financially]. They can't afford to pay a premium. Or they cannot afford to pay their co-pay for visits or co-pay for medications. So they avoid coming to the doctor unless they actually are extremely sick and go to the ER instead. And the reason is because if they go to the ER, if they don't have that co-pay, they can still be seen. But if they go to the doctor visit, they have to pay that co-pay. We have one patient that has gone to the ER in the last 12 months 28 times.

While going to the ER has no co-pay for HSN and MassHealth patients, the financial costs to the state and hospitals are extremely high. The ER is a very expensive form of care relative to preventive care. But the "high" co-pay for patients to see their physician offsets the less expensive costs borne by the insurance provider. Because many patients (immigrants and non-immigrants alike) do not understand this, they are unaware of how their type of health service use financially affects the system, which ultimately has an impact on health care costs for all involved. Furthermore, because HSN and MassHealth patients are low-income, their preference to use the ER versus their provider illustrates how their limited financial resources also presents structural barriers that influence their behaviors when seeking health care, also illustrating stratified citizenship in the health care system on the basis of income.

This type of health care barrier also broadly demonstrates the politics of health reform in terms of consumers' lack of understanding regarding how the health care system financially works. Essentially, immigrants (and other residents) in Massachusetts had access to coverage without comprehending where that coverage could be used, what types of services could be obtained, and who bore the financial costs for those services. Lack of effective government-provided and structural access to information about Chapter 58 for newly insured patients limited their ability to make cost-effective use of the system. Implicit in the implementation of Chapter 58 is that residents must also share the responsibility and risk for their health care. Although the state government does its part by providing subsidized coverage options, residents are responsible for seeking necessary assistance in order to apply for and learn where, when, and how to use that coverage.

Given the complexity of the larger U.S. health care system, income and education level affected some Massachusetts residents' understanding of their health coverage and where to use it. Past research has shown that individuals with lower levels of income and education have less health literacy than those with higher levels (Kutner et al. 2006). In turn, Massachusetts residents' choices for care (i.e., opting for the ER instead of the doctor's office) could increase government health care costs, which in turn might encourage legislators to reshape health policy to be more fiscally beneficial for the government rather than patients. This also leads the government to shoulder additional responsibility for those costs when residents are ill informed. And, such decisions might again be stratified by citizenship with negative consequences for vulnerable populations like non-citizens and low-income individuals, which was the case after the 2008 recession. Because of the complexity of the U.S. health care system, some respondents asked whether the Massachusetts government was intentionally using vague language in its documents or requiring extensive documentation to deter eligible state residents from actually enrolling in and using their coverage. Doing so would mean less health care costs for the state. While it is unclear if that was the case, this highlights an important issue about the politics of health reform: legislators and government employees play a key role in shaping the type of information disseminated to the public about particular policies and how they are enacted. Lack of clear (and language-accessible) information creates barriers for patients, which reduces their ability to receive quality care, the original intent of the Chapter 58 reform. This is especially the case for patients who are unable to understand the formal English in which the enrollment materials are written, as this is another form of bureaucratic disentitlement that illustrates stratified citizenship in terms of language and socioeconomic status.

Conclusion

Despite being included in Massachusetts's Chapter 58 reform, immigrants experienced various barriers to applying for and using health coverage that demonstrate stratified citizenship and the politics of health reform. Many of these barriers were forms of bureaucratic disentitlement that informally precluded immigrants from accessing health care benefits for which they were formally eligible. Yet, in spite of these various barriers, respondents from all groups felt that Massachusetts immigrants had access to better care compared to elsewhere. But, respondents discussed how local and federal immigration enforcement directly influences immigrants' willingness to use the health care services.

Since I conducted this research, Massachusetts fully complied with ACA implementation. Given federal restrictions excluding many immigrants under the ACA, the state revised Chapter 58 to ensure that previously covered immigrants would retain coverage post-ACA (Joseph 2016). Thus, relative to other ACA-compliant and non-compliant states, Massachusetts immigrants still had more coverage options regardless of documentation status. However, that coverage was still delimited by documentation status and income. Undocumented immigrants were still vulnerable, as HSN allocations continued to be reduced with more eligible "legal" state residents gaining more coverage under the ACA. On June 1, 2016, Massachusetts implemented legislation that would discontinue the state's annual $30 million contribution to HSN. The same legislation also proposed reducing HSN income eligibility from 400% FPL to 300% FPL, reducing the retroactive eligibility period from 6 months to 10 days, and implementing deductibles for HSN patients with incomes of 150% FPL and above (Mass.gov 2016; Mass Legal Services 2016). These changes are another example of how the state continued to stratify citizenship in terms of health care. Immigrants' legal (in)eligibility on the basis of documentation status, but also in terms of income (which is the case for citizens as well), demonstrates how these individuals are not fully included in the body politic. Amid the politics of health reform, these individuals were considered to be expendable whenever budget concerns arise. The costs for low-income immigrants and citizens' health care were shifted from the state government to these individuals, making them more financially responsible for their health care. HSN health care facilities like BHC were also affected, as they could no longer rely on the state government to compensate them. Essentially, these facilities were expected to take on more financial responsibility for providing much-needed care to these populations, who often cannot go elsewhere. At the same time, this cost shifting placed more of the risks of health care usage on these individuals and facilities, in asking them to fund associated health care costs. Because these individuals and facilities were already under-resourced, the risks were greater for accessing and providing care respectively as both try to afford these new costs. Local health advocacy and immigrant organizations expressed grave concerns that these changes will negatively affect HSN recipients' health care access and the quality of care they receive at HSN facilities. Federally ineligible immigrants who had few coverage options, given their exclusion from the ACA and inability to meet new HSN income requirements, lost their coverage from the program. But those who remained financially eligible faced the challenge of paying deductibles. These changes also affected low-income citizens who had HSN to complement their MassHealth coverage. They too experienced less coverage in the post-ACA era.

Nationally, while the ACA would have expanded coverage to nearly 32 million Americans, the reform literally and figuratively demonstrated stratified citizenship in action. The health care that most immigrants and some citizens received nationally via the ACA and in Massachusetts under Chapter 58 demonstrated what sociologist Donald Light (2012) refers to as "categorically unequal" health care. Through its legal exclusion of most immigrants and de facto exclusion of eligible citizens who lived in non-compliant states (that have denied Medicaid expansion), documentation status, income, race/ethnicity, and state of residence played a significant role in determining who benefitted from the policy (Capps and Fix 2013; Hall and Rosenbaum 2012). Despite some notable progress through the reform, studies also indicated that previous disparities were exacerbated on the basis of the aforementioned factors, with low-income and ethno-racial minorities at greater risk of remaining un-insured, especially in non-compliant states (Artiga et al. 2015; Garfield and Damico 2016). In both compliant and non-compliant states, individuals were expected to assume some, if not all, of the responsibility and risk for their participation in the health care system, with or without coverage. While compliant states provided subsidized coverage, it was up to residents to enroll in and use that coverage. And cost concerns under the ACA also meant that the risk for not using health services was higher. In non-compliant states, residents were completely responsible and assumed all the risks for their health care. In both Massachusetts and nationally, there was an upward trend of devolution of responsibility and risk for public resources from state and federal governments to individuals, who were expected to shoulder the burden.

Because of this responsibility and risk devolution at federal and state levels, the stratified citizenship and health care disparities at the national level reflect those that continued to unfold in Massachusetts. Because the state was perceived as a model for health care, other (compliant) states may follow suit in attempts to address their own fiscal constraints. The contribution of this chapter is that its qualitative examination of the Massachusetts model for immigrants effectively highlights stratified citizenship in action, and how that stratification can change over time. Of course, the consequences of this stratification are more dire for immigrants, many of whom are low-income and ethno-racial minorities, which leaves them triply disadvantaged in public policy.

Therefore, MA may serve as both a model and cautionary tale for the nation in the wake of ACA implementation. It serves as a model because it demonstrates that through subnational politics of health reform, populations that are federally excluded from health and other social services can be included at the local level. Though undocumented immigrants were legally excluded from the health exchanges and MassHealth programs, they had access to HSN. Similarly, the state granted middle-income, short-term LPRs eligibility to receive coverage under Commonwealth Care (now known as ConnectorCare) using state funds, as this group was otherwise ineligible. Yet, Massachusetts remains a cautionary tale because it demonstrates that, despite mandating and making health coverage available to many individuals, this coverage is stratified along documentation status, income, and ethno-racial lines, either explicitly or implicitly. This stratification also means that the state's coverage cannot guarantee its residents' actual use of health services. Though the state reduced its uninsurance rate, some Massachusetts residents, especially those who are immigrants, low-income, and with less education, have experienced difficulty finding providers who accept their coverage. Marrow and Joseph (2015) also argue that the intersection of federal immigration and welfare policy with local health policy further stratified Massachusetts residents by citizenship, making that reform less effective for immigrants. The state's ongoing reduction of the HSN budget alongside the removal of short-term LPRs from Commonwealth Care in 2009 especially illustrate the political expendability of immigrants (and low-income individuals) in times of fiscal budgetary concerns. And when considering how the national politics of health reform also stratified the U.S. population by documentation status and state of residence, the barriers I found in Massachusetts are likely to remain and become exacerbated, particularly for immigrant, low-income, and minority populations (Portes et al. 2012; Zuvekas and Taliferro 2003).

Furthermore, lower enrollments of (eligible) immigrants and Latinos during the initial ACA national rollout indicated that language and difficulty understanding how to navigate the health care system serve as forms of bureaucratic disentitlement. These barriers also highlight the significant role that health care navigators and community organizations played in assisting individuals, who were newly eligible for coverage under the ACA, with enrollment procedures and use of health services around the country. Even citizens who were previously uninsured or whose first language may not be English exhibited similar implicit barriers to care in the post-ACA era, given the complexity of the U.S. health care system (Garfield and Damico 2016). And in non-compliant states where both eligible citizens and federally ineligible immigrants were excluded from ACA provisions, the barriers to care were compounded, making it difficult to access coverage and care.

In closing, the Massachusetts and national ACA examples illustrate the non-static aspect of public policies. That is, policies can shift over time due to political opposition, changes in leadership, and the social climate directed toward specific groups. As a result, interpretation of these policies, or the outcomes of such policies, must be considered in light of the local and national sociopolitical context in which the policy is written and implemented. More specifically, when considering the Massachusetts reforms, which were implemented under a conservative governor but have become less generous under subsequent progressive and conservative governors amid budget constraints, the policies have become less beneficial for immigrant and low-income residents at the local level. But, nationally, compared to compliant states that had no provisions for immigrants, or non-compliant states that excluded both immigrants and citizens, Massachusetts—like California—is still considered a best-case scenario. At the same time, increasing anti-immigrant sentiment in public and political discourse has also yielded more anti-immigrant subnational policies and increasing harshness toward immigrants around the country. This climate alongside no federal immigration reforms means that local inclusive (health) reforms, like those in Massachusetts, are not fully effective while immigrants elsewhere remain excluded. Non-policy recommendations like partnerships between immigrant-friendly health care facilities and local (multilingual and multicultural) organizations conducting outreach and enrollment assistance to diverse communities are essential for reducing some of the barriers discussed. But, such efforts require funding, which is difficult to come by in the current political context where immigrants especially and other vulnerable populations are politically expendable. In the absence of policy reforms to more proactively include these populations, their explicit and implicit exclusion continued under the ACA, meaning that the barriers identified in this chapter will remain and likely intensify across the country.

ACKNOWLEDGMENTS

The author would like to thank the co-editors and other contributors of this volume for their extensive feedback on previous drafts of this chapter, as well as the Robert Wood Johnson Foundation for grant support of the study.

NOTES

1 The ACA increased federal funding to federally qualified health centers (FQHCs) that provide primary care for "medically underserved populations" (Searles 2012; Sommers 2013). But, the ACA reduced funding to the Disproportionate Share Hospital Program (DSH), which increased Medicaid payments to safety net hospitals that serve Medicaid and uninsured patients as more Americans became insured (Warner 2012).

2   Under the individual mandate, U.S. citizens and long-term legal permanent
    residents (LPRs) were required to have insurance or pay a fine, and premiums
    were subsidized for low-income earners. The fine was waived for those ineligible
    for public coverage and unable to afford insurance in the exchange (Blumberg and
    Clemans-Cope 2012).
3   This is likely because physicians can opt out of seeing Medicaid patients.
4   This is a pseudonym.
5   The one uninsured Brazilian immigrant I interviewed had her MassHealth cover-
    age discontinued because of failure to submit her re-enrollment documentation.
    The one uninsured Dominican immigrant was undocumented.
6   See Castañeda (this volume) for more on this.
7   See López (2005) and Lipsky (1984) for more on "bureaucratic disentitlement."
8   Secure Communities (S-Comm) automatically sends the fingerprints of ar-
    rested individuals to the FBI and ICE to determine if the person is subject to
    deportation. If so, ICE asks the local jail to hold the individual for 48 hours to be
    interviewed by ICE, which then makes a decision regarding deportation based on
    criminal history, immigration history, and duration of stay in the United States
    (Secure Communities website).

REFERENCES

Artiga, Samantha, Jessica Stephens, and Anthony Damico. 2015. *The Impact of the Coverage Gap in States Not Expanding Medicaid by Race and Ethnicity*. Menlo Park: Kaiser Family Foundation.

Blue Cross Blue Shield Foundation of Massachusetts (BCBS). 2013. *Health Reform in Massachusetts: Expanding Access to Health Insurance Coverage— Accessing the Results March 2013*. Boston: Blue Cross Blue Shield Foundation of Massachusetts.

Blumberg, Linda, and Lisa Clemans-Cope. 2012. *Reconciling the Massachusetts and Federal Individual Mandates for Health Insurance*. Boston: Blue Cross Blue Shield Foundation of Massachusetts.

Capps, Randy, and Michael Fix. 2013. Immigration Reform: A Long Road to Citizen-ship and Insurance Coverage. *Health Affairs* 32(4): 639–642.

Garfield, Rachel, and Anthony Damico. 2016. *The Coverage Gap: Uninsured Poor Adults in States that Do Not Expand Medicaid—An Update*. Menlo Park: Kaiser Family Foundation.

Gottlieb, Nora. 2015. State, Citizenship, and Health in an Age of Global Mobility—A Comparative Study of Labor Migrants' Health Rights in Germany and Israel, in *The Meaning of Citizenship*. Edited by Richard Marback and Marc W. Kruman. Detroit: Wayne State University Press.

Hacker, Karen, Jocelyn Chu, Lisa Arsenault, and Robert P. Marlin. 2012. Provider's Perspectives on the Impact of Immigration and Customs Enforcement (ICE) Activ-ity on Immigrant Health. *Journal of Health Care for the Poor and Underserved* 23: 651–665.

Hall, Mark A., and Sara Rosenbaum. 2012. The Health Care Safety Net in the Context of National Health Insurance Reform. In *The Health Care "Safety Net" in a Post-Reform World*. Edited by Hall and Rosenbaum. New Brunswick, NJ: Rutgers University Press.

Health Law Advocates. 2013. Legal Immigrant Access to Health Care. www.healthla wadvocates.org.

Joseph, Tiffany D. 2016. What Healthcare Reform Means for Immigrants: A Comparison of the Massachusetts and Affordable Care Act Health Reforms. *Journal of Health Policy, Politics, and Law* 41: 101–116.

Kutner, Mark, Elizabeth Greenberg, Ying Jin, and Christine Paulsen. 2006. *The Health Literacy of America's Adults: Results from the 2003 National Assessment of Adult Literacy*. National Center for Education Statistics, Washington, DC.

Light, Donald. 2012. Categorical Inequality, Institutional Ambivalence, and Permanently Failing Institutions: The Case of Immigrants and Barriers to Health Care in America. *Ethnic and Racial Studies* 35: 23–39.

Lipsky, Michael. 1984. Bureaucratic Disentitlement in Social Welfare Programs. *Social Service Review* 58: 3–27.

Lockwood, D. 1996. Civic Integration and Class Formation. *British Journal of Sociology* 47: 531–550.

Long, Sharon, and Karen Stockley. 2010. Sustaining Health Reform in a Recession: An Update on Massachusetts as of Fall of 2009. *Health Affairs* 29: 1234–1241.

Long, Sharon, Karen Stockley, and Kate Willrich Nordahl. 2013. Coverage, Access, and Affordability under Health Reform: Learning from the Massachusetts Model. *Inquiry* 49: 303–316.

López, Leslie. 2005. De Facto Disentitlement in an Information Economy: Enrollment Issues in Medicaid Managed Care. *Medical Anthropology Quarterly* 19: 26–46.

Marrow, Helen B. 2012. Deserving to a Point: Unauthorized Immigrants in San Francisco's Universal Access Healthcare Model. *Social Science and Medicine* 74: 846–854.

Marrow, Helen B., and Tiffany D. Joseph. 2015. Excluded and Frozen Out: Unauthorized Immigrants' (Non)Access to Care after Health Care Reforms. *Journal of Ethnic and Migration Studies* 41: 2253–2273.

Mass.gov. 2016. Announcement about Health Safety Net Changes. April 6, 2016. www .masshealthmtf.org.

Mass Legal Services. 2016. Blowing a Hole in the Health Safety Net: EOHHS Notice of Proposed Rules. www.masslegalservices.org.

Maxwell, James, Dharma Cortés, Karen Schneider, Anna Graves, and Brian Rosman. 2011. Massachusetts Health Care Reform Increased Access to Care for Hispanics, But Disparities Remain. *Health Affairs* 30(8): 1451–1460.

Park, Lisa Sun-Hee. 2011. *Entitled to Nothing: The Struggle for Immigrant Health Care in the Age of Welfare Reform*. New York: New York University Press.

Patel, Kavita, and John McDonough. 2010. From Massachusetts to 1600 Pennsylvania Avenue: Aboard the Health Reform Express. *Health Affairs* 29(6): 1106–1111.

Portes, Alejandro, Patricia Fernández-Kelly, and Donald W. Light. 2012. Life on the Edge: Immigrants Confront the American Health System. *Ethnic and Racial Studies* 35(1): 3–22.

Pryor, Carol, and Andrew Cohen, eds. 2009. *Consumers' Experience in Massachusetts: Lessons for National Health Reform*. Menlo Park, CA: Henry J. Kaiser Family Foundation.

Rosenbaum, Sara. 2012. Reinventing a Classic: Community Health Centers and the Newly Insured. In *The Health Care "Safety Net" in a Post-Reform World*. Edited by Marc A. Hall and Sara Rosenbaum. New Brunswick, NJ: Rutgers University Press.

Searles, Christopher. 2012. Beyond Health Care Reform: Immigrants and the Future of Medicine. *Ethnic and Racial Studies* 35: 135–149.

Secure Communities Website. www.ice.gov.

Sommers, Benjamin D. 2013. Stuck between Health and Immigration Reform-Care for Undocumented Immigrants. *New England Journal of Medicine* 369(7): 593–595.

Warner, David C. 2012. Access to Health Care Services for Immigrants in the U.S.A.: From the Great Society to the 2010 Health Reform Act and After. *Ethnic and Racial Studies* 35(1): 40–55.

Zuvekas, Samuel H., and Gregg S. Taliaferro. 2003. Pathways to Access: Health Insurance, The Health Care Delivery System, and Racial/Ethnic Disparities, 1996–1999. *Health Affairs* 22(2): 139–153.

4

Stratification through Medicaid

Public Prenatal Care in New York City

ELISE ANDAYA

It's a busy day on the women's health floor at Beaumont Hospital,[1] a public hospital in one of the boroughs of New York City. The four clinics providing gynecological, prenatal, and post-partum care are filled with women awaiting their appointments, some with a male partner, family member, or a small child in tow. A few spill out to the plastic chairs lining the hallway, while others line up outside offices to see the financial counselor, the nutritionist, or the cashier. The population served here is primarily Afro-Caribbean: Many are recent immigrants with limited English who work largely in low-paid home health care and childcare positions. There is also a large number of first- or second-generation women from the Anglophone Caribbean who are employed in a broader range of service positions: retail, food service, child care, and home health care aides. "These are working people," a harried but kind administrator tells me as his lead-off sentence in our introductory meeting. I sense both a little defensiveness and some pride in his tone, and I guess that he is used to defending his work and his patients in a national context that greatly undervalues medical service to the poor and the undocumented. Indeed, virtually everyone I speak to is covered by Medicaid: Some enter the hospital prenatal care system already covered by the program, a few take advantage of Medicaid's higher income threshold for pregnant women to transfer from employer-based plans, and others—usually those previously uninsured because of their documentation status—receive Medicaid coverage onsite through New York State's guarantee of free prenatal care for all female residents.

Public prenatal care provides a unique view of how the health care system works for low-income people following the 2010 passage of the

Affordable Care Act (ACA). When President Obama first raised the flag of health care reform in the United States, many supporters imagined an unprecedented opportunity to reform America's patchwork health insurance system into a national, single-payer program like those in place in many other countries, both "developed" and "developing." By assuring all U.S. residents health coverage, regardless of employment status, income level, region, gender, race/ethnicity—and for some, documentation—these supporters hoped that health care reform would provide the basis for a new and inclusive health care system that would undo the deeply stratified system of the past. The end result, as is universally acknowledged, was very far from this ideal. Despite the ACA's effort to expand health coverage and access, long-standing social hierarchies were ossified in the law. As this volume argues, the ACA in many cases simply reconstituted preexisting patterns of exclusion, reinforcing long-standing moral divisions between the "righteous" and the "undeserving." A key question for observers, therefore, is whether—and to what extent—the ACA succeeded in changing ideologies and experiences of health citizenship for the huge number of U.S. residents who were previously uninsured or underinsured.

Building on the growing anthropological literature on health citizenship (e.g., Biehl 2013; Briggs 2002; Farmer 2001; Fassin 2007; Holmes 2013), the concept of stratified citizenship draws attention to the fact that all (health) citizens are not created equal; even among those legally included within the state's health compact, some people's claim to health services may be considered more deserving than those of others (Horton 2004; Willen 2012). As a consequence, they may receive better quality health care, be attended in a more timely fashion, or may simply experience more care and respect in their health encounter than those people who are considered less worthy health citizens.

This chapter argues that a focus on stratified citizenship must not end with analyses of the effects of the *lack* of health coverage. It must also take account of how different *forms* of health coverage—in this case, Medicaid—can also contribute to experiences of health inequality. Discussions of Medicaid under the ACA have tended to focus on the consequences of state decisions around expansion, tracking the health effects for those newly covered and for those in non-expanding states who continue to be ineligible for coverage. This is critical and urgently needed research. However, given that Medicaid expansion accounted for more than half of the population newly insured under the ACA, as well as the centrality of Medicaid to the success of health care reform, it behooves us to ask not only about access to care, but also about the *experience* of "health citizenship" for those who were covered under the program.

Had the ACA been designed as a national single-payer system, all U.S. residents would have been incorporated as equals into the same health care system. However, the compromise battled out over the ACA—to expand health insurance coverage through Medicaid expansion, insurance marketplaces, and the individual mandate—effectively maintained the long-standing division between "consumers" of private health insurance and Medicaid "recipients." A large body of social scientific research has documented the negative valuation given to public assistance in the United States, as well as the tendency to attribute neediness to personal moral failings rather than structural inequalities (Gilens 2009; Hays 2003; Katz 1990; Wacquant 2009). While attitudes toward Medicaid and Medicaid enrollees are less well-studied, it is clear that those covered under Medicaid face a cultural landscape in which public aid (as opposed to the "private" government aid that middle- and upper-class families receive in the form of tax deductions for mortgages and marriage) is inextricably entangled with judgments about citizenship and moral worth.

Of particular interest, then, is not only whether Medicaid coverage translates into better health and access to care in states that accepted Medicaid expansion. Observers must also ask whether Medicaid expansion resulted in a broader experience of health equality for those in the program or, alternatively, whether it simply increased the pool of people who are positioned as less deserving health citizens because of their form of health coverage. This nuanced analysis of the effects of the ACA is data that ethnographers are well-positioned to contribute. Yet such a focus can be problematic for social liberals, in large part because of a justified fear that any criticisms of the program will be co-opted by its opponents to argue for dismantling it and devolving health coverage to individual private health insurance. I therefore wish to state emphatically my support for the Medicaid program; the expansive health coverage it offers to low-income Americans is critical to their well-being and is clearly preferable to either remaining uninsured or "choosing" the frequently expensive and limited employer-based plans that are the only other alternative for many people in low-wage and unstable jobs. Rather than undermining Medicaid, I intend this chapter to add to other voices calling to strengthen and improve the program to ensure good health care and good health experiences for its millions of enrollees.

New York City's public prenatal care clinics are a particularly interesting site to explore issues around the stratification of health citizenship, precisely because of its long-standing commitment to providing health care to its residents. Of the estimated 1.9 million residents of New York State newly enrolled in health insurance since the Marketplace opened in October 2013, the vast majority—more than a million individuals—signed up for Medicaid.[2] As of March 2016, more than 6.5 million people were enrolled in Medicaid or the Children's Health Insurance Program, representing a 16% increase over the average monthly enrollment in Medicaid/CHIP prior to the passage of the ACA (KFF 2016). Given New York State's 2015 population of 19.7 million, this means that close to a third of its residents received health coverage through Medicaid/CHIP. In addition to accepting Medicaid expansion, New York provides free health coverage to all pregnant women up to 223% of the federal poverty level, regardless of their migratory status. Public prenatal care in New York thus creates what I am calling a temporary "zone of inclusion," during which all women are legally entitled to full access to all health care (not simply to pregnancy-related services) from conception to 60 days postpartum.

Yet this chapter argues that the experiences of Medicaid-covered pregnant women underscore the distinction between *inclusion* in health care and *equality* of health citizenship, where the former indexes juridical rights to health coverage and the latter signals experiences within forms of health coverage. Drawing on my own and others' ethnographic research in New York City's public hospital–based prenatal clinics, I focus on two primary contributors to experiences of stratified health citizenship: long clinic wait times and extensive Medicaid-required prenatal counseling. I suggest that in many cases, experiences of health inequality are in fact the unintended—although not inevitable—consequences of political and social commitments to inclusion. The fact that issues of health inequality are so apparent in a relatively progressive and socially liberal state like New York suggests such tensions are both entrenched and widespread.

Methods

This material is based on ongoing research in a prenatal clinic of Beaumont Hospital as part of a broader project examining access to prenatal health care among women who work in the low-wage service sector. Data collection was ongoing at the time of writing: beginning in September 2015, I spent two days a week observing in one of Beaumont's prenatal clinics, tracking patient flow through appointments, recording wait times, and engaging in informal conversations with patients, clinic staff, and providers. I conducted formal interviews with 55 Medicaid-covered pregnant women to ask about health care coverage, perceptions of their health care quality and access, availability of leaves and benefits while working, and experiences of working in service labor while pregnant. Reflecting the demographic composition of the clinic, virtually all of the participants identified as African American or as Afro-Caribbean, all worked in service-sector labor, and were 18 years or older. Interviews lasted between 15 and 45 minutes and were audiotaped with informants' permission. When informants were uncomfortable with being audiotaped, I took notes during the interview and wrote detailed field notes immediately thereafter. In addition, I interviewed five prenatal care providers (obstetricians and midwives) who work in various public hospitals in New York City. Like all ethnographic work, these observations are shaped by their context; Medicaid-covered pregnant women receiving care in a private clinic or non-pregnant Medicaid enrollees receiving other services may well report very different experiences. Yet attention to sites in which patients almost entirely suffer the "conjugated oppression" (Bourgois 1988) of poverty, minority status, and, for some, lack of documentation, can shed light on the broader dynamics of health coverage for the poor after the ACA.

Zones of Inclusion: Public Health Care in New York City

New York City has a long and distinguished history of providing public health care to its residents. The city's system of public municipal hospitals is the oldest and historically the most extensive in the country; several currently operating public hospitals (including Beaumont) emerged from almshouse charities instituted in the eighteenth and nineteenth centuries. Legally bound to accept all persons in need of health care, public municipal hospitals served a wide swath of city residents in the first part of the twentieth century. One of the distinctive features of the city's pre-Medicaid public health system was its generous subsidies for the "medically indigent," those people who were not considered destitute but for whom health care payments would have constituted a significant financial burden. Underscoring the commitment to health care for all, a study conducted shortly prior to the 1965 inauguration of Medicaid showed that 40% of the city's hospital patients met municipal standards for medical indigence. After the implementation of Medicaid, New York set the highest Medicaid eligibility threshold of all states, surpassing the next-highest state (California) by a third, simply by matching its already-existing medical indigence standards (Opdycke 1999). As Sandra Obdycke argues, these generous eligibility criteria "expressed the broader idea that free health care was not just a charitable arrangement for very poor, but a need and right of ordinary citizens" (1999, 139). Thus, she points out, while Medicaid made health care truly accessible for the first time for millions of people around the country, New York City's extensive network of public hospitals and clinics, charitable institutions, and private teaching hospitals meant that health care access for city residents was already close to universal. Although financial support for public health care institutions has been threatened over the decades by declining federal contributions to Medicaid, the city's budget crisis in the 1970s, and shifts toward managed care and cost-control mechanisms in the 1980s and 1990s, public hospitals in New York have long stood as zones of inclusion where all could receive care.

Yet inclusion did not mean equality; the city's system of public hospitals also reflected and reproduced deep social hierarchies. In the division between public and private hospitals, public hospitals served as safety nets—chronically underfunded and oversubscribed facilities that took in patients that private hospitals refused to admit, whether because of economic status, moral "failings," or type of illness. Reliant largely on the shifting fortunes and commitments of the city, and despite the efforts of many well-intentioned and dedicated health workers and administrators, conditions over the long decades were generally serviceable at best and, at worst, grim if not outright dangerous (Obdycke 1999). Although officials and other observers had long recognized the financial and moral problems of allowing private hospitals to shunt poor or undesirable patients to a cash-strapped public system, political tensions around any radical transformations of the system meant that public hospitals remained the lower rung of a two-tier system. Even the introduction of Medicaid, expected to provide an influx of much-needed money to the public system, in fact produced competition between private and public hospitals as the former scrambled to attract patients with Medicaid dollars while refusing to care for patients with no means to pay for their services. In many ways, this situation remains largely unchanged today, as public hospitals strive to bring in patients with health coverage (usually Medicaid) to cover patients unable to pay for medical services and to otherwise supplement their always-insufficient budgets.

New York's public hospitals also developed expertise in prenatal and obstetric care early because unwed mothers, with their taint of moral corruption, comprised one of the groups frequently turned away from private hospitals. Bellevue, America's oldest public hospital, opened the country's first maternity ward in 1799. The demand for prenatal care was such that Bellevue opened the country's first school for midwives in 1911 to provide free six-month training for women, particularly new immigrants, who could not afford traditional nursing school or who would not have met the criteria for entry (Obdycke 1999). The commitment to inclusion through supporting publicly funded prenatal care continued through the twentieth century. In 1986, in the face of growing data demonstrating that declining Medicaid thresholds were negatively impacting the health of low-income pregnant women, the U.S. Congress established the PCAP (Prenatal Care Assistance Program) to reimburse states for providing health care to pregnant women whose income exceeded Medicaid eligibility standards but who had no other form of insurance. In 1989, new legislation required all states to cover pregnant women up to 133% of the federal poverty level. That same year, New York State enacted its own version of PCAP to cover pregnant women with incomes up to 200% of the federal poverty level. Although PCAP was reimbursed through the state Medicaid program (and PCAP patients are temporarily entitled to all of the same benefits), New York departed from the federal guidelines by electing not to require immigration documentation as a precondition for the program.

New York's inclusive prenatal health policy thus allows qualified health institutions to provide prenatal care to all low-income women, regardless of insurance or documentation status, without fearing that they will have to absorb the costs of caring for the uninsured. Although about half of the women I interviewed came to the hospital already covered by Medicaid, the remainder entered the hospital system because they were uninsured, undocumented, or, in a few cases, carried expensive employer-based health insurances, and knew that public hospitals will provide them with free care by enrolling them into Medicaid/PCAP. The importance of this moral and political commitment to care cannot be understated, particularly given that rates of late prenatal care (defined as care initiated at or after 13 weeks of gestation) or no prenatal care among poor and minority women continue to be far higher than public health officials would like (New York State Department of Health 2013).[3] The concern about the timely initiation of prenatal care reflects official recognition of the ongoing class and racial/ethnic disparities in birth outcomes, as well as the appalling fact that rates of maternal mortality in the United States—largely correlated with poverty, minority status, lack of access to prenatal care, and co-morbidities during pregnancy—doubled between 1990 and 2013, from an estimated 12 deaths per 100,000 births to 28 deaths per 100,000 births (Agrawal 2015). Yet, given the historic tensions between New York's commitment to inclusion with respect to *access* to care and entrenched inequalities with respect to *experiences* of health care, it is unsurprising that such conflicts continued under the ACA. In the following section, I draw on my own ethnographic research, as well as those of other anthropologists working in New York City's public hospitals, to consider this tension in more detail.

Health Inclusion versus Health Equality

The waiting room is relatively quiet on this Wednesday morning, although the line of women waiting to check in for their appointments is beginning to build as the sole receptionist on duty works steadily to open electronic check-in records, process paperwork, answer the telephone, and direct patients to the correct suite. A pregnant woman approaches the desk; she just needs to have her bloodwork done today and can be sent straight to the laboratory, but she wants to ask her provider a question. The receptionist tells her to take a seat and goes back to the examination rooms to alert the provider, who is currently seeing another patient.

Forty minutes pass. Finally, the woman approaches the desk again to request the return of her clinic identification card that is required for all medical appointments at this hospital. "On Monday, I was here at 9:30 a.m. and didn't leave until 7 p.m.," she declared, "They ain't gonna do that to me again." I offer to go to the provider's office to retrieve the clinic card, but when I do so, the provider indicates that she has time to talk to the patient. Despite my concern that both might be feeling aggrieved (the patient by her wait, and the provider by needing to fit in an unscheduled patient), I hear them greet each other warmly as the door closes behind them.

The patient leaves the provider's office about ten minutes later and stops by the front desk for a WIC (Special Supplemental Nutrition Program for Women, Infants, and Children) form, since medical confirmation of pregnancy and expected date of delivery are required for enrollment into this federally subsidized food program. A nurse must fill out this paperwork, and the receptionist hesitates, saying, "It's going to take a while, and I know you can't wait." The woman responds, "It's not that I *can't* wait today. It's that everywhere you go here you've got to wait. You go to [financial] clearance, you've got to wait; you go the nutritionist, you wait; you see a nurse, you wait; you want a WIC form, you wait." Shaking her head, she reiterates, "I was here 9:30 to 7 on Monday and I can't do that again." The receptionist looks at her sympathetically, and says quietly, "I understand. You're justified in feeling that way."

Examining ideologies around health-related deservingness with respect to undocumented migrants, Sarah Willen has argued that social scientists studying health inequalities must consider the complicated relationship between *entitlement* to health care, practical questions around health care *access*, and "situationally specific, vernacular, and *moral* debates around health care *deservingness*" (2012, 806). Deservingness, she argues, is the "flip side" of rights; whereas arguments about rights to health care are made in juridical language that presumes universality and equality, debates about moral deservingness are context-dependent, relational (vary according to personal or historical relationships to the group in question), and conditional upon presumed or actual characteristics of the individual or group.

This conceptual clarification between access, entitlement, and deservingness is useful in elucidating the tensions experienced by those who receive health care coverage under Medicaid/PCAP. Medicaid has long been one of the most popular government programs (Sanger-Katz 2014). Repeated surveys have found that expansion of the program was one of the most approved components of the ACA, particularly in the Democratic states (KFF 2012)—a rather unsurprising finding given that the alternative for many low-income people would be either employer-based insurance, with limited coverage and high co-pays and deductibles, or remaining uninsured. Yet, although Medicaid generally ranks well against private insurance in respondents' assessments of the affordability and quality of health care, it lags in the categories of "seeing the doctors you want, without having to wait too long" and "having doctors treat you with care and respect" (Sanger-Katz 2014). Thus, on the one hand, Medicaid coverage is deeply desired by the majority of low-income Americans, who see it as important to their ability to access and afford health care. This is an argument about rights and the importance of inclusion into health citizenship. Yet, on the other, the answers of respondents also suggest that they do not experience a sense of health *equality*, as indicated by their perception that people with Medicaid coverage are subjected to lengthier wait times and are less likely to receive "care and respect" from their providers than are those with private insurance.

Attention to these findings is critical, since negative experiences in the health care system can lead to poorer health outcomes or even discourage individuals from seeking care (e.g., Holmes 2013). While Medicaid certainly facilitates health access, at least for prenatal care, ethnographic researchers in hospital prenatal clinics in New York City have argued that these are prime sites in which low-income, minority, and migrant patients are socialized into experiences of unequal health citizenship (Bridges 2011; Gálvez 2011). Thus, in Willen's schema, while pregnant patients are legally entitled to prenatal health care and are usually able to access it, in so doing they may also encounter discourses and practices that question whether they are deserving of "free" health care. Sometimes these moral judgments are overt; in her research on racialization in prenatal care at "Alpha Hospital" in New York City, Khiara Bridges

(2011) notes that clinic staff frequently evoked an archetypical figure that she calls the "wily patient," who is simultaneously unintelligent and yet also capable of shrewdly manipulating hospital and state resources to her benefit. This figure, she argues, overlaps substantially with that of the "welfare queen," a racialized and classed epithet that questions the individual's deservingness of public assistance. Such accusations tended to be voiced by low-level workers (reception staff and PCAs, who take patients' vital signs prior to their provider visit) rather than providers (see also Marrow 2012), and were partly attributable to the fact that these comprised the "front-line" of patient relations; they interacted most directly with frustrated and disgruntled women without any authority to intervene in the situation. However, Bridges also points out that this front-line staff shared many of the same socioeconomic characteristics as their low-income patients. Questioning the legitimacy of patients' entitlement to public aid, she argues, thus served as powerful boundary markers through which they distinguished between themselves—the working "deserving poor"—and women they constructed as lazy, unemployed, and otherwise morally undeserving.

Such overt hostility has not been my experience at Beaumont. Whether due to a different clinical culture, or because the staff and their patients often share roots in the Caribbean with their patients, the interactions I observed between patients and clinic staff at Beaumont were generally cordial, despite occasional behind-the-scenes complaints about some patients or providers. Nevertheless, I concur with other researchers that these public prenatal clinics frequently become sites that produce and reproduce experiences of unequal health citizenship. That this frequently occurs *despite* the good intentions and hard work of many clinic workers, care providers, and hospital administrators underscores its deeper structural roots in entrenched institutional and social policies. In what follows, I examine two often-interconnected mechanisms by which such experiences of health inequality are produced: waiting and Medicaid-required prenatal interventions.

Waiting

One of most striking aspects of the several public hospital-based prenatal clinics I observed or visited around New York City was the sheer number of waiting women. Providers in different facilities confirmed this impression of delay, noting that women not infrequently waited hours for a provider visit that might only last 15 minutes. At Beaumont, women endured these wait times patiently, alternately sleeping, playing with their phones, listening to the health educators' presentations on breastfeeding and safe infant sleeping practices, or glancing at the television set that was tuned to "Hospital TV," an endless loop of informational segments on diabetes, surgical wound care, and the dangers of antibiotic-resistant bacterial infections. Only when wait times became an hour or longer did women start to stir and complain quietly under their breath. When overt conflicts between staff and patients did arise, they were almost exclusively around women's frustrations at long delays: in one case, a woman who had been waiting almost three hours to be seen for her 1:40 appointment complained loudly to the desk staff before sliding back into her seat, muttering under her breath, "I have to go to work. They don't respect my time!"

Research on state social service institutions in the United States and elsewhere has identified pervasive beliefs about the disposability of poor people's time and the disciplinary power of waiting for services (Auyero 2012; Edin and Lein 1997). Based on research in state welfare institutions in Argentina, Javier Auyero (2012) underscores the taken-for-granted nature of waiting and the assumption that the poor *should* wait for the services that they are receiving "for free." Drawing from Bourdieu, he argues that this "doxa of waiting" socializes the poor into expectations of government services as well as into their inferior place in the political community. Experiences of lack of control over time, as well as the frequently opaque reasons for delays, he suggests, are part of the production of experiences of unequal citizenship. In one example of this lack of control, a midwife at Mayfield, another public hospital in New York City, described her hospital's scheduling practices: Whereas women receiving care at private clinics select future appointments according to their own availability, women attending Mayfield Hospital were assigned appointment days and times without concern for women's preexisting schedules. When I asked about the rationale for these scheduling practices, she responded, "Part of it is that it's a busy hospital. We have about 3,000 births a year, so you know, I guess they can't take everyone's preferences and schedules into account. But I think a huge part is that women are seen as charity cases—you know, you're getting health care for free so you should just be grateful for what you get. Their time isn't valued." Appointments were assigned similarly at Beaumont; although women could, and sometimes did, ask for appointments to be re-scheduled around work and other obligations, this usually meant additional waiting while PCAs searched for new appointment openings. Many women, already eager to leave, simply decided to re-arrange their other commitments around their prenatal appointment rather than engage in potentially fruitless waiting.

Such practices highlight Auyero's point that among low-income recipients of government services, time is an important locus of both conflict and acquiescence (2012, 27). The language of time, or the "disrespect" for time, is one idiom in which women articulate their sense of unequal treatment in the system. Yet ultimately, there was little they could do besides express their dissatisfaction; only occasionally did I see a woman leave because of the long wait times, and these departures usually occurred after a woman had already been waiting for hours. Usually, the effort of coming to the clinic and the time already invested meant that women ultimately acquiesced to the seeming necessity of waiting. Of course, waiting for the doctor, and the accompanying recognition that doctors' time is considered more valuable than that of their patients, is an experience shared by many privately insured patients as well. Yet, in my experiences of privately insured prenatal care in New York City, wait times never approached those frequently experienced by women in public prenatal care facilities, and women were more vocal about expressing their displeasure when delays did extend beyond that which was considered reasonable. By contrast, the Mayfield midwife suggests, women in public hospital clinics are expected to wait patiently because, as "charity cases," they are not considered active health care consumers who may take their "business" elsewhere—although they sometimes did. Rather, they are passive "Medicaid recipients," who should demonstrate their gratitude for care by waiting without complaint. Indeed, while some women I interviewed expressed indignation when I asked about wait times, many others just shrugged and said that they expected to have to wait. Thus, as Auyero points out, waiting both produces and reproduces unequal citizenship: health care experiences are shaped by women's previous expectations about what health care (or other social services) should provide and how those in the system should be treated.

Yet I do not wish to imply that long wait times are deliberately inflicted on women as a way of achieving political subordination. Rather, waiting is "a strategy of domination without a strategist" (Bourdieu and Wacquant 1992). In the case of prenatal care, I suggest that waiting—and the consequent experiences of unequal health citizenship—is the often-unintended consequence of policies designed to ensure pregnant women's *inclusion* in, and access to, prenatal health services. For example, the chronic underfunding of public hospitals is a critical factor, one that must be addressed if Medicaid expansion is to adequately serve all new enrollees. The volume of patients served, and the frequently inadequate material and human resources with which to serve them, is a major contributor to delays. Another important factor is the commitment of public prenatal clinics to seeing all patients on the day that they come in, if at all possible, even if they arrive late. One provider at Beaumont pointed out that this commitment was unique to public clinics. In most private settings, women who arrived more than 30 minutes late for their appointment would in all likelihood be rescheduled so as not to inconvenience other patients. For women at Beaumont, keeping appointment times was frequently a problem; the reception staff often had to inform women that they were late for their appointment, and many of the women I interviewed reported having been late to, or having missed, two or more appointments. (Lateness was usually blamed on transportation, a common problem in an area of the city in which most women depend on one or more buses that are frequently late, overcrowded, or otherwise unreliable, particularly in inclement weather.) In almost all cases, their late arrival was accommodated. However, in order to maintain patient flow, Beaumont's current policy is to see patients in the order that they arrive rather than by their scheduled appointment time. This means that if a number of patients arrive late for morning appointments, patients who do arrive on time for appointments later in the day suffer the effects of these delays. Thus, the hospital's goal of inclusion—seeing all women whenever possible rather than rescheduling their appointments to another day—was one contributor to some patients' experience of health inequality that they described as "disrespect" for their time and other commitments.

The hospital administration was well aware of women's dissatisfaction with these long delays, and was actively trying to improve patient flow (I was surprised and rather touched to see the genuine distress expressed by one high-ranking administrator about the issue). Near the beginning of my fieldwork, for example, in an effort to curtail lengthy delays for those with afternoon appointments, the prenatal clinics had moved from a de facto first come, first served policy regardless of appointment time, which had encouraged all women to arrive early in the morning in order to be seen as quickly as possible, to a system whereby women were only able to check in 30 minutes prior to their scheduled appointment. I also observed an administrator conducting a time study, during which she followed various patients throughout their prenatal visit to log times and observe reasons for delays. As this chapter neared publication, a few providers began instructing reception staff to reschedule patients who came late to appointments as a means of both controlling patient flow and, as one said, to "try to teach patients to come on time." However, there was no set policy about how late was too late to be seen; determinations were dependent on the provider, her good will, and the number of patients still waiting to be seen. This unannounced change of policy and its ambiguity, as well as the effort that many women felt they had expended to get to the clinic, in fact usually produced further tensions and conflict for the beleaguered desk staff who were given the unwelcome duty of informing women that they would not be seen.

Thus, in the context of oversubscription and underfunding, stratified citizenship—experienced in part as long delays for services—was partly an unintended consequence of state and institutional policies that sought to include all women in prenatal health care in the context of limited resources. In the next section, I examine another contributor to both lengthy prenatal appointments and experiences of unequal health care treatment: the requirements of Medicaid-covered prenatal care.

Public Prenatal Care: Discipline and Nurturance

Women's interactions with public prenatal care in New York are in many ways very different from the typical experiences of women covered by private insurance. As part of its commitment to care, New York State's Medicaid regulations require that all pregnant women have access to a diverse array of social and medical services. As a consequence, Medicaid-covered women are brought far more thoroughly into the ambit of state medical and social oversight than their privately insured counterparts. Their first prenatal visit is generally the longest, and women are told to expect to be in the hospital for several hours (in practice, women often spent five hours and sometimes longer at this first appointment). Prior to their appointment with their medical provider—usually the least time-consuming of the day's meetings—new patients receive financial clearance from their Medicaid insurer, a process that must often be repeated before every visit, or, if uninsured, patients are enrolled into PCAP. They take an HIV test and are screened by a nurse for any social, emotional, economic, or health concerns that might pose a danger during the pregnancy. During their pregnancy, they are counseled about HIV and nutrition, again, and may be referred to the social worker or in-house psychologist if mental health support is deemed necessary. These visits are intended to "educate" women about recommended diet, exercise, and sexual practices, and also to establish risk categories by inquiring about past and present sexual or domestic violence, conjugal relationships, household finances, exposure to environmental toxins (such as the lead paint still present in many older apartment buildings), and so forth.

The extensive oversight over pregnant women receiving public prenatal care sharply underscores the Janus-faced nature of discipline and nurturance. While this tension between the disciplinary and nurturing aspects of prenatal care exists in many other global sites (Andaya 2013, 2014; Ivry 2009), in the United States the disciplinary aspect falls more heavily on women receiving public prenatal care, who are constructed as being at higher medical and social risk, than on women with private coverage. On the one hand, these requirements clearly intend to provide women perceived as potentially at risk with services that they need in pregnancy and beyond. As such, these policies are part of the state's commitment to include all pregnant women in health care. Some women do indeed experience these encounters with clinical and social services as a useful source of information or a sign of institutional care (e.g., Fraser 1995), and in some cases they may also provide important information that guides clinical services. On the other hand, it is striking that these additional screening and counseling visits are rarely offered to women with private insurance, let alone required of them.

Ethnographers of New York's public prenatal care (Bridges 2011; Gálvez 2011), as well as some providers I interviewed, have questioned the quality of some of these services and their fit with the reality of women's lives, suggesting that in many cases these perfunctory consultations simply existed to "check the boxes" of Medicaid requirements rather than improving prenatal health or care delivery. In her work, Bridges (2011) argues that Medicaid-covered prenatal care is fraught with racialized and classed policies—such as the requirement for multiple HIV tests—that frame poor women as a single population of medically and socially high-risk patients regardless of their reported risk factors. For some women, questions about topics such as the quality of their marital relations, referrals to a nutritionist, or the expectation that they submit to multiple tests for sexually transmitted infections—requirements that are restricted only to those individuals who are enrolled in Medicaid rather than private insurance—may thus be experienced as onerous, time-consuming, and intrusive. Women have limited ability to opt out; as with welfare, acceptance of Medicaid-subsidized prenatal care also requires that women accept the surveillance that comes with it. This is not to cast aspersions on the health care workers that provide these services, many of whom work diligently to serve their patient population. It does, however, underscore the ideological underpinnings of Medicaid-covered prenatal care and its driving assumptions about low-income women, as well as how it nurtures and disciplines both pregnant women and hospital providers and facilities (who must adhere to Medicaid requirements) in ways that profoundly shape the patient/provider relationship.

In addition to justifying increased state-medical oversight in the name of risk, these additional tests and consultations contribute to the length of patients' visits. Privately insured patients are subject to fewer routine clinical and social service requirements in general. However, when additional services are medically advised, testing and counseling are often performed outside the prenatal clinic and can be scheduled at a time that suits the patient. By contrast, in many hospital-based public clinics, virtually all clinical and social services are performed "in-house," which often leads to delays as women all queue for the same required providers. Women sent to see the nutritionist may be confronted with a sign that she has gone to lunch and will not return for another hour.

Similarly, women seeking to begin prenatal care must have confirmation of pregnancy performed through a test at the hospital lab, usually waiting an hour or more for the results before they can schedule a prenatal appointment.

Such institutional policies reflect again the twin processes of nurturance and the social and fiscal discipline to which both Medicaid-covered pregnant women and Medicaid-accepting hospitals are subject. In part, by providing in-house services to fulfill Medicaid requirements, hospitals hope to provide women with a number of services in the same physical location, eliminating their need to travel or seek out other facilities. In addition to facilitating the recommended or required consultations, this also reflects a concern that women will not carry out the required testing or counseling if they must find their own sources. Economic concerns are also at play; as one health provider told me, cash-strapped public hospitals want to keep counseling and testing within their facilities in order to be able to bill for these services.

Whatever the motivation, the consequences are that women spend lengthy periods of time not just waiting to see their health care provider, but also fulfilling—or waiting to fulfill—the many additional requirements of public prenatal care. Of course, women often resist ideologies that position them as passive subjects of "charity care," as the Mayfield midwife put it. Some women at Beaumont sought to re-shape clinic hierarchies, and ultimately the clinic experience, by cultivating friendly relationships with some of the staff. Women not infrequently moved between different public prenatal clinics if they did not like the care or the time delays at one institution, sometimes re-appearing at their former clinic after a negative experience in their second site. A provider at Greenwood, a public hospital in another borough of New York City, noted that women who had received prenatal care at this facility would not infrequently show up in the emergency room of the nearby private hospital in advanced stages of labor. These health-seeking strategies, aimed at ensuring a birth at a private hospital, illustrate the circulation of knowledge about ways to sidestep Medicaid constraints (since all emergency rooms, public or private, are legally bound to offer service regardless of insurance status). Further, it reflects dominant cultural beliefs about the superiority of care at private facilities and women's efforts to obtain such care for themselves and their newborns. Although hospital staff considered such practices problematic and undesirable for reasons relating to continuity of care, fiscal bureaucracy, and the unnecessary burdening of emergency facilities, they must also be contextualized within women's constrained attempts to navigate health care in the context of America's stratified health citizenship.

Conclusion

Anthropologists of reproduction have long argued that attention to ideologies and practices around pregnancy and birth shine a bright light on broader social tensions (Ginsburg and Rapp 1995). Building from this observation, I suggest that public prenatal care offers a prime opportunity to consider the difference between health inclusion and health equality, and the consequences of this distinction for Medicaid-covered individuals under the ACA. In ensuring access to health coverage for millions of the previously uninsured, the ACA was an important step toward closing the gaps in America's still-fractured system of health coverage. Yet, at the same time, its failure to dismantle the public/ private division in health coverage places into question the degree to which health reform transformed ideologies of health citizenship in the contemporary United States. We need more attention to the ways that health citizenship is shaped by type and quality of health coverage, not simply by its presence or absence. My observations in prenatal care, echoing those of other researchers of public prenatal care in the United States, suggest that while inclusion in the Medicaid rolls may enfranchise enrollees through facilitating access to health care, they may not feel that such inclusion necessarily provides a sense of health equality, insofar as equality means receiving the same care and respect accorded to those with private insurance. More research is needed to elucidate the policies, practices, and institutions that successfully expand health citizenship among individuals and communities, as well as the entrenched practices that reproduce hierarchy and stratification.

Further, while I applaud New York's commitment to provide care to all pregnant women, this prenatal zone of inclusion also has temporal limits. Pregnancy creates a liminal period that temporarily suspends juridical categories that otherwise dictate who is and is not eligible for health coverage. Like virtually all liminal periods (Turner 1969), this inclusion is temporary, lasting only until 60 days after pregnancy. At this point, women and infants are reincorporated into the social body through new or existing categories of stratified health citizenship, including non-citizenship. Low-income women and infants eligible for Medicaid are inscribed into state registers. Higher-income women, whose coverage under Medicaid's elevated threshold for pregnant women may be ending, can sign up for individual health plans, return to employer-based plans, or remain uninsured, although their infants may continue to be eligible for public insurance given higher eligibility thresholds for children. Similarly, the U.S.-citizen infants of undocumented women will be enrolled into children's Medicaid plans. Their undocumented mothers, however, will recede into the background, returning to their previous insurance-ineligible status.

New York State's prenatal health policies thus provide one state-level illustration of a broader national concern, whereby women and children move "in and out of rights," as Jennifer Burrell (2010) has put it in a different context, according to state policies and factors such as gestational status, documentation, income, age, and state residence. Although I can only nod to this important point, the withdrawal of health coverage after the end of pregnancy reveals the state's interest in fostering some lives and rights while ignoring others; previously uninsured women are of state concern only as the producers of citizen-fetuses. Pregnancy is constructed as a state of emergency that requires temporary exemptions to the law, but when no longer pregnant, women lose their ability to make claims on the state for health care except as emergency care or as mothers of citizen-children. Prenatal health care thus underscores the temporal and shifting landscape of health coverage, as well as the stratification of bodies and persons within hierarchies of national and health citizenship. Tracing the repercussions of the uneven treatment of pregnant women across U.S. states, and the way this shapes health care–seeking practices, represents a fruitful avenue for future research on the interplay between (health) citizenship, rights, and deservingness under contemporary health reform.

I wish to end by reiterating that my intention is not to undermine Medicaid or its expansion. Rather, this is a call to consider the ways in which we can support a robust Medicaid program that can provide quality health care and health care experiences to its millions of enrollees. The election of Donald Trump, who campaigned on promises to repeal the ACA, only underscores the urgency of this call. It seems likely that much, if not all, of the federal money that had supported Medicaid expansion under the ACA will disappear. By the 2016 election, the nation's uninsured rate had dropped to its lowest recorded levels; the greatest decreases in rates of uninsured were among poor and near-poor adults who received health coverage through Medicaid expansion (Cohen, Martinez, and Zammitti 2016). While the fate of these newly covered individuals will vary greatly depending on their U.S. state of residence, it is probable that many will return either to uninsured status or to employer-based plans with high deductibles, premiums, and co-pays.

The threat of rollbacks highlights the importance of continued research into health equality and experiences of health citizenship among lower-income people. Even under the ACA, marketplace insurance plans did not always offer the quality health care that the architects of the ACA had imagined. In a 2016 study, the McKinsey Center for U.S. Health Reform found a steady decline in the array of physicians and facilities covered by marketplace insurance plans. Six years after the passage of the ACA, most of the plans available through the marketplaces looked more like Medicaid networks—albeit with high deductibles— than they did employer-based insurance (Sanger-Katz 2016). Faced with health care networks more limited than those available through most employer-based plans, many enrollees in marketplace plans said they felt like "second-class patients"—an experience very familiar to many Medicaid enrollees (Rosenthal 2016).

Such developments should spur further discussion about stratified health citizenship and the crucial role that Medicaid plays in providing health care to millions of people who would otherwise be uninsured or underinsured. As a post–Obama health care era takes shape, we must call on federal, state, and local legislatures to support Medicaid, adequately fund the public health institutions that serve lower-income populations, and incentivize more providers to take Medicaid. In the case of prenatal care, this will ensure not only more provider options and more timely service for pregnant women, but also better working environments for providers in public facilities who, in turn, may be more likely to continue serving these populations. Just as important, we must critically re-think Medicaid delivery and many of the assumptions that structure Medicaid coverage, particularly in prenatal care, to consider how Medicaid can ensure not only inclusion in health care, but also equality of health citizenship. Such reflective and reflexive analysis can contribute both to broader discussions about Medicaid and health citizenship in the United States today, as well as to practical institutional and local policies that can support Medicaid enrollees, providers, and institutions in a changing federal and state landscape. Given the recent fiftieth anniversary of the federal Medicaid program, this is an opportune time to examine the ongoing inequalities of public/private health coverage in the United States.

ACKNOWLEDGMENTS

I am profoundly grateful to the women who generously shared their experiences with me, and to the administrators, doctors, and clinic staff at Beaumont Hospital who made me feel welcome and facilitated my research at the clinic. This research was conducted with the support of a faculty research grant from the University at Albany (SUNY).

NOTES

1   All names of individuals and institutions are pseudonyms.

2   Of Medicaid recipients enrolled after the passage of the ACA, more than 90% were uninsured when they applied. Yet, despite national attention to changes in Medicaid eligibility guidelines, the degree to which changes in eligibility guidelines contributed to growth in enrollments is an open question. Even prior to the ACA, New York State boasted relatively generous Medicaid policies, covering even childless adults up to 100% of the federal poverty level. Indeed, data collected by Governor Cuomo's budget office demonstrate that as of February 2015, 96% of new enrollees would have been eligible for Medicaid even prior to the ACA. Far more important than increased eligibility appears to be the effect of wide-scale outreach and publicity about the program and, crucially, the availability of application counseling through in-person consultation, call centers, and web support. Of all new Marketplace applications in New York, only 22.5% were completed without help from a certified application counselor, a health navigator, a broker, or a call to the Marketplace call center.

3   In 2013, 13.1% of non-Hispanic black women and 8.1% of Hispanic women in New York City received late or no prenatal care as compared to only 3.7% of non-Hispanic white women (New York Department of Health 2013).

REFERENCES

Agrawal, Priya. 2015. *Maternal Mortality and Morbidity in the United States of America.* In Bulletin of the World Health Organization: World Health Organization.

Andaya, Elise. 2013. Conceiving Statistics: The Local Practice and Global Politics of Reproductive Healthcare in Havana. In *Health Travels: Cuban Health (care) On and Off the Island*. Edited by Nancy J. Burke. Berkeley: University of California Press.

———. 2014. *Conceiving Cuba: Reproduction, Women, and the State in the Post-Soviet Era*. New Brunswick, NJ: Rutgers University Press.

Auyero, Javier. 2012. *Patients of the State: The Politics of Waiting in Argentina*. Durham, NC: Duke University Press.

Biehl, João. 2013. *Vita: Life in a Zone of Social Abandonment*. Berkeley: University of California Press.

Bourdieu, Pierre, and Loïc JD Wacquant. 1992. *An Invitation to Reflexive Sociology*. Chicago: University of Chicago Press.

Bourgois, Philippe. 1988. Conjugated Oppression: Class and Ethnicity among Guaymi and Kuna Banana Workers. *American Ethnologist* 15(2): 328–348.

Bridges, Khiara. 2011. *Reproducing Race: An Ethnography of Pregnancy as a Site of Racialization*. Berkeley: University of California Press.

Briggs, Charles L. 2002. *Stories in the Time of Cholera: Racial Profiling during a Medical Nightmare*. Berkeley: University of California Press.

Burrell, Jennifer. 2010. In and Out of Rights: Security, Migration, and Human Rights Talk in Postwar Guatemala. *Journal of Latin American and Caribbean Anthropology* 15(1): 90–115.

Cohen, Robin, Michael Martinez, and Emily Zammitti. 2016. *Health Insurance Coverage: Early Release of Estimates from the National Health Interview Survey, January–March 2016*. Washington, DC: National Center for Health Statistics, U.S. Department of Health and Human Services.

Edin, Kathryn, and Laura Lein. 1997. *Making Ends Meet: How Single Mothers Survive Welfare and Low-Wage Work*. New York: Russell Sage Foundation.

Farmer, Paul. 2001. *Infections and Inequalities: The Modern Plagues*. Berkeley: University of California Press.

Fassin, Didier. 2007. *When Bodies Remember: Experiences and Politics of AIDS in South Africa*. Berkeley: University of California Press.

Fraser, Gertrude. 1995. Modern Bodies, Modern Minds: Midwifery and Reproductive Change in an African American Community. In *Conceiving the New World Order: The Global Politics of Reproduction*. Edited by Faye D. Ginsburg and Rayna Rapp. Berkeley: University of California Press.

Gálvez, Alyshia. 2011. *Patient Citizens, Immigrant Mothers: Mexican Women, Public Prenatal Care, and the Birth Weight Paradox*. New Brunswick, NJ: Rutgers University Press.

Gilens, Martin. 2009. *Why Americans Hate Welfare: Race, Media, and the Politics of Antipoverty Policy*. Chicago: University of Chicago Press.

Ginsburg, Faye, and Rayna Rapp, eds. 1995. *Conceiving the New World Order: The Global Politics of Reproduction*. Berkeley: University of California Press.

Hays, Sharon. 2003. *Flat Broke with Children: Women in the Age of Welfare Reform*. New York: Oxford University Press.

Holmes, Seth. 2013. *Fresh Fruit, Broken Bodies: Migrant Farmworkers in the United States*. Berkeley: University of California Press.

Horton, Sarah. 2004. Different Subjects: The Health Care System's Participation in the Differential Construction of the Cultural Citizenship of Cuban Refugees and Mexican Immigrants. *Medical Anthropology Quarterly* 18(4): 472–489.

Ivry, Tsipy. 2009. *Embodying Culture: Pregnancy in Japan and Israel*. New Brunswick, NJ: Rutgers University Press.

Kaiser Family Foundation (KFF). 2012. Kaiser Health Tracking Poll: July 2012. kff.org.

———. 2016. Total Monthly Medicaid and CHIP Enrollment. State Health Facts. kff.org.

Katz, Michael B. 1990. *The Undeserving Poor: From the War on Poverty to the War on Welfare*. New York: Pantheon Books.

Marrow, Helen B. 2012. Deserving to a Point: Unauthorized Immigrants in San Francisco's Universal Access Healthcare Model. *Social Science & Medicine* 74(6): 846–854.

New York State Department of Health. 2013. *Percent Early and Late or No Prenatal Care, by Race and Resident County, New York State–2013*.

Opdycke, Sandra. 1999. *No One Was Turned Away: The Role of Public Hospitals in New York City since 1900*. New York: Oxford University Press.

Porter, Dorothy. 2011. Health Citizenship: Essays in Social Medicine and Biomedical Politics. Berkeley: University of California Press.

Rosenthal, Elisabeth. 2016. Sorry, We Don't Take Obamacare. *New York Times* (May 15), Sunday Review.

Sanger-Katz, Margot. 2014. Medicaid, Often Criticized, Is Quite Popular with Its Customers. *New York Times* (October 9), The Upshot.

———. 2016. Think Your Obamacare Plan Will Be Like Employer Coverage? Think Again. *New York Times* (August 19).

Turner, Victor. 1969. Liminality and Communitas. In *The Ritual Process: Structure and Anti-structure*. London: Routledge.

Wacquant, Loïc. 2009. *Punishing the Poor: The Neoliberal Government of Social Insecurity*. Durham, NC: Duke University Press.

Willen, Sarah 2012. Migration, "Illegality," and Health: Mapping Embodied Vulnerability and Debating Health-related Deservingness. *Social Science & Medicine* 74(6): 805–811.

Implementation along the Red/Blue Divide

The Affordable Care Act, President Barack Obama's signature legislative achievement, catalyzed a new level of polarization in national politics. The law passed along party lines with the support of a Democratic president but no Republican votes in Congress. The structure of the law—and American federalism more generally—split major responsibilities for health care reform implementation between federal and state governments. As a result, partisan political divisions led to profound geographic differences in the law's implementation. In most "red states," those with Republican-dominated executive and legislative branches, the law was only ever partially implemented. In "blue states," those with Democratic majorities, the law was fully, and often enthusiastically, implemented. Analyzing the law along the "red/blue divide" shows that there are at least "two Americas" that are split ideologically, politically, and demographically. One major cleavage was the division between those who believe in expanded social protections, including for health, and those who do not believe that it is the role of the government to offer or encourage health coverage. As the chapters in this section show, people made sense of these divisions when talking about the ACA by using the language of deservingness, individualism, dependence, and responsibility.

Unlike all other high-income and most middle-income countries, the United States has never made universal health coverage a social right. Instead, health care is delivered and paid for through a complex patchwork of federal and state programs, alongside private outlays like employer-sponsored insurance and out-of-pocket spending. Medicare, a federal entitlement, covers most people who are older than 65 and those who have met the program's criteria for disability. Medicaid is administered through a state/federal partnership with shared funding and administrative responsibilities. States are also responsible for regulating the insurance sold within their borders. This sharing of responsibilities between the national and state governments is usually referred to as *federalism*.

The Affordable Care Act expanded the role of the federal government through the individual and business mandates, new national insurance regulations, and changes to Medicaid. But the law also required a lot of the states: They had to decide whether or not to create an exchange, enforce new insurance regulations, and expand Medicaid (Jones, Bradley, and Oberlander 2014, 98). When the U.S. Supreme Court decided in 2012 to make the Medicaid expansion to working adults below 138 percent of the federal poverty level optional, states gained even more leverage over implementation. Predictably, many red states refused to expand Medicaid—though more ended up expanding every year, following public pressure and after the financial benefits became obvious. Many red states also enacted policies that obstructed ACA implementa-

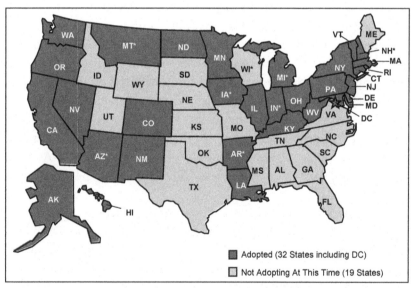

Figure S2.1. Kaiser State Medicaid Expansion Decisions Map
Current status for each state is based on KCMU tracking and analysis of state executive activity. *AR, AZ, IA, IN, MI, MT, and NH have approved Section 1115 waivers. WI covers adults up to 100% FPL in Medicaid, but did not adopt the ACA expansion. Source: "Status of State Action on the Medicaid Expansion Decision," KFF State Health Facts, updated January 1, 2017; kff.org.

tion, such as imposing strict requirements on enrollment assisters and by suing the federal government. As the chapters in this section detail, the "coverage gap" that was created by the decision not to expand Medicaid left many poor adults with no viable option for insurance, despite the passage of the law. Red states were also home to vibrant opposition movements that called for repealing and replacing the law. The partisan rancor over the ACA can be difficult to puzzle through because it does not align with simple ideological differences between the parties. Exchanges—the regulated marketplaces that sell private insurance plans—seem like an idea that Republicans would embrace, as evidenced by past Republican support for exchange-like initiatives. These are based in market principles of competition and choice, and the federalist structure of the law provides leeway for states to develop their own exchanges, rather than commit to a one-size-fits-all approach. Democrats liked that exchanges made a push toward universal coverage, regulated insurance plans, and provided financial assistance for low-income people. Though exchanges were supposed to have been a bipartisan policy compromise, there was widespread Republican opposition to them and this opposition actually increased over time, rather than subsiding (Jones et al. 2014).

There were also many compelling reasons for red states to accept Medicaid expansion. First, Medicaid improves health, particularly for the most economically vulnerable and those in worse health status. Second, the uninsured have serious access issues that emergency care alone cannot remedy. Finally, Medicaid expansion would have brought federal dollars into state coffers. States would spend far less on the expansion than they received in federal funds; thus, expansion clearly represented a net benefit to state economies (Frakt and Carroll 2013).

But rather than embracing exchanges and Medicaid expansion, many red states adamantly refused to cooperate with ACA implementation. This produced several acute ironies. For instance, red states, which typically favored greater state's rights, defaulted to the federal exchange Healthcare.gov, thus effectively increasing the role of the federal government. Blue states enthusiastically embraced health reform, even when they did not have nearly as many uninsured people to begin with. The states that needed health reform the most—who have the largest numbers of uninsured—were the most against it. Texas, Florida, and Georgia

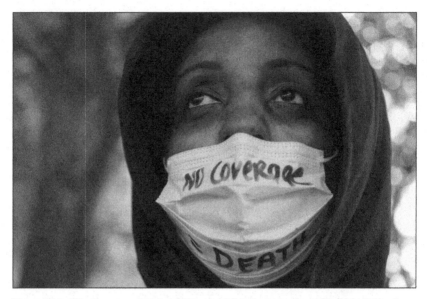

Figure S2.2. "No Coverage = Death." Kamalah Fletcher wears a medical mask over her face saying "No Coverage = Death" during a protest in support of Florida lawmakers expanding the eligibility criteria for Medicaid as called for under the Affordable Care Act, Thursday, January 8, 2015, in Miami. The Supreme Court ruled in 2012 that Medicaid expansion is an optional part of the Affordable Care Act. (AP photo/Lynne Sladky)

topped the list of states with the highest uninsurance rates (KFF 2016). After health reform, the red/blue divide mattered more, not less.

In order to understand the red/blue divide, the chapters in this section, as in the previous section, argue that we must pay attention to how the ACA intersected with existing inequalities and created new ones. Most prominently, racial politics and class cleavages mattered acutely in ACA implementation. As Mulligan argues in her chapter, the subtext to political debates about the ACA was "dog whistle politics" and resentment (Haney López 2014; Morone 2016). Red state politicians followed a well-worn pattern in American politics of manipulating white resentment and opposing a social program that, if fully implemented, would have led to greater racial and social equality. Mulligan shows how residents of Florida (a red state) and Rhode Island (a blue state) navigated coverage decisions on insurance exchanges and how some made sense of their exclusion from coverage through the prism of resentment. Scred vividly documents that frequent changes to insurance status are the rule, not the exception, for working-class people in the United States. She illustrates geographic differences in the experience of being uninsured across five states, arguing that the 2012 Supreme Court decision on Medicaid exacerbated "geographically-driven gaps between the healthcare 'haves' and 'have nots.'" Brunson begins her chapter with a quote from a Texas health administrator claiming: "*People in Texas are uninsured because they want to be. Texans don't want health insurance.*" Brunson contextualizes this statement within Texas's red state political climate and then illustrates how social class differences have come to matter even more among the uninsured in the state as the poorest fall into the coverage gap.

REFERENCES

Frakt, Austin B., and Aaron E. Carroll. 2013. Sound Policy Trumps Politics: States Should Expand Medicaid. *Journal of Health Politics, Policy and Law* 38(1): 165–178.

Haney López, Ian. 2014. *Dog Whistle Politics: How Coded Racial Appeals Have Reinvented Racism and Wrecked the Middle Class.* New York: Oxford University Press.

Jones, David K., Katharine W. V. Bradley, and Jonathan Oberlander. 2014. Pascal's Wager: Health Insurance Exchanges, Obamacare, and the Republican Dilemma. *Journal of Health Politics, Policy and Law* 39(1): 97–137.

KFF (Kaiser Family Foundation). 2016. State Health Facts. kff.org.

Morone, James A. 2016. Partisanship, Dysfunction, and Racial Fears: The New Normal in Health Care Policy? *Journal of Health Politics, Policy and Law* 41(4): 827–846.

5

Segmented Risks

Eligibility and Resentment on Insurance Exchanges

JESSICA M. MULLIGAN

A young white man in his early twenties struggled to get his wife's wheelchair out of the trunk. He urged his two kids to hurry up. The Florida sun pierced through low-flying clouds. Cicadas hummed loudly. The man wore jeans, sweat dampened his T-shirt, and his face flushed under a straw hat. Once his wife was finally situated in the wheelchair, he looked up, scrunched his eyes at us and shouted:

"What are you guys doing? Are you with that Obamacare? Are you Obama?"

The comment was directed at two white researchers sitting under a tent at a folding table in front of a community health center. It was June 2014, a few months after the first open enrollment season for obtaining health coverage on the newly created Affordable Care Act (ACA) insurance exchanges. It was mid-morning, hot, and most people who saw us nodded, but kept their distance. Some were polite and warned that it was going to rain. Our sign raised concern even if it was a little opaque. It read, "Volunteers Wanted for a Research Study. Expanding Access to Care: Insurance Exchanges and the Impact of Health Reform."

Our contact at the health center vetoed an earlier version of the sign because it said Obamacare. Better not to mention Obama, she advised us. The health center was the home of enrollment efforts in this rural county. It housed the only navigators around, trained and state-certified enrollment assisters who could help people pick out an insurance plan and access federal tax credits. But the navigators scrupulously avoided any mention of Obama.

The man who rushed past us, late to his wife's appointment, got the message though: "Obama can stick it up his ass," he said.

* * *

This is not the reaction that framers of the Affordable Care Act were hoping for. Ironically, this man is exactly who the law was supposed to help: an uninsured, low-income, part-time worker.

After the family was inside, his wife checked in, and he had cooled off in the air-conditioned waiting room, he came back out and chatted with us. With the stress of getting to the appointment on time subsiding, he was animated and friendly. He explained that his wife was on Medicare for disability, but he was uninsured. He worked two fast food jobs part time to support the family. One offered coverage, but it was too expensive and covered too little. The family's income was low enough that he would have qualified for Medicaid in a state that had opted to expand the program to low-income adults. But since he lived in Florida, he fell into the coverage gap. He had checked out his options with a navigator, but the plans were just too expensive. He was adamant that Obamacare was not for him. He did not blame the state legislature, the governor, or the Republican strategists who decided not to expand Medicaid to millions. He blamed Obama.

Race and more particularly what legal scholar Ian Haney López (2014) has called "dog whistle politics" undoubtedly shaped this white southern man's understanding of whether or not the new health care law was for him. Dog whistle politics refers to "coded racial appeals that carefully manipulate hostility toward nonwhites" (ix). Like a dog whistle, this mode of communication can be imperceptible to some audiences. When the Speaker of the House Paul Ryan characterizes the ACA as a program for "takers," or Florida governor Rick Scott invokes states' rights as a reason to reject Medicaid expansion, they dog whistle. This coded rhetoric, that does not seem to be overtly about race, mobilizes white racial fears to reject social programs that are perceived as benefiting minorities.[1] Without a concept like dog whistling, it is difficult to understand how a law that so closely resembled Republican health reform proposals from the previous two decades would elicit feelings strong enough to cuss at strangers. The visceral rejection of

Obamacare only makes sense when contextualized within the racial politics of the United States (Hughey and Parks 2014; Morone 2016).

But it wasn't just white folks who let us know that the law left them out. Later that day an uninsured African American woman named Mary with multiple health bills that she couldn't afford to pay explained to us: "Obamacare is for people with money and that's not me." She too worked in the fast food industry and had looked at her options on the exchange, but because her income was very low, she did not qualify for help purchasing coverage and she fell into the gap. Had Mary's income been a little bit higher, or had money been no issue, then she would have been able to purchase a plan on the exchange. So for her, this program that was supposed to help low-income Americans buy coverage was seen as being just for rich people. Her only hope for getting needed care was to qualify for disability.

A couple of months later in Rhode Island, a white woman named Erica who enrolled in a marketplace plan (discussed further below) explained that she almost didn't go down to the enrollment office to find out what was available even though she was uninsured and has a chronic medical condition that requires regular doctor visits. She too assumed the law wasn't for her, because in this case, she thought that it was just for low-income people, a label she didn't identify with. She had a college degree and was getting back on her feet after a period of being unemployed. She thought the ACA only provided help for the poor, a category in which she did not place herself.

These stories of non-belonging point to the ways in which Obamacare was experienced in highly stratified ways. The program had very different meanings and impacts for differently situated individuals and families. In this chapter, I argue that these differences derived from three overlapping sources: (1) the contradictions of using means-tested, actuarially rated programs to increase insurance coverage rather than universal access; (2) the move by Republican-dominated states not to expand Medicaid and therefore deprive millions of access to insurance and medical care; and (3) racial politics that structure how many white people made sense of the law. I will draw on the concepts of dog whistle politics and white resentment to argue that repeated attempts to repeal and disrupt the implementation of the law must be understood as part of a long history in the United States of strategic opposition to programs that are perceived as benefiting communities of color (Haney López 2014). Though these sources of different experiences seem quite distinct from one another, they actually overlap considerably. By making the provision of help to pay for coverage income dependent and using certain actuarial categories (age, geography, smoking status, and family size) to price coverage, while explicitly prohibiting others (preexisting conditions and gender), designers of the law guaranteed that experiences of the ACA would vary tremendously depending on one's personal circumstances. This highly technical eligibility grid is usually not well understood by people applying for coverage. And so, they utilize other, more familiar frameworks for making sense of who does and does not benefit from the law: dog whistle politics and resentment. Republican lawmakers who have opposed the implementation of the law and the expansion of Medicaid have very skillfully deflected blame for the law's shortcomings onto the Obama administration and away from state policymakers who have obstructed its implementation.

This chapter examines how a program that was supposed to lessen inequality tapped into deep concerns with social stratification and even created new forms of inequality in its implementation. The question "is this for me?" is ultimately about belonging and inclusion in a social program that aimed to dramatically expand access to health insurance in the United States.[2]

Methods

The ethnographic stories in this chapter come from fieldwork conducted from 2013 to 2016. Beginning with the first open enrollment period for the Affordable Care Act, I carried out interviews and observations with residents of Florida and Rhode Island who gained access to insurance coverage through the law or who remained uninsured (I have conducted 80 interviews and observed more than 185 enrollment interactions). In Rhode Island, I sat in on enrollment interactions at the state-run insurance exchange and community-based enrollment events. I used these observations as an opportunity to recruit interview participants who I then contacted several months after the initial observation. In Florida, the methods differed largely because there is no state-based exchange and therefore no comparable customer service center to observe. Instead, with the help of two colleagues, we collaborated with a community health center in a rural county in central Florida. The health center was the main site for enrollments through the navigator program. There, we set up a table outside the health center (as described above) to recruit newly insured and uninsured residents for interviews about their experiences trying to access coverage. Interviews were open-ended and focused on family background, work and education history, insurance coverage, and health status. Field notes and interviews were transcribed and subjected to thematic analysis.

Florida and Rhode Island provide useful contrasting case studies because the approaches that state governments took to implement the ACA were so different. Florida opposed implementation of the law, promulgated policies that make it difficult for navigators to assist with enrollments, and refused to expand Medicaid coverage to poor adults. Rhode Island was an enthusiastic implementer of the law, creating its own state-based insurance exchange, expanding Medicaid, and fostering opportunities for all kinds of people to assist with enrollments.

In this chapter, I draw on a small selection of interviews from Florida and Rhode Island where people explained the ways in which health reform did or did not benefit them. The first two stories focus on means testing and actuarial categories for people who were eligible to purchase coverage on the exchange. The third story recounts the experience of someone who fell into the Medicaid coverage gap in Florida. I start with means testing and actuarial categories because these are the criteria that determine eligibility. For people who are eligible for coverage and experience it as affordable, resentment and dog whistling did not come up in the interview. But for people whose location on the eligibility and actuarial grid placed coverage out of reach, like the young man whose story opened this chapter, blame and resentment colored their stories of seeking out coverage.

Means Testing, Actuarial Categories, and Belonging

The president repeatedly told the public that "if you like your coverage, you can keep it. Nothing will change." So for the more than 80% of people who had insurance coverage when the law was passed, they were advised that the law was not for them. The ACA coverage expansions were targeted at those who were formerly priced out of insurance or excluded because of pre-existing conditions. However, policy choices made in the design and implementation of the ACA ensured that there was no one unified experience of the program.

In addition to statutory eligibility criteria,[3] the ACA distributed access to coverage through two important components of its design: (1) means testing for access to subsidies and (2) actuarial variables of age, family size, smoking status, and geography that set the price for coverage. Means testing and pricing by actuarial variables ensured that, even for those who were eligible for coverage, experiences of the law varied dramatically according to income, age, and place of residence. The result was a complex and difficult to understand eligibility infrastructure, enhanced monitoring and surveillance of individuals and families,[4] and problems mobilizing a broad base of support for the law.

Collecting data that located individuals and families on eligibility and pricing grids formed the scaffolding of the electronic system known as the exchange. Accurately determining eligibility and pricing was the major purpose of the electronic application. One of the first questions in applying for coverage was: Do you already have access to insurance? If so, and if it was deemed "affordable" by official definitions, then you were not eligible to receive help buying coverage on the exchange. Other questions that applicants must answer were about place of residence, family size, whether they were incarcerated, income, and employment.

Initial evidence from the first two years of enrollment suggested that qualifying for subsidies was essential to making coverage attractive: One study found that on the federal marketplace only 2% of eligible individuals over 400% of poverty ($46,680) bought on the exchange (Andrews 2015). Individuals and families were eligible for Medicaid if their income fell below 133% of the federal poverty line, they were in an eligible immigration status, and they resided in an expanding state. Those between 100% and 400% of poverty qualified for premium assistance in the form of a tax credit that gradually phased out as income increased. Between 100% and 250% of poverty cost-sharing assistance was also available (to reduce out-of-pocket spending at the point of service in the form of deductibles, co-insurance, co-pays, etc.). This eligibility and means testing grid was very difficult to understand, and what it actually meant in

TABLE 5.1. Eligibility Grid

Premium Subsidies, by Income, in 2014 and 2015

Income % Poverty	Income Range for the 2014 Benefit Year ($)		Income Range for the 2015 Benefit Year ($)	
	Single Individual	Family of Four	Single Individual	Family of Four
Under 100	Less than 11,490	Less than 23,550	Less than 11,670	Less than 23,850
100–133	11,490–15,282	23,550–31,322	11,670–15,521	23,850–31,721
133–150	15,282–17,235	31,322–35,325	15,521–17,505	31,721–35,775
15–200	17,235–22,980	35,325–47,100	17,505–23,340	35,775–47,700
200–250	22,980–28,725	47,100–58,875	23,340–29,175	47,700–59,625
250–300	28,725–34,470	58,875–70,650	29,175–35,010	59,625–71,550
300–400	34,470–45,960	70,650–94,200	35,010–46,680	71,550–95,400
Over 400	More than 45,960	More than 94,200	More than 46,680	More than 95,400

Source: Kaiser Family Foundation, Kff.org
Alaska and Hawaii have different poverty guidelines. Note that tax credits for the 2015 benefit year are
calculated using 2014 federal poverty guidelines, while tax credits for the 2014 benefit year are calculated using
2013 federal poverty guidelines.

terms of coverage and price depended on income, family size, and the plan under consideration.

Means testing has long been controversial in the design of public programs. In poverty relief programs that are stigmatized, means testing is often used to sort the "deserving" from the "non-deserving" poor (Katz 2008). When means testing exists, bureaucratic processes must be applied to sort eligible from non-eligible applicants, and eligibility must be periodically reassessed. Income-based eligibility standards also introduce technical problems with the way income is calculated[5] and contributes to "churn," wherein changes in eligibility status mean moving in and out of public programs, which can disrupt continuity of services and coverage. For people receiving ACA tax credits to make their insurance premiums more affordable, the credits were based on estimates of how much one expected to make in a year. If an individual or family made more or less than the estimate, they may have had to pay back subsidies they were not eligible for or may have received additional tax refunds. In an era of extreme unstable employment, flexible work schedules, and underemployment, this way of administering help for paying for insurance was administratively challenging. Furthermore, the negative impacts of income-based tax credits (churning between coverage types, owing additional money at tax time, and the stress and uncertainty of making an estimate for the upcoming year) were disproportionately experienced by low-wage workers and those in poverty. Higher-income workers were unlikely to receive subsidies and hence were shielded from the tax impacts of the law. Means testing often leads to stigmatization as certain programs are identified with being poor. In the stories below, we see how beneficiaries talked about and navigated this stigma. Despite all of these drawbacks, means testing is often favored by policymakers as a way to limit public spending to those truly unable to pay, or to populations considered more "deserving" (Katz 2008; Goode 2002).

The other major grid for mapping how the law was understood so differently by differently situated individuals is to look at the actuarial variables through which rates were set. By actuarial variables, I mean the categories that insurance actuaries were statutorily permitted to use to estimate risk and set the price of coverage for plans offered on ACA insurance exchanges. Individuals buying on the exchange received different prices for their insurance plans depending on these actuarial variables. The law mandated that only four variables could be used, which was generally understood as being beneficial to women and people with preexisting conditions, since before the ACA both of these variables were also used in rate-setting. The four allowed actuarial variables were:

- Age 3:1 bands. Younger people paid less in most states, but the largest ratio or band by which the rates could differ was 3:1. In other words, the oldest person could not pay more than 3 times what the youngest person paid.
- Geography. Rates were allowed to vary geographically in recognition of differing costs of doing business in different geographical areas.
- Tobacco use 1.5:1. Smokers could pay up to 50% more for a plan than non-smokers.
- Individual or Family. Family size was also used to calculate rates.

Together, eligibility criteria, means testing, and actuarial variables formed the largely invisible official grid for recognizing and processing differences on the insurance exchange. But how did individuals and families make sense of and move through this official grid? I turn to two examples from my fieldwork to illustrate how people actually navigated enrollment bureaucracies and how they talked about whether or not the law was "for them."

Passing the Means Test: Wendy and Mike (FL)

Wendy (45) and Mike (52) lived in a doublewide trailer near the Gulf of Mexico on land inherited from Wendy's dad. The living room was under construction; there was only subfloor and the ceiling was covered in plastic drop cloth. We sat at a small table pushed up against a wall in the already renovated kitchen, where the tile, stainless steel appliances, and cabinets were all new. "You wouldn't believe this place when we got here," Mike said. "It was a total mess, but we're bringing it back."

Mike worked in HVAC (Heating, Ventilation, and Air Conditioning) and even installed some of the cooling systems at the Cape Canaveral NASA launch complex when he was younger. He had learned the hard way about the value of insurance. He got cancer at age 29, after having turned down his employer's insurance thinking he would never get sick. Emergency Medicaid covered most of the cancer treatment, but he required regular testing and medication as a result of his illness.

As someone with a skilled trade, his jobs usually offered coverage, but he was currently working as an independent contractor. He was pretty sure that he had lost a few jobs as a result of his medical needs. He usually worked for very small companies and the addition of one person who used a lot of medical services could quickly push the premiums up for everyone.

Wendy worked waitressing and cleaning jobs and has spent most of her life uninsured. They had been together for 15 years, but Wendy and Mike had only recently gotten married. Wendy had not been eligible to join the plans that Mike had received from his employers.

Mike said he did his homework when it was time to sign up for Obamacare coverage. He had qualified for disability due to a work-related injury, but decided not to take Medicare. The plan he could get on the exchange was better and that way Wendy would be covered too. After the tax credits they received, the premium for two people was

$2.77 a month with very limited cost sharing.[6] Mike and Wendy quali-
fied for a plan with significant subsidies because their income fell in the
sweet spot of just over 100% of the poverty level; had it been much lower,
they might not have qualified for any help on the exchange. And since
they lived in Florida—a non-Medicaid-expanding state—Wendy would
still be uninsured.

Though it was affordable, their coverage was not without challenges.
When we first met Wendy and Mike, they were at the community health
center trying to get referrals authorized. Mike was surprised when he
learned that the most affordable plan on the exchange also had a very
limited network. He couldn't go to any doctor who accepted his insurance carrier; he had to access primary care at the Community Health
Center and the insurance company had to authorize referrals for specialty care. "I didn't mean to sign up for a Medicaid plan that you get
at a clinic," he told us. We talked about all the bad things being said
about Obamacare on cable news and Mike said he was skeptical of
how the press was talking about the law. But, he was also sensitive to
how their plan made them different from other people who have insurance through his carrier, Humana.

Wendy and Mike's understanding that Obamacare "benefitted them"
was largely a product of the means testing variables that determined
their eligibility for tax subsidies and cost-sharing reductions. They
were middle-aged, which means that their premiums were higher, but
their income was so close to 100% of poverty that they were eligible
for help that covered almost the entire cost of their coverage. Mike
considered himself to be highly educated about insurance. And when
it came to price, he was. But he also had to make a decision with very
incomplete information. He had tried to get help from the customer
service line, but spoke to someone in a different state who couldn't give
him information that was informed by his local health care landscape
and insurance options. He didn't initially realize that this means-tested
program would give him access to insurance that was slightly different than what he had used previously with employer-based coverage.
There were more rules that restricted utilization, a very limited network, and, as he pointed out on his card, it clearly said Humana-HMO.
While most doctors accepted Humana in his area, they did not want

the HMO plan; once a receptionist told him that the doctor would not take Obamacare, thereby clearly marking his form of insurance as separate from other plans.

Some scholars have discussed insurance as a technology that obliges people to calculate their risks and engage in responsible decision-making to meet their household needs (Baker and Simon 2002). And though Mike did attempt to responsibly calculate the costs of his different coverage options (Medicare versus the ACA exchange plan), his primary concern was familial, not financial. Wendy and Mike are interesting because, for them, getting covered was a way of caring for one another, particularly in light of previous illness experiences and their coverage histories; Mike did not sign up for Medicare thinking it would leave Wendy uncovered. He was very worried about her health, as years of being uninsured had taken their toll. For them, insurance was especially important because they had been turned away from care before. "Even at the hospital?" I asked because in the U.S. hospitals are supposed to stabilize anyone who comes in with an emergency.

Wendy explained a recent incident: "I'd been coughing a lot and went to the hospital and they didn't do anything. They said it was fine; it was from smoking."

Mike added, "as long as your heart is good and your pulse is good, they tell you to go see a doctor."

Wendy said, "They didn't explain anything to me about why I can't breathe! There is something going on. 'You're not dying—see you later,' more or less. They didn't even look at me. They put me in the back and then escorted me out the door and told me I'm fine. I will never go there again. I was really mad. I was so mad."

I asked, "Do you think they did that because you don't have insurance?"

Wendy answered, "I know they did that because I don't have no insurance. They wouldn't even prescribe me an antibiotic. I got an antibiotic [given to her by her daughter] and it helped. It took it away."

* * *

Their experiences being sick and uninsured, together with the lack of treatment at local emergency departments, made getting covered particularly appealing to Wendy and Mike.

Wendy and Mike also cared for one another in how they used their new coverage; they accompanied one another on multiple trips to the community health center to get their authorizations processed. For Wendy and Mike, the new insurance bureaucracies created to administer Obamacare at times exhibited the callousness that is common in bureaucracies charged with aiding the poor (Gupta 2012; Lipsky 1984). But other times, Wendy and Mike expressed relief and were grateful that health reform had passed; they understood that there might be bumps in the road during the first year of implementation.

Overall, Mike and Wendy benefited from the means testing criteria used in the Affordable Care Act (though they were not fully aware of how good a deal they got based on their location on the eligibility-actuarial grid). They were, however, aware that they were on a plan that was different and marked because of its association with Obama. Next I'll turn to another interviewee who navigated the enrollment process (with help) and got connected to coverage that she was satisfied with. She too benefited from her location on the means testing and actuarial grid, even though she perceived herself as being high income and non-poor.

Insurance for a Flexible Economy: Erica (RI)

When we spoke at a café in the upscale shopping center, Erica was 39 and just starting a new job. Growing up, her father owned a jewelry factory, which was then an important industry in Rhode Island. Erica studied jewelry design at the Rhode Island School of Design (RISD) and worked in the industry for about a decade. During that time, jewelry manufacturing largely moved off-shore, with U.S.-based personnel responsible for the design work. Erica's career was repeatedly thrown off course by globalization; she had to navigate a rapidly changing economy that included the erosion of the manufacturing base in Rhode Island, increasing job insecurity, the rise of contract and temporary work, and the disappearance of benefits.

Eventually Erica tired of the insecurities in jewelry manufacturing and wanted a change, so she followed her cousin's lead and decided to become a pharmaceutical rep. She lamented that she made the jump a bit late; the glory days of lavish parties and golf outings were over. At the time she made her move, there were fewer blockbuster drugs and more regulations. She also worked for a subcontractor, not the actual manufacturer. It's a way to get out of offering health care and other benefits to employees, she explained.

Erica had a preexisting condition. She was diagnosed with thyroid cancer at 19, and needed regular medical care, checkups, and maintenance medication. This experience made her savvy about insurance, even turning down a job she really wanted once because the health benefits were so poor.

She was very happy with the Blue Cross plan she bought on the exchange in Rhode Island—it was affordable at $70 a month in premiums (including dental) with a $250 deductible. In fact, she wanted to keep it even if her new employer offered a plan. She was pleasantly surprised, considering she almost didn't try to sign up for coverage on the exchange; she only tried after hearing about it from a neighbor, because she originally thought it was only for low-income people, not people like her.

Erica had a college degree and experience in health care. Nonetheless, she did not feel comfortable choosing an insurance plan online. She went to the contact center in Providence for in-person assistance and talked through the various plan options with her enrollment assister. I observed multiple individuals in this situation—they met the educational profile of someone who should have been able to do their shopping alone online, but they simply were not comfortable making such a big decision in isolation.

Irregular jobs and working on commission also made it difficult for her to predict her income for 2014. She received a large tax credit, but took the risk of having to pay part of her subsidy back if her income increased substantially (and she hoped that it would). For most people with unstable or seasonal employment, multiple part-time jobs, or who work on commission, the income portion of the application is very difficult to complete. Small changes in income make big and often counterintuitive differences. For example, if Wendy and Mike made much less, they would not have qualified for any help in Florida; instead, they would fall into the coverage gap. Although Erica was happy with her plan and the eligibility and actuarial calculus worked out for her, she was still not convinced that this was a program for people like her.

She always assumed that she would have a job that offered coverage, but in her career, that kind of stability was elusive.

The big factors that structured belonging for Wendy, Mike, and Erica were eligibility criteria and actuarial pricing. Mike and Erica were able to afford coverage because insurance plans were no longer able to exclude those with preexisting conditions. Wendy was able to qualify because together with Mike, their income was just high enough to get them over the 100% of poverty line (an arbitrary and largely accidental determinant of who can sign up for coverage in non–Medicaid expanding states like Florida). They all felt that the program had some stigma they were ambivalent about but were willing to work through given how much they valued insurance.

For other people who I spoke to—like the man in the parking lot described at the start of the chapter—their sense of whether Obamacare was "for them" can only be understood by looking at how racial politics and white resentment have transformed social welfare programs and attitudes about government in the United States. Importantly, the people who most relied on dog whistling or resentment politics when explaining why the law was not for them were also the people whose location on the eligibility and actuarial grid priced them out of coverage.

The Coverage Gap and Dog Whistling

National policy debates about the Affordable Care Act were racialized well before the Supreme Court's 2012 decision that the individual mandate was constitutional and the Medicaid expansion was optional. The widespread othering of Obama by Tea Party and conservative activists so that he appeared as a threat to white Americans is one register in which racialization occurred (Enck-Wanzer 2011). The coining of the term "Obamacare" was likewise an act of racialization; Ian Haney López argues that this term exemplifies how dog whistle politics currently work in the United States. On the surface, the term "Obamacare" doesn't seem to be overtly racial, but subliminally it evokes racial reactions: "here comes a black man to get government involved raising taxes on you in order to fund even more giveaways to minorities" (2014, 206). Political scientists have also shown by using nationally representative poll data that during the Obama presidency, racial attitudes such as resentment and ethnocentrism became more strongly associated with opposition to health reform (Maxwell and Shields 2014; see also Tesler 2012).

But the area that has been the most racially charged and has had the most profound negative consequences for the well-being and life chances of the poor has been the decision by Republican-dominated states not to expand Medicaid. This decision must be seen as part of a longer history of welfare programs that devolved decisions about funding and coverage to the states in recognition of racial politics. For example, when domestic and agricultural workers who were disproportionately people of color were excluded from Social Security, minimum wage legislation, and workers' compensation programs in the 1930s, this was explicitly a trade-off to gain political support from Southern politicians (Katznelson 2005). The decisions of state leaders not to expand Medicaid has followed this well-worn pattern in American racial politics: Oppose the expansion of programs that would benefit the poor and minorities, but do so in the language of state's rights and limited government (Brown-Nagin 2014; Hughey and Parks 2014).[7] It is no coincidence that 91% of people who fall into the coverage gap live in the South (Garfield and Damico 2016). Avoiding any explicit mention of race while promulgating policies with racially disparate impacts is the definition of dog whistle politics (Haney López 2014).

A further consequence of non-expansion is that whites, who would have been helped by the law if they lived in an expanding state, instead see their continued lack of coverage as evidence that the law is a bad one. It also generates resentment and the perception that "others," i.e., people of color and women, are benefiting from the law, as we will see in Kenny's narrative below.

Resentment in the Coverage Gap: Kenny (FL)

Kenny rented a townhouse in a gated community outside Tampa where the orange tree groves were being turned under to build more tract homes. As we entered the house, Kenny pointed out a contraption of sticks and cardboard, duct taped to the bottom of the screen door to keep out snakes.

I met Kenny and his wife at a Community Health Center where they were trying to find a doctor. They had recently moved back to Florida after living in Virginia for a decade Kenny was a veteran in his early forties who described himself as 10% disabled. He had mostly worked in sales: cars, real estate, and medical equipment and sometimes he slipped into his sales voice while he spoke.

The first question he asked before we even sat down at the kitchen table was: "Are you-all Democrats? You're not trying to enroll me in one of those Obamacare plans are you? He's the worst president ever." Kenny also said he understood that Obamacare made sense for black people—"I am a statistics guy. I know for a fact that 60% of them have HIV. So then, yeah that plan would make sense."

Kenny was fired from his most recent job. "I was fired on March 28 and the Obamacare deadline was March 31, you figure it out." He left work on a Friday with his boss trying to find out about insurance plans for him, and on Monday, he was fired. "The current healthcare.gov mandate is what's killing jobs. I'm not preaching off of the news, I lived it first-hand."

Kenny clearly made sense of Obamacare through the prism of the politics of resentment: He wasn't angry with the boss who fired him, or about the erosion of opportunities for guys with a high school diploma, or at Wall Street for the real estate bust; he was mad at Obama.

But, importantly, resentment doesn't tell the whole story. Despite Kenny's ideological opposition to the law, he did try to buy coverage for his family. In Virginia, he was eligible for "rebates," but the premiums were still $350 a month with a $6,000 deductible. He concluded that Healthcare.gov plans are junk; there wasn't anything worth paying for. Kenny was angry, but he also could not afford a plan on the exchange and had no good alternatives. When he lost his job and moved to Florida, his income fell below 100% of poverty and so he fell through the coverage gap created by the Supreme Court decision in 2012 that made the Medicaid expansion optional.

Kenny has a daughter, which made it extra stressful to be uninsured. He explained, "Kids seem to get sicker. When she got sick, I googled for an answer. And thank God for everything that it worked out. . . . I'm just praying that I get a good job that comes with insurance soon." In this example, Kenny would have signed up for a plan in an act of caring for his family even if it was Obamacare. But when the eligibility and actuarial calculus did not work in his favor, he was quick to blame the president and use a racial frame to make sense of how he was losing out.

Letting Die

Writing of the failure of the Indian government to eradicate poverty, Akhil Gupta argues that extreme poverty should be theorized as a "direct and culpable form of killing" (2012, 5). Advocates of Medicaid expansion have likewise argued that the refusal to expand Medicaid is a direct and culpable form of killing. One estimate puts the number of avoidable deaths that can be attributed to opting out of Medicaid expansion somewhere between 7,115 and 17,104 (Dickman et al. 2014).

Take the case of Amy. She was a 42-year-old uninsured white woman with COPD, who I interviewed in Florida. She could not afford the inhaler she needed to regulate her breathing. Instead of regularly using this $300 a month inhaler, she decompensated, had episodes where she could not breathe and her boyfriend had to call an ambulance. "When they put the breathing mask on me," Amy explained, "I always feel like I'm being strangled or choked. I'm terrified of that mask." Amy had co-occurring mental health issues and a personal history of abuse and trauma that all contributed to the panic attacks. These attacks and the unmanaged COPD that was shortening her life are the outcome of dog whistle policies that refuse to expand medical coverage to poor adults. Amy is a non-Hispanic white, a group that made up 46% of those in the coverage gap nationally, while 49% of adults who fell into the gap were black or Hispanic (Garfield and Damico 2016).

The upshot of dog whistle politics—in addition to perpetuating racism—is that anti-government language provides a neutral sounding cover for a decision that has brutal, deadly consequences. The refusal to expand Medicaid shortens the lives of the poorest adults in the state, and this impact was disproportionately experienced by people of color. Seduced by anti-government rhetoric, white people like Kenny advocated for their own exclusion from health care. And now, with a Trump presidency, the 20 million people who gained access to coverage under the Affordable Care Act may very well lose that coverage.

Conclusion

The Affordable Care Act provoked stark partisan attacks and just as adamant defenses. Despite the way the political lines were drawn, it's actually quite difficult to classify the law ideologically. One reason for this ideological confusion is that the law amalgamated a commitment to expanding access to care (historically, a liberal goal) with conservative commitments to a privatized insurance system that preserved the economic status of physicians, hospitals, insurance companies, and pharmaceutical manufacturers. The law mandated that individuals purchase private coverage on a market, but with income-dependent subsidies and coverage virtually for free for those below 138% of poverty in a state that has opted to expand Medicaid. Behind the scenes, various financial instruments spread out (i.e., socialize) risk, for example, high-risk corridors, re-insurance, and risk-based payments (Goodell 2014).

In a 2011 article in the *University of Pennsylvania Law Review*, insurance scholar Tom Baker argued that health care in the United Sates "is on track to become a form of social insurance" (1579). By social insurance, he meant that it was "compulsory, easily available, and the price must bear some relation to the ability to pay" (1579). He went so far as to say that the Affordable Care Act "embodies a new social contract of health care solidarity through private ownership, markets, choice, and individual responsibility, with government as the insurer for the elderly and the poor" (1577).

It's hard to square Baker's vision of how the ACA was likely to work with the raucous polemic surrounding its implementation. There have been dozens of votes in Congress to repeal the law (Pear 2015). President Obama was routinely called a socialist during his time in office. How can that represent a new social contract? To be fair, Baker could not anticipate that the Supreme Court in 2012 would make the Medicaid expansion optional, thereby ensuring that millions of the most needy in many of the states with the highest rates of uninsurance would fall into newly created coverage gaps. Nonetheless, I find the suggestion that the ACA is essentially a social insurance program deeply problematic. Certainly the ACA came closer to universal access than we had ever been and used various levers to bring people into coverage. But, this means-tested program was experienced in very unequal terms by differently situated individuals.

One of the most important forces working against the legacy of Obamacare as social insurance is that there was no shared sense of the social created through the law. Instead, for many the law was viewed through the prism of the politics of resentment. In her work on the politics of resentment, Marlia Banning explains, "backlashes against feminism and civil and racial rights direct attention away from root, material causes of anxiety and distress and toward others construed as advantaged, as getting something for nothing." Within this political structure of feeling, experiences like losing one's income can "fuel shame, anger, and resentment" (Banning 2006, 83). If dog whistling is useful for making sense of political discourses that deny access to coverage in the putative name of smaller government, resentment gets at the more intimate ways that people make sense of whether the law is for them. Though the two examples of resentment discussed here were from the Florida field site, there is no mistaking that resentment is not just a southern phenomenon. A small minority of project participants from the very blue state of Rhode Island also expressed views that were antigovernment and critical of recipients of public aid (even as these individuals also received public aid). The election of Donald Trump likewise evidences that resentment is a widespread structure of feeling that can be activated and fanned in the pursuit of political power.

In the interviews, the politics of resentment (or dog whistling), eligibility, and actuarial categories, past experiences with insurance and illness, and attempts to care for loved ones mediated how people understood whether or not the law benefited them. Kenny's views were definitely shaped by the politics of white resentment, but he also went on the exchange and tried to find a plan, which ultimately was unaffordable. Obama became the repository for his blame. However, if Florida had pursued the Medicaid expansion, Kenny's whole family would have been covered for free. Given Wendy and Mike's socioeconomic status, they qualified for considerable help, and though they were critical of all the bureaucratic hoops they had to jump through to get specialty care, Mike was able to see an urologist, get a sleep study, and replace his C-Pap mask which he had been keeping together with tape. Erica was happy that she could access affordable coverage, especially in the face of more contract and sales work with no benefits. She was not as aware though of the actuarial and eligibility categories operating in the background that would increase sharply what she paid for coverage if her income ever increased.

The Affordable Care Act's approach to expanding coverage only makes sense when contextualized within shifts to public service provision and insurance that have been occurring over the last 30 years. Enabled by ideologies that value individual responsibility over social responsibility, insurance schemes have increasingly moved away from broadly pooling risk and toward greater individualization through risk segmentation (Ericson, Barry, and Doyle 2000).[8] Insurance products are no longer designed to completely insulate or protect people from risk, but instead to transfer risk onto individuals in order to foster certain behaviors, like maintaining health, avoiding unnecessary care, or prudently managing one's finances (Baker and Simon 2002). As Kenny noted, the plans being sold on healthcare.gov left him with considerable financial exposure.

The ACA curtailed some insurance company practices that had grown so extreme they were undermining the entire health care system, with almost 48 million people uninsured in 2011 (KFF 2012). The law took on some risk segmenting practices, like exclusions for people with preexisting conditions, excision, and gender-based rating. It also created high-risk corridors, re-insurance, and risk-based payments to counterbalance the widespread unpooling of risk on the individual and small-group markets (Goodell 2014). *And yet*, the policy choice of relying on means testing for eligibility and actuarial variables for pricing meant that the experience of the law remained deeply stratified. This stratification was often interpreted through dog whistle politics and resentment as some (women, people of color) were perceived as benefiting from the law at the expense of others (white men). Resentment was further amplified when households faced considerable stress in trying to meet the call to assume more financial and moral responsibility for medical coverage and health care outcomes. This highly segmented approach to reforming the health care system has proven politically contentious and it is hard to imagine how a law that generated almost as many unique experiences as there were people trying to enroll could ever gain widespread popular support.[9]

ACKNOWLEDGMENTS

Thank you to Kyle Kusz (University of Rhode Island) and Paula Mead (University of South Florida) who helped gather data in Florida. Thank you to Rebecca Martin for sharing your insight about the health delivery system in Florida. Thank you to Sarah Horton, audiences at Syracuse University, the University of Chicago, the Providence College Interdisciplinary Faculty Seminar on Systems, and participants in the School for Advanced Research Seminar, Social Citizenship: Stratification, Risk & Responsibility in Health Care Reform for helpful comments on earlier versions of this chapter. Student researchers at Providence College, and especially Stephanie Arriaga, also assisted with data collection, transcription, and analysis. Funding for the research was provided by the Committee on Aid to Faculty Research, the School of Professional Studies, and the Health Policy and Management Program at Providence College. Thank you to the Rhode Island health exchange and the community health center in Florida for their transparency and openness to research.

NOTES

1 See Paul Ryan's "A Better Way Up from Poverty" (2014) for an explanation as to why he used the terms "makers" and "takers." Rick Scott (2015) explained that he was rejecting Medicaid expansion in the name of protecting states' rights and even went so far as to sue the federal government. For further evidence of how this kind of language was used in Florida, see the James Madison Institute's list of "25 Reasons NOT to Expand Medicaid," www.jamesmadison.org. Reason number 25 is that "the dependency cycle will expand." This document shaped how legislators talked about the Medicaid expansion, and links to the list were tweeted by Florida lawmakers.

2 Though the law expanded access to insurance, it was never intended to achieve universal coverage. Even in states like Rhode Island where it was fully implemented, some immigrants, those who continue to find coverage unaffordable, those churning between eligibility statuses, those who encountered unresolved technical difficulties in the enrollment process, and those who opted out of coverage for personal or political reasons remained uninsured. Other chapters in this volume document and analyze how immigration status impacted access to coverage. Certain categories of immigrants are statutorily excluded from the insurance exchanges and/or Medicaid expansion—these categories include those who have not met the five-year mark for being in the country with an authorized legal status (for Medicaid) and those who are undocumented. In this chapter, I focus on those people the law was supposed to bring into coverage rather than those the law intentionally excluded.

3 To be eligible for coverage, an individual could not be on Medicare, must live in the United States, could not be incarcerated, and must be in an eligible immigration status (Healthcare.gov 2016). To be eligible for financial assistance, an individual must have met the income requirements and not have had access to affordable coverage through another government program or an employer.

4 Enhanced monitoring of individuals and families was carried out in order to ensure their ongoing eligibility through requirements like having to report any changes in income or family status immediately to the exchange and linking the exchange database to the IRS to verify income, process penalties, and verify that tax credits were estimated correctly. Goode (2002) points out how welfare reform in 1996 had similar impacts as women were increasingly surveilled to ensure they were eligible for benefits and not cheating the system (see also Morgen et al. 2010).

5 The question of what should be included in an assessment of ability to pay can be quite complex and might include wages, gifts, financial assets like savings, non-financial assets like real estate or automobiles, non-wage income like alimony or social security payments, etc. For the ACA, the decision was made to use income or what is known as MAGI (Modified Adjusted Gross Income) (Healthcare.gov 2016).

6 Mike and Wendy's household also consisted of Mike's adult daughter and her new baby, but they did not count in how the ACA defined family size and income.

7 Opponents of Medicaid expansion employed well-worn rhetoric about states' rights, block grants, and responsibility when advocating for policies with disproportionately negative impacts on women and people of color. Anthropologists studying the punishing rhetoric and material consequences of welfare reform in the 1990s documented how policymakers and the media likewise demonized poor women with children, portraying them as the undeserving poor (Goode 2002; Kingfisher 2001).

8 Neoliberal changes to insurance contribute to insurance functioning as a generator of difference: Insurance becomes "a difference machine, constituting a world of fragmented interests in increasingly refined calibrations of deselection" (Ericson, Barry, and Doyle 2000, 555; see also Baker and Simon 2002). Some of these shifts that have been occurring in the insurance industry for decades include strategies that increase segmentation and unpool risk (Ericson et al. 2000; French and Kneale 2012). Insurance firms evaluate past claims experiences in search of ever more precise classifications of risk based on actuarial variables such as age, gender, place of residence, diagnoses, credit history, income, and so on. These risks, once classified, are then used to sort insureds into different risk pools that range from high to low risk with varying insurance products and distinct premiums and deductibles. Counterintuitively, in highly segmented markets, high-risk pools can be very profitable for insurance companies. The notion that insurance is a consumer product and that people should buy coverage that is individualized to their circumstances is an indicator that insurance is understood as a consumer rather than a social good. Much attention was paid on conservative media sites, for example, to the fact that maternity care and contraception were deemed essential benefits that every insurance plan must cover. Conservatives argued that men shouldn't pay for maternity care since they won't use it.

9 This is a long-standing criticism of means-tested programs, which are often quite politically vulnerable when they only cover the poor or other groups like women and children.

REFERENCES

Andrews, Michelle. 2015. Many People Entitled to Hefty Subsidies Still Opt Against Coverage. *Kaiser Health News.* kaiserhealthnews.org.

Baker, Tom. 2011. Health Insurance, Risk and Responsibility After the Patient Protection and Affordable Care Act. *University of Pennsylvania Law Review* 159(6): 1577–1622.

Baker, Tom, and Jonathan Simon. 2002. *Embracing Risk: The Changing Culture of Insurance and Responsibility.* Chicago: University of Chicago Press.

Banning, Marlia E. 2006. The Politics of Resentment. *Journal of Rhetoric, Culture, & Politics* 26(1–2): 67–101.

Brown-Nagin, Tomiko. 2014. Two Americas in Healthcare: Federalism and Wars over Poverty from the New Deal-Great Society to Obamacare. *Drake Law Review* 62(1): 981–1015.

CDC. 2013. Health Insurance Coverage: Early Release of Estimates from the National Health Interview Survey, 2012. www.cdc.gov.

Dickman, Sam, David Himmelstein, Danny McCormick, and Steffie Woolhandler. 2014. Opting Out of Medicaid Expansion: The Health and Financial Impacts. *Health Affairs.* healthaffairs.org.

Enck-Wanzer, Darrel. 2011. Barack Obama, the Tea Party, and the Threat of Race: On Racial Neoliberalism and Born Again Racism. *Communication, Culture & Critique* 4: 23–30.

Ericson, Richard, Dean Barry, and Aaron Doyle. 2000. The Moral Hazards of Neo-Liberalism: Lessons from the Private Insurance Industry. *Economy and Society* 29(4): 532–558.

Ericson, Richard Victor, Aaron Doyle, and Dean Barry. 2003. *Insurance as Governance.* Toronto: University of Toronto Press.

French, S., and J. Kneale. 2012. Speculating on Careless Lives: Annuitising the Biofinancial Subject. *Journal of Cultural Economy* 5: 391–406.

Garfield, Rachel, and Anthony Damico. 2016. The Coverage Gap: Uninsured Poor Adults in States that Do Not Expand Medicaid. *Kaiser Family Foundation Issue Brief.* kff.org.

Goode, Judith. 2002. From New Deal to Bad Deal: Racial and Political Implications of U.S. Welfare Reform. In *Western Welfare in Decline.* Edited by Catherine Kingfisher. Philadelphia: University of Pennsylvania Press.

Goodell, Sarah. 2014. Health Policy Brief: Risk Corridors. *Health Affairs* (June 26). healthaffairs.org.

Gupta, Akhil. 2012. *Red Tape: Bureaucracy, Structural Violence, and Poverty in India.* Durham, NC: Duke University Press.

Haney López, Ian. 2014. *Dog Whistle Politics: How Coded Racial Appeals Have Reinvented Racism and Wrecked the Middle Class.* New York: Oxford University Press.

Healthcare.gov. 2016. Are You Eligible to Use the Marketplace? www.healthcare.gov.

Hughey, Matthew W., and Gregory S. Parks. 2014. *The Wrongs of the Right: Language, Race, and the Republican Party in the Age of Obama.* New York: New York University Press.

Katz, Michael B. 2008 (2001). *The Price of Citizenship: Redefining the American Welfare State.* Philadelphia: University of Pennsylvania Press.

Katznelson, Ira. 2005. *When Affirmative Action Was White: An Untold History of Racial Inequality in Twentieth Century America.* New York: W.W. Norton and Company.

KFF (Kaiser Family Foundation). 2012. *The Uninsured: A Primer.* Kaiser Commission on Medicaid and the Uninsured.

Kingfisher, Catherine. 2001. Producing Disunity: The Constraints and Incitements of Welfare Work. In *The New Poverty Studies.* Edited by Judith G. Goode and Jeff Maskovsky. New York: New York University Press.

Lipsky, Michael. 1984. Bureaucratic Disentitlement in Social Welfare Programs. *Social Service Review* 58(1): 3–27.

López, Leslie. 2005. De Facto Disentitlement in an Information Economy: Enrollment Issues in Medicaid Managed Care. *Medical Anthropology Quarterly* 19: 26–46.

Maxwell, Angie, and Todd Shields. 2014. The Fate of Obamacare: Racial Resentment, Ethnocentrism and Attitudes about Healthcare Reform. *Race and Social Problems* 6: 293–304.

Morgen, Sandra, Joan Acker, and Jill Weigt. 2010. *Stretched Thin: Poor Families, Welfare Work, and Welfare Reform.* Ithaca, NY: Cornell University Press.

Morone, James A. 2016. Partisanship, Dysfunction, and Racial Fears: The New Normal in Health Care Policy? *Journal of Health Politics, Policy and Law* 41(4): 827–846.

Pear, Robert. 2015. House G.O.P. Again Votes to Repeal Health Care Law. *New York Times.* www.nytimes.com.

Ryan, Paul. 2014. A Better Way Up from Poverty. *Wall Street Journal* (August 15).

Scott, Rick. 2015. Governor Rick Scott to Take Legal Action Against Obama for Stopping Federal Funds to Force State Further into Obamacare. www.flgov.com.

Stack, Carol B. 1997. Beyond What Are Given as Givens: Ethnography and Critical Policy Studies. *Ethos* 25(2): 191–207.

Tesler, Michael. 2012. The Spillover of Racialization into Health Care; How President Obama Polarized Public Opinion by Racial Attitudes and Race. *American Journal of Political Science* 56(3): 690–704.

6

Uninsured in America

Before and After the ACA

SUSAN SERED

Two Stories

Denise

Denise and her husband have worked hard—and overcome many obstacles—to build a good life together in central Illinois. The best job Denise ever had was at the Caterpillar machinery plant, where she worked for eight years. During that time, she enjoyed excellent benefits, including good health insurance with dental care and full coverage for their three children. When she became pregnant in 1991, she was working in the plant's paint shop. The work involved cleaning out the insides of large iron vats. Leaning into a vat, she bumped her stomach into a handle, causing a miscarriage. At the same time, the ongoing strain of the paint shop work injured her back. Her doctor told her to stay home from work until she felt fully recovered from both the miscarriage and the back injury. But before the doctor released her for work, Caterpillar insisted that she return to the plant. She was fired when she told them that she was still unable to work.

After the Caterpillar job, Denise worked at a series of jobs as a nurse's assistant, a profession that she loves. However, these jobs involved lifting patients for bathing and toileting, which exacerbated her back problems. None of these jobs lasted for long and none provided health insurance. By the 2010s the medical bills had piled up and Denise did not see a way out. But then, "The year [2013] Obamacare was announced we got it right then."

In 2015 Denise's health was good; she was steadily employed as a nurse's aide at a job where she felt valued; she had become active in her church's choir and youth ministry; and she and her husband had a lovely home where they looked after rotating cohorts of grandchildren.

Bridget

Bridget, a white woman in her early thirties, used to work as a nurse's aide. While the salary was low and the job did not provide health insurance, it paid enough for her to rent an apartment for herself and her children. Then her life fell apart. A decade ago she took the fall for her former husband's drug dealing (he bullied and threatened her into acquiescing) and she went to prison. When she came out, she committed the unforgiveable Mississippi sin of falling in love with a black man, and her family cut her off. In 2015 she and her boyfriend were living as squatters in a collapsing, semi-abandoned building. She wanted to work, but due to her prison record could no longer obtain employment as a nurse's aide. And she'd lost custody of her children and thus her own eligibility for Medicaid.

A diabetic, Bridget no longer had access to medical care. "I manage it by keeping candies and juice in the house for when I feel I need it, when my fingertips are numb [that is, she feels her blood sugar is too low]. When it's bad I go to the hospital. They give me a shot." Several months before the 2015 interview she suffered a second-trimester miscarriage. Though she should have been eligible for free prenatal care, she somehow fell through the cracks. Bridget did not know whether this was a result of an error she made in following through on the registration process, whether the person with whom she spoke at the hospital did not know that she should be eligible due to the pregnancy, or whether—given the racial background—the clerk simply failed to facilitate her registration.

Methods

During the years 2003 and 2004 I traveled to Texas, Mississippi, Illinois, Idaho, and Massachusetts to meet working individuals and families who were scraping by without health insurance (Sered and Fernandopulle 2005). Listening to the stories of white, black, Hispanic, urban, rural, suburban, young, middle-aged, and near elderly women and men, I identified a spiral in which jobs that did not provide health insurance led to untreated health problems which in turn led to lay-offs, declining employability, medical debt, evictions and loss of homes, more serious illnesses, and even death. At the time I wondered how the people I had met could possibly exit this death spiral. The results of that project were published in 2005 as *Uninsured in America: Life and Death in the Land of Opportunity*. In 2007, a second edition with updates on the people portrayed in the book came out.

Over the next decade Americans experienced deep economic recession, a housing crisis, anti-union ("right to work") legislation in some states, cutbacks in social services, mass incarceration and—on the other side of the roster—the Affordable Care Act. In the wake of these changes, I wanted to learn how the uninsured people I had interviewed in 2005 and 2007 were faring. In 2015, I returned to the communities that I had visited 12 years earlier. I looked for 145 people in the five states[1] and was able to re-interview 82 people. In sum, I discovered:

- Twenty-eight people were insured through their employer or spouse's employer, though outside of Massachusetts that insurance typically did not include coverage for spouses or children.
- Seventeen people were on Social Security Disability and therefore covered by Medicare. Many of these men and women would likely have been able to continue working if they had been able to access consistent medical care *and* if they had been able to find jobs that allowed for some level of accommodation for workers with minor physical limitations, repetitive stress injuries, normal declines in physical strength related to aging, or chronic but not incapacitating illnesses.
- Thirteen people were covered by Medicaid, with the largest Medicaid contingent living in Illinois.
- Twelve people were covered by Medicare by virtue of being age 65 or older; several of those people also have Medicaid as supplemental insurance.
- Eleven people purchased insurance on the ACA Marketplace (exchanges), with several of them receiving some level of subsidy through the ACA and/or financial assistance from their employers for the purchase.
- Ten people were uninsured at the time of the re-interview, though many more had been uninsured for most of the preceding 12 years. Texans were especially likely to be uninsured.
- Ten people were ascertained to be dead (I found death certificates or obituaries). All ten died prematurely: seven in their fifties, one in the sixties, and two in their early seventies.

Bridget's and Denise's experiences exemplify the most striking finding of the reprise tour: Geographically driven gaps between the health care "haves" and "have nots" (which the ACA sought to redress) were exacerbated by the 2012 U.S. Supreme Court ruling, *NFIB v. Sebelius*, which allowed states to opt out of the ACA's Medicaid expansion. (See the Introduction to this volume.) In states that did not expand Medicaid (including Idaho, Texas, and Mississippi), people like Bridget continued to struggle to access even basic health care services. In states that did expand Medicaid (including Illinois and Massachusetts), large numbers of people—like Denise—were able to access the medical care that made it possible for them to engage in work, family, and community.

States that Have Not Expanded Medicaid
Politics of Resentment, Texas-Style

The still-uninsured people whom I re-interviewed disproportionately lived in Texas, which also was the state with the highest rate of uninsured people nationwide. Texas's dismal record reflected lower than the national average rates of employer-based insurance as well as the state's refusal to expand Medicaid. With several exceptions (including low-income elderly and disabled people on Medicare), adults without dependent children were not eligible for Medicaid regardless of income (Texas Medical Association 2016). Adults with dependent children were eligible for Medicaid only if their household income did not exceed 15% of poverty level. This amounted to less than $3,000 a year for a family of three.

During my return trip to the Rio Grande Valley, I was able to re-interview 16 of the 26 people I'd met a decade earlier. In 2015, four people were covered by Medicaid as a supplement to Medicare (three were on Disability, one was over 65); no one qualified for Medicaid as primary insurance. Another four people were uninsured in 2015. All four fell into the "coverage gap" (see chapter by Mulligan in this volume). In other words, when they applied for insurance on the exchange, they were told that their incomes were too high to qualify for Medicaid but too low to qualify for subsidies.

The experiences of the Martinez family were typical. Maria worked full-time in a food service job that provided health insurance for her but required a biweekly payment of $250 to cover her children. Her biweekly income was $500, so she had to turn down the coverage. Her husband, Enrique, was a truck driver whose employer did not offer insurance, but he earned too little to qualify for a subsidized premium on the exchange. For a short time their youngest child was eligible for Medicaid (CHIP), but then Enrique's income went up (marginally) and the child no longer qualified. In 2013 Enrique spoke with an ACA enrollment specialist who helped him apply for an exemption from the penalty for not having insurance. In 2014 he forgot to re-apply and had to pay $190 in fines ($95 for himself and $95 for their 21-year-old child). In the meantime, he took medication for high blood pressure when the border with Mexico was safe enough for him to cross over to buy medication there (a situation that was increasingly rare in this era of drug cartels and border fighting).

Five Texans were insured via the exchange (two of those received limited subsidies from their employers for insurance) and three were insured through employers—certainly a step up from when I first met them. However, all eight of these Texans were unhappy with their insurance. The Texas people who purchased insurance on the exchange could only afford the lowest premium / highest deductible "bronze" plans that often ended up costing the poorest Americans more than higher premium "silver" or "gold plans" (Sered and Proulx 2011). Texans I interviewed told me they could not use their insurance because the deductible was too high (in some cases as high as $7,000 / year) or co-insurance or copayments were too expensive.

Rosa, an energetic and articulate middle-aged woman, was insured but still owed tens of thousands of dollars for past medical treatments. As a consequence, she had a bad credit record, which meant she could not get loans for her children's college tuitions. Shortly after I originally met her she had a hysterectomy, but without insurance she never went back for a post-surgical checkup. In 2015, she was worried about severe breast pain and out-of-control diabetes. (Her mother died of diabetes.) She also had a tumor in her kidney, which she was supposed to have checked every two years, but it had been six years since the last scan. The problem was that because of her low salary she "chose" a bronze plan with a low monthly premium (all that she could afford) and thus was stuck with a $4,500 annual deductible and $1,000 co-pay for hospitalization. To her dismay, Rosa had realized that she could not actually use her health insurance because she could not afford to spend enough to reach the deductible.

Unfortunately for Rosa, women's health services were hit hard by budget cuts in Texas during the past three legislative sessions. And, in 2012, Texas refused federal money for the women's reproductive health program (expanded Medicaid), which had a 9 to 1 federal-state match. What made her story particularly compelling was that she herself was a health care advocate with a deep understanding of policy issues, yet she was stuck with an insurance plan that most definitely did not meet her needs.

Most people whom I interviewed were unaware that the coverage gap was a product of their own state government's refusal to accept federal money to expand Medicaid. Consistently, they blamed "Obamacare" for this situation. One middle-aged woman who worked full-time and was the primary caregiver of her elderly, ill mother complained bitterly that she only got three days of sick leave each year and she needed to spend a significant portion of her income to pay for an aide to stay with her mother while she was at work. "I don't see that Obamacare helped my mother [get coverage for an aide]. My parents were punished for saving their money. Because they have money they saved they don't get jack shit."

The existence of coverage gaps, together with the ubiquitous high-deductible plans pitched to low-income families, created barriers and hostilities, with many people feeling (with some justification) that other categories of people received greater benefits. In Texas, where the Republican party had poured enormous resources into billboards and radio and television ads denouncing "Obamacare," and where, according to Rosa, politicians needed to "prove" that they were more conservative than their potential challengers. People's frustration was directed toward President Obama rather than toward the state governor and legislature that turned down the expansion and set the Texas Medicaid eligibility thresholds far below the income of even the poorest paid workers. State politics, thus, were not only compromising access to care but fueling a politics of resentment.

In Texas as well as in Mississippi and Idaho, objections to the ACA and other "government hand-outs" often were framed in terms of race, sometimes explicitly, sometimes implicitly (see chapter by Mulligan, this volume). A friendly and boisterous Texas man in his thirties shared his thoughts with me over an abundant "Texas size" lunch. Bragging that he owned numerous guns, he told me, "I buy a new one every six months just to piss off Obama." His anger at Obama infused his attitude toward the ACA: His former employer, he said, laid off half its employees because of Obamacare, and he himself was now paying twice as much for worse insurance. The problem, he explained, was "them—the immigrants coming across the border just to work the system." (Ironically, this man was a grandson of Mexican immigrants.)

Who Does and Who Does Not "Deserve" Health Care: Idaho-Style

In northern Idaho I looked for 37 people and re-interviewed 20. Two had Medicaid (they moved to Washington State to get medical coverage); five had Medicare through Disability; two had Medicare because they were over age 65; seven were insured through their employers (two of them moved to Pennsylvania in part to get health insurance and one married a woman from Washington and was insured through her employer).

Only three Idahoans had purchased insurance through the exchange. One of them, Al—a farmer in his early sixties—was embarrassed to admit to liking "Obamacare." Moriah Nelson, Outreach and Enrollment Manager at the Idaho Primary Care Association Direct, explained that in rural parts of Idaho there is "a cultural ideology that is anti-Obamacare, anti-government help. Some people wouldn't take Medicaid even if it were available." But Al certainly had benefited from expanded health care access. Diagnosed with lung cancer a number of years ago, he had not been able to obtain health insurance before the ACA because of his preexisting condition. During those years, hospital bills were as high as $300,000 annually, leaving him in horrendous debt. In 2015, he paid $12 per month for insurance through the exchange and his doctor was satisfied that "there are no new tumors." Al was one of the lucky few. Many Idahoans struggled to find affordable health care. Approximately 95% of Idaho businesses employed fewer than 50 workers (Idaho Department of Labor 2013), exempting the businesses from the ACA mandate to provide health insurance.

Idaho did not take the Medicaid expansion. As a consequence, Medicaid was only available to children, pregnant women, parents of children under the age of 19, disabled people, and the elderly. Even within those categories not many Idahoans met the Medicaid criteria: A family of four must earn less than $650 per month to qualify (Idaho Department of Health and Welfare 2016). Idaho also suffered from one of the lowest per capita rates of doctors in the country (United Health Foundation 2016). Consequently, some Idaho physicians were selecting the better-paying patients; some restricted the number of Medicaid patients they treated; some did not take any Medicaid or uninsured patients. Physician shortages were especially felt in the rural counties where oftentimes the nearest doctor or hospital was a considerable distance away on winding mountainous roads.

Marla and Peter, parents of three healthy kids, exemplified how Idahoans faced these challenges. Marla and Peter were uninsured when I first met them and remained uninsured until a year before the interview. This was challenging because Peter had some serious health problems, including a blood disorder, ulcerative colitis, and glaucoma. Throughout his adult life Peter had worked steadily for a company that he liked and liked him, but did not provide health insurance. For a number of years Marla ran a home-based elder care business. When their kids reached school age, she found an office job, but it too did not provide health insurance. During those years, to take care of her family's health needs, Marla drove them to doctors all over the northern part of the state—sometimes putting hundreds of miles on the car. At each office she would accumulate a manageable bill that they tried to pay off over time. Typically, the doctor would not see them again until they fully paid the bill.

Knowing they needed health care coverage, Marla began to work for another small business owner who agreed to pay half of their monthly health insurance premium. But the remaining half was so high that after it was deducted from her salary she ended up taking home about $5 / hour. She and Peter looked into Obamacare, but they earned too much for a subsidy and couldn't afford the insurance without it. A year before our recent interview she moved to a better job with somewhat better insurance. Her premium then was down to $250 per month, but the deductible was $3,000 per person and there were hefty copays and co-insurance. Marla and Peter were lucky. They were relatively young when I first met them; they were white, articulate, and middle-class in their appearance; their jobs were not overly dangerous; Marla was incredibly resourceful; and they managed to avoid any major health crises during their uninsured years.

Lenny was a different story altogether. When I first met Lenny in 2003 he seemed in shock at how quickly he went from being known as someone who had always worked and looked after his family to being someone who needed the assistance of the county indigent committee. The son of an Idaho logger, Lenny began working to help support himself and his two brothers when he was 14. At the age of 23 he took a job working underground at the Sunshine Mine, where he stayed for 30 years. In those days Sunshine was a unionized mine where workers enjoyed a union-negotiated package of health and retirement benefits. "Benefits were the reason people went to the mines. Sunshine was a good mine as far as pay, it paid well and they had the best insurance, they covered you, your wife, and all your kids 100%, dental, optical everything."

In the mid-1980s silver prices fell. In order to help save the mine and hold onto their jobs, the miners took cuts in pay and insurance, and began paying part of their own premiums. In 2001 the mine closed permanently, and Lenny, along with his co-workers, lost their health insurance and other benefits. Calling on all his friends and relatives for help, he lined up a job installing telephone lines. The rub was that it took 60 days on the job to get the insurance. Thirty days after he began the job, he fell down on the pavement in full cardiac arrest. Paramedics flew him to Spokane to a cardiac unit. Lenny's recovery was far better than anyone expected, but he was saddled with enormous medical bills. A year later, he was sent to the hospital for a bypass operation, angioplasty, and eventually open-heart surgery. The bills for his various surgeries, consultations, medications, and treatments were over $140,000—a sum that might as well be one billion dollars in terms of Lenny ever being able to pay it. His sole income at the time was the $400 per month pension he received from Sunshine. Fortunately, the administrator of the county indigent committee went out of her way to facilitate Lenny's application for assistance. As she told me at the time, she was happy to be able to help "hard-working" people like Lenny and his wife who "deserve" help. "They're long-time residents. They've paid taxes for a long time. They're good people."

In 2015 Lenny looked healthy and happy. Due to the cumulative injuries and illnesses of work in the mines, he'd become eligible for Disability not too long after I originally met him and he'd been able to take care of his health issues. Savvy about the history and importance of labor unions, Lenny emphasized that he would like to see the government doing more for people.

In contrast to Lenny, his girlfriend Lucy, in her late sixties, believed that the government was already doing too much—and for the wrong people. After her long marriage to a minister (whom she doubted "had a real calling") ended, Lucy took a job at Wal-Mart. She made a point of telling me that she liked working at Wal-Mart and that—unlike Lenny—she couldn't see herself puttering around the house all day. But "at my age" standing on her feet at work was not easy. And she was resentful of the customers she saw who "get welfare and food stamps and use it to buy cigarettes and alcohol." (In fact, food stamps could not be used for cigarettes and alcohol. They could not even be used for toilet paper or toothpaste.) Unlike Lenny, who, in her estimation, deserved the assistance he received from the County. "These are the people who get a free ride from Obama." For this reason, she added, she was opposed to Obama and Obamacare.

Anger expressed by low-income workers like Lucy toward people poor enough to qualify for Medicaid or other government assistance was a common theme in the non-expansion states. In particular, working people who did not qualify for Medicaid but whose incomes limited them to the lowest-premium/highest deductible plans expressed anger that they could not use the "Obamacare" that they paid for while other people—people who did not work—got Obamacare for free. Rubbing salt into the wounds, several people told me that they themselves or someone they knew had to pay a fine for not purchasing health insurance, while other people got "handouts from Obama."

Mississippi Disability

In the Mississippi Delta and surrounding counties I was able to locate only 13 of the 28 people whom I sought. Given Mississippi's consistent last-place national rank in terms of most measures of population health (Mississippi has the lowest life expectancy in the country [KFF 2009]), it is difficult to imagine that the missing people are doing particularly well. Of the people I found, only one remained uninsured, but that number masked a grimmer reality. One was dead; three had Medicaid—a high number in light of Mississippi's exceptionally stingy Medicaid eligibility threshold; three were covered via Social Security Disability; one had Medicare because he was over 65 (this person also had Disability); and six now had insurance through an employer or a spouse's employer (two of these six now live in other states). No one in Mississippi had purchased insurance on the exchange.

Mississippi's decision to decline Medicaid expansion negatively affected an estimated 280,000 residents (Healthinsurance.org 2016). And political opposition to the ACA made it difficult for information about enrollment to reach people. Roy Mitchell of the Mississippi Health Advocacy Program estimated that another 300,000 or so residents were eligible for insurance on the marketplace but either did not know about it or had been discouraged from signing up. Together with the chronic shortage of primary care providers in rural areas, the situation was grim for many residents of the state.

In Mississippi, race is always relevant. Neighborhoods remain racially segregated, personal identities revolve around race, and state policies are racially driven. Blacks disproportionately live in states that have not expanded Medicaid. In fact, of ten states with the largest black populations, only Maryland and Delaware expanded Medicaid (Ferris 2014). According to a report by the Urban Institute, of all of the non-expansion states, Mississippi would have seen the second largest decrease of uninsurance for black residents (68.2%, just behind Louisiana's 68.4%) if the state had accepted the Medicaid expansion (Clemens-Cope, Buettgens, and Recht 2014).

Mississippians have high rates of chronic illness and of injuries: 26.9% of blacks and 21.4% of whites, rates well above the national average, reported fair or poor health status (KFF 2015). During all of my Mississippi visits I heard stories of people whose illnesses or injuries went untreated or were improperly treated, and who eventually became too disabled to work. These stories were reflected in the wider statistics: Mississippi was part of a cluster of states (Arkansas, Alabama, Kentucky, Maine, and West Virginia) in which 7% or more of the population aged 18–64 received Social Security Disability payments (Social Security Office of Retirement and Disability Policy 2011).

When I originally met Daniel in 2003, he was 61 years old and living in a pleasant working-class African American neighborhood. He explained to me that injuries he'd "collected" during more than 40 years of construction work had taken a toll on his body and he'd been unable to work for the past two years. In particular, he was afraid to climb ladders, both because of the numbness in his fingers (he suspected the numbness was the result of falling off a ladder on the job) and because of deteriorating vision in his one good eye (he suspected that glasses could help, but he couldn't afford them). Although he was a skilled carpenter, over the years Daniel often had to take unskilled jobs because labor was considered replaceable in the Delta: "Well you have to [take any job] if you're going to get paid. So they gonna try to keep you down."

Like most of the construction workers he knew, Daniel had spent years flip-flopping on and off health insurance. When he'd been lucky, he'd had jobs that lasted seven or eight months in which he was employed by a firm large enough to offer insurance to employees. When he'd been less lucky, he'd worked for smaller contractors or picked up some income doing home repairs as an independent laborer. In these situations, health insurance had never been an option. Consequently, Daniel never had the recommended surgery on his back following a serious injury incurred installing heavy pipes on a Navy base. Nor did he have physical therapy—or any treatment except for pain medication—for the neck he broke when he fell off a ladder working on a bathroom. Daniel mentioned a doctor whom he thought of as his primary provider during the periods when he had health insurance. But the last time he tried to go to this doctor he was uninsured and the doctor wouldn't see him unless he paid $50 up front. Daniel didn't have the money, and didn't see the doctor.

Shortly after he stopped working, Daniel filed for disability insurance. The process did not go smoothly. To begin with, when he was sent for a doctor's exam as part of his disability application, he was asked the name of his regular doctor so that forms could be sent to him in order to verify Daniel's medical history. Not only had Daniel not seen a doctor in years, but the only doctor he could name was the one who several months earlier had refused to see him.

The medical examination performed by the disability physician seemed to have been cursory at best. A few months later, Daniel was informed that his request for disability insurance was turned down. As is typically the case, he was not told why he had been turned down. The Social Security office did, however, give him the names of several lawyers in the area that he could hire to represent him at a hearing if he chose to appeal the decision. The arrangement is that, if the appeal is successful, the lawyer will receive a percentage of the money Daniel would receive from Social Security—money intended to serve as living expenses for someone unable to work.

When I returned in 2015, Daniel was no longer living in the pleasant family-friendly neighborhood. A local teenager told me that Daniel was most likely living in the trailer park "back behind Wal-Mart" and offered to drive over with me to look for him. Together with my new young friend, I entered a dilapidated trailer park in which random scatterings of derelict and inhabited trailers were scattered across muddy patches of land.

A few weeks later I caught up with one of the women I'd originally met in Daniel's old neighborhood and she put me in touch with Daniel's niece, who helped me reach Daniel by phone. Unable to speak clearly, Daniel handed the receiver to a woman who introduced herself as his caregiver. She confirmed that Daniel indeed lives in the trailer park and that she helps him out because he became too disabled to care for himself. Ironically, she took on this under-the-table caregiving job in order to make money for food and rent while she is waiting to be accepted onto Disability. She is not "really" disabled, she told me, but she needs to get onto Disability so that she can get insurance and take care of her diabetes.

For millions of Americans, Social Security Disability has become the sole social welfare program to which they can turn for help. Since 1996, when Congress passed the Personal Responsibility and Work Opportunity Act, welfare eligibility is strictly limited to a lifetime cap of five years. In the post-PRWORA era, the number of people on Social Security Disability has increased at more or less the same rate as the number of people receiving welfare has decreased. Eligibility for Disability requires

that the applicant either be blind or have a physical or mental impairment that prevents engaging in any *"substantial gainful activity"* and that
the condition has lasted or is expected to last 12 months or to result in
death (Nadel, Wamhoff, and Wiseman 2003/2004). In American society,
where glowing health is seen as virtuous, the label of "disabled" comes
with the price of admitting to weakness, to failure, to personal flaws,
to being placed below "normal" Americans who are healthy enough to
work and "contribute to society" through paying taxes and other activities of citizenship. Bolstered by long-standing cultural beliefs regarding
the moral virtues of work (Weber 2002 [1905]), those unfortunates who
cannot work (or cannot work "sufficiently"), risk losing their place in the
social fabric—as well as their access to normative (employment-based)
health insurance. In our culture of "healthism" (Crawford 1980), disability is the ultimate outcome and exemplar of stratified citizenship.

States That Have Expanded Medicaid

Illinois: Modest Improvements

In south-central Illinois—a mixed region of small industrial cities and
of rural towns—I looked for 31 people and re-interviewed 21. None
were uninsured. Four were covered by Medicaid (two had Medicaid as
a supplement to Medicare); six were on Medicare through Disability;
eight were covered by Medicare because they were over age 65 (most
had just recently turned 65 so were newly covered by Medicare); four
were insured through their employers; one purchased insurance on the
exchange.

In many ways, the ACA was a success in Illinois. Illinois residents
who previously were denied insurance because of preexisting conditions or denied benefits because they reached the insurance company's
"lifetime limits" were able to obtain coverage. Illinois accepted the Medicaid expansion, which had a substantial impact throughout the state.
According to navigators in Danville, Decatur and Champaign-Urbana
almost all applicants were eligible either for Medicaid or subsidies on
the exchange.

Despite these successes, nearly everyone I met during my return
trip to Illinois was dissatisfied with their coverage. Even those few re-
interviewees whose status had remained relatively stable for most of the

past decade found that out-of-pocket costs (deductibles, copays, and co-insurance), referral requirements, and coverage limitations changed without their knowledge or agreement. People I interviewed often were confused and frustrated with these inconsistencies, felt that they personally were being "screwed over," and often blamed their doctors for insurance company policies that providers dislike as much as patients did. One woman in her sixties summed up the ambivalence of Illinois residents like this: "Around here Obama's either the Devil or one step above God."

Like in other states, high deductible insurance plans baffled residents. Hal, a man with advanced university degrees, worked full-time for nearly all of his adult life. Like many of the other Illinois men I met both in 2003 and again in 2015, Hal had received insurance through his employer for most of his life. Then, right about when I first met him, he had been laid off and rehired by the same company as an independent contractor without benefits. This kind of change, he understood, was happening all over the state. A few years later he landed another job that provided insurance, but then the company collapsed and he lost the insurance. Jill, his wife, worked full-time for a large company but she too was employed as an independent contractor through a staffing agency. The agency offered insurance, but it was far too expensive for Hal and Jill.

In 2015 Hal was old enough for Medicare but Jill was not. Stretching their budget as far as they could, they signed up through the exchange for a plan to cover Jill and their two young adult children. For that plan they paid $500 per month with a $6,000 deductible per person per year. A month before our last meeting, Jill had been in the hospital for a week and they were facing a bill that they could not pay. Hal explained, "It's been a financially risky dance to try to make sure everyone is covered." Hal was a highly educated and well-informed man, yet (and he and I discussed this) he bought into the notion that there is a stigma to "government hand-outs." (For more on Medicaid and stigma see Andaya, this volume.) When I told him that his daughters, both of whom have disabilities, may have been eligible for Medicaid, he said, "I don't want to take advantage of a system made for people less fortunate than I am. Jill makes a good salary." Yet he (retired) and Jill (nearing retirement) had a grand total of $200 in savings.

Hal and Jill's reluctance to accept "government hand-outs" may well have been motivated by factors in addition to altruism. Denise, met at the beginning of the chapter, was in poor health, uninsured, and virtually unemployable when I'd initially met her twelve years ago, but was covered by the ACA in 2015, and was happy, healthy, and employed. But when I commented, "So you must be happy for Obamacare," she explained that, "It's not like real insurance. When you go to the hospital they are not interested in me. They look at you in a different way and they send you home, but if you had real insurance they'd put you in the hospital."

Massachusetts: It Works (If You Work)

In Massachusetts, where most of the people I originally interviewed were college graduates, I looked for 22 people and was able to re-interview 13. Of those, seven were covered by their employers; two people (both self-employed) purchased insurance through the exchange; two were covered by Medicaid; no one was on Disability or Medicare; and two were currently uninsured. In 2006, Massachusetts enacted a health care reform similar to the ACA, and by 2015 close to 98% of residents were insured. (For more on Massachusetts see Joseph and Shaw, this volume.) Because Medicaid eligibility was expanded up to the levels at which residents were eligible for highly subsidized coverage on the exchange, there was no significant coverage gap in the state.

Several groups stood out among the people who benefited from the health care reform: near elderly women whose husbands retired before them (previously, if the woman was covered as a dependent through her husband's employer, she risked becoming uninsured when he retired and enrolled in Medicare); young adults up to age 26 who could stay on their parents' insurance; and self-employed people who had real options on the exchange.

Yet some problems persisted. The Affordable Care Act, like the Massachusetts reform, built on (rather than unified) fragmented assortments of for-profit, not-for-profit, local, state, and federal programs and institutions. Individuals were tasked with figuring out what coverage they were eligible for and re-enrolling when their life circumstances (marriage, divorce, widowhood, reaching age 26 or 65, gaining or losing a job, etc.) changed. Significantly, the two uninsured Massachusetts re-interviewees had been insured but lost their coverage when their job or school situation changed and they had not yet, as one put it, "got around to signing up again."

While nearly all Massachusetts residents were insured, an increasing number (post-ACA) were saddled with plans with high deductibles and co-insurance. Advocates were concerned that moves to open state borders to insurance companies may exacerbate these problems. Thus, the ACA coming several years after the Massachusetts reform, has had both positive and negative impacts in the state.

Some people who were eligible for coverage remained uninsured or churned on and off insurance because they did not understand the multiple forms they needed to fill out or because they were homeless, transient, or did not have their names on their mailbox (frequently the case in housing projects). And there were some neighborhoods (in particular neighborhoods with many immigrants) and demographics (young, male, Hispanic) that had not yet benefited from the reform (though the state maintains a health care program for people not eligible for Obamacare because of their immigration status) (Blue Cross Foundation 2013).

Jodi, an educated woman in her mid-forties, walked me through the previous 12 years of (mostly) ups and (a few) downs in her family's health care story. When we met in 2003, both she and her husband worked part-time and neither had insurance. Shortly after our initial interview her husband landed a job with insurance and she and the kids were covered. A few years later they divorced. When the couple split up her husband kept the kids on his insurance. "I had a crisis when I was dumped from his insurance without their telling me." Well-connected to the professional communities of Massachusetts, she found a pro bono lawyer who helped her get on COBRA through her former husband's insurance.

Then he committed suicide and she and the kids lost their insurance. She then found a job that covered 80% of her premium but nothing for the kids. "It was very costly." Then the company "downsized" and she was laid off.

When the health care reform was enacted in Massachusetts, she and the kids were able to enroll in Medicaid. While this wasn't perfect (for example, it didn't pay for the out-of-state emergency room visit when one of the kids sprained an ankle while visiting his grandparents), it provided coverage that allowed her to finish college while working part-time. In 2015, she had a full-time professional job and she and the kids had excellent insurance through her employer. Her opinion of the Massachusetts health care reform and the ACA: "Relief. I don't have to worry. Super helpful. Thank you, Obama."

Conclusion

Throughout this chapter I have identified people by the coverage status they reported at the time of the 2015 interview. It is critical to understand, however, that not a single person I interviewed in 2015 had remained in the same health care coverage status and situation for more than a few years at a time. Due to the patchwork nature of health care coverage, Americans experience breaks in coverage when they change their jobs, marital status, health status, or hometown.

While the overall number of uninsured Americans had decreased significantly post-ACA, the health care landscape remained stratified into holders of "Cadillac" policies, those covered by decent insurance (typically through employers), people who could only afford low-premium / high-deductible "lousy" policies, people deemed eligible for some sort of government-funded coverage, and the unlucky class—the health care "untouchables"—whose employment, immigration, or social status pushed them outside of the system altogether. Unfortunately, the Supreme Court ruling to allow states to decline Medicaid expansion further contributed to inequality in access to health care nationally.

For nearly everyone I met in my return trips to four of the five states—Idaho, Texas, Mississippi, and Illinois—the name Affordable Care Act obscured the reality that even with health insurance, health care was hardly affordable for most Americans. Even those few re-interviewees whose status had remained relatively stable for most of the past decade found that out-of-pocket costs (deductibles, copays, and co-insurance), referral requirements, and coverage limitations changed without their knowledge or agreement. People I interviewed often were confused and frustrated with these inconsistencies, felt that they personally were being "screwed over," and often blamed their medical providers or racial "others" for policies decided upon by insurance companies or state governments.

The enormous resources that many Republicans poured into attacking Obamacare seemed to have lulled many Americans into forgetting that the Affordable Care Act was no more than a political compromise between middle-of-the-road Democrats and right-of-center Republicans. Though it included many good provisions and a certain expansion of health care coverage, the ACA was never designed to overhaul the U.S. health care landscape. We still had a smorgasbord of donut holes, coverage gaps, and nonsensical limits on rehabilitative services rather than a rational, unified system. We still linked health care coverage to employment, reinforcing cultural tendencies to valorize work and stigmatize those who cannot work—and pushing large numbers of Americans into Disability. Even as we kept in place the ties between employment and normative health care coverage, we continued to exempt large categories of employers (for example, businesses employing fewer than 50 workers) from providing insurance. With its gold, silver, and bronze plans, the ACA continued to treat health care access as a personal "choice" and to allow private insurance companies the power to allow or disallow treatments. And we still saw substantial racial disparities in access to health care and in health care outcomes.

While we cannot know the precise trajectories that led to the early deaths of at least ten of the original uninsured interviewees, their premature demises surely signify the ultimate consequences of our national failure to treat health care as a basic, universal human right.

ACKNOWLEDGMENTS

Travel for the follow-up project was funded by a Suffolk University Faculty Development Grant. In each state many local experts, providers, and advocates helped me understand the bigger picture of health care delivery. In Mississippi I'd particularly like to thank Roy Mitchell and Jarvis Dortch, Mississippi Health Advocacy Program; Marcus Davenport, Health Help Mississippi, Greenville; Stephanie Taylor and Lori Latham, Community Mental Health Center (CMHC), West Point; Linda Dixon Rigsby and Sherry Rainey, Mississippi Center for Justice;

Dr. Walter Gorton, Belzoni; Jonelle Husain, Mississippi State University. In Texas I'd particularly like to thank Ramona Casas, ARISE; Edith Silvas, Methodist Hospital, Houston; Yvonne Gutierrez, Planned Parenthood; Brad Klos and Rachel Udow, MHP Salud; Christian Muñoz, Nuestra Clinica de Valle; Carmen Boudreau, University of Texas Health Science Center; Dr. Laura Guerra-Cardus, Children's Defense Fund–Texas; Liz James, Lesbian Health Initiative of Houston. In Idaho I'd particularly like to thank Terri Sterling, ICAN; Charlotte Ash, Snake River Community Clinic; Ken Whitney, Jr., Mayor of Troy; Dr. Richard Thurston, St. Maries Volunteer Clinic; Donald Duffy, Panhandle Health District; Moriah Nelson, Idaho Primary Care Association; Pam McBride, Clearwater Valley Hospital, Orofino; Ashley Piaskowski, Heritage Health, Coeur d'Alene; Dr. Ted Epperly, Idaho Healthcare Coalition and Family Medicine Residency of Idaho; Stephen Weeg, Board Chair, Idaho Health Insurance Exchange.

In Illinois I'd particularly like to thank Cheryl Rome, VA Illiana Health Care System; Karen Schneller, Decatur Memorial Hospital; Linda Fasik, Community Health Improvement Center, Decatur; Claudia Lennhoff, Champaign County Health Care Consumers; Julie Pryde, Champaign Urbana Public Health District; Jenny Trimmell and Melissa Rome, Vermilion County Health Department; Mona, Maggie and Lupe, Francis Nelson Health Center; Kathy Waligora, EverThrive Illinois. In Massachusetts I'd particularly like to thank Hannah Frigand, Suzanne Curry, Kate Bicego, and Brian Rosman, Health Care For All; Rob Restuccia and Reena Singh, Community Catalyst; Patricia Edraos and Liz Sanchez, Massachusetts League of Community Health Centers.

NOTE

1 I have changed the names and identifying details of all study participants. This project has been approved by the Suffolk University Institutional Review Board.

REFERENCES

Blue Cross Foundation. 2013. Reaching the Remaining Uninsured in Massachusetts: Challenges and Opportunities. bluecrossfoundation.org.

Clemens-Cope, Lisa, Matthew Buettgens, and Hannah Recht. 2014. Racial/ Ethnic Differences in Uninsurance Rates under the ACA. Urban Institute. www .urban.org.

Crawford, Robert. 1980. Healthism and the Medicalization of Everyday Life. *International Journal of Health Services* 10(3): 365–388.

Ferris, Sarah. 2014. Blacks Falling Behind Under Obamacare. *The Hill*, December 16. thehill.com.

Healthinsurance.org.2016. Mississippi Medicaid. www.healthinsurance.org.

Idaho Department of Health and Welfare. 2016. About our benefit service. www .healthandwelfare.idaho.gov.

Idaho Department of Labor. 2013. Idaho Fringe Benefits Survey 2013. https://labor .idaho.gov/.

Kaiser Family Foundation (KFF). 2009. Life Expectancy at Birth (in years). kff.org.

———. 2015. Percent of Adults Reporting Fair or Poor Health Status, by Race/Ethnicity. kff.org.

Nadel, Mark, Steve Wamhoff, and Michael Wiseman. 2003/2004. *Disability, Welfare Reform, and Supplemental Security Income.* Social Security Bulletin 65(3). Social Security Administration Office of Policy.

Sered, Susan Starr, and Rushika Fernandopulle. 2005. *Uninsured in America: Life and Death in the Land of Opportunity.* Berkeley: University of California Press.

Sered, Susan, and Marilyn Delle Donne Proulx. 2011. Lessons for Women's Health from the Massachusetts Reform: Affordability, Transitions and Choice. *Women's Health Issues* 21(1): 1–5.

Social Security Office of Retirement and Disability Policy. 2011. Annual Statistical Report on the Social Security Disability Insurance Program, 2011. www.ssa.gov.

Texas Medical Association. 2016. "The Uninsured in Texas." www.texmed.org.

United Health Foundation. 2016. America's Health Rankings. americashealthrankings .org.

Weber, Max. 2002 (1905). *The Protestant Ethic and the "Spirit" of Capitalism.* Penguin.

7

"Texans Don't Want Health Insurance"

Social Class and the ACA in a Red State

EMILY K. BRUNSON

> You don't want to study that. This is Texas. People in Texas are uninsured because they want to be. Texans don't want health insurance.
> —Texas health administrator

Shortly after moving to Texas I had an opportunity to speak with a senior administrator at the Texas Department of State Health Services. As part of our conversation, he asked me what I planned to research next. I stated that I was very interested in identifying a local project and mentioned the possibility of studying the experiences of people who lack health insurance. His immediate response, quoted above, shocked me. Not only did I consider it dismissive of a significant issue—at the time Texas had the highest rate of uninsured persons in the country—I also thought that it was blatantly untrue. The vast majority of the literature I had read suggested that a lack of health insurance, and all of the difficulties that come with it, was anything but a choice (for a few examples see Becker 2004, 2007; Horton and Barker 2010; Sered and Fernandopulle 2005).

At the same time, this official's statement did make me reconsider my approach when I began my research on this topic. Instead of focusing my recruitment in venues where I expected to find people without health insurance, places like food banks or community health clinics, I made a concerted effort to identify and recruit uninsured persons throughout my research area, including wealthier persons who might—as the public health official implied—be making a purposeful choice to be uninsured. This approach, combined with longitudinal data collection, has allowed me to examine how the Affordable Care Act (ACA) affected not just poor, marginalized persons but also non-marginalized and wealthier individuals and families.

In this chapter I draw on the experiences of three Texas women who—while all uninsured at the start of the research project in 2013—varied with regard to their incomes and levels of social capital. By comparing and contrasting the experiences of these women, I examine the commonalities and disjunctions in how they experienced living without health insurance and how their situations were impacted, or not impacted, by the ACA. In this way, this chapter is not so much about describing individuals' experiences with the ACA generally, or in a small, local area of Texas specifically, but rather how and why people can experience the same legislation in varied and contrasting ways because of their social position and specifically their social class.

Social Class in the United States

Class can be a nebulous concept. For the purposes of this chapter, I define class as a socially constructed identity based on a combination of economics and social capital, i.e., individuals' incomes as well as the types of social networks they can draw upon for support. In the United States today, as has been true throughout U.S. history, a spectrum of economic and social capital exists. While movement along this spectrum is possible, being poor, being wealthy, or being somewhere in between influences how people think and talk about themselves and others, as well as how people act. The differences that stem from these processes result in the perpetuation of different social classes.

According to Ortner (2006), current U.S. society can be divided into four groupings: the lower class, the lower middle class, the upper middle class, and the upper class. Ortner characterizes the lower class and the lower middle class as "working class," meaning that they do not own any of the means of production and that they earn their livings primarily through some type of manual labor. According to Ortner, the lower class is separated from the lower middle class by being poorer, but also by being non-white. Of course, the majority of lower class individuals are white and many non-whites belong to other classes (Rank 2004), but, as Ortner suggests, there is a strong element of racism that plays into perceptions of the lower class in many parts of the United States. In comparison, the upper middle class is not working class per se. While they also do not typically own the means of production, at the same time they do not usually perform manual labor. Instead, they act as administrators and managers, their jobs are often salaried, and they have more wealth compared to members of the lower middle class. The upper class, according to Ortner, is typically comprised of white, Anglo-Saxon Protestants (WASPs) who possess "old money"; they are also the owners of the means of production. As for the middle middle class, Ortner suggests this category does not exist, that it is either a "modest self-label for the upper middle class or a covering label for the lower middle class" (p. 71).

Despite the fact that classes, and class differences, exist in the United States, this is not generally recognized in the public discourse. Traditionally, most Americans have viewed themselves as part of the "middle class," so many in fact that the United States is widely considered to be a "classless" society. This fallacy was and is made possible by a widespread set of beliefs and practices that exist in the United States, as Sered and Fernandopulle (2005, p. 15) describe: ["Middle class" Americans] shared American values of family and hard work, they saw themselves as upwardly mobile, and they believed themselves the social equals of almost all other Americans. Perhaps most important, millions of middle class Americans followed the same clothing fashions, chose the same hairstyles, spoke in similar accents, shared the same standards of 'beauty,' and—at least superficially— looked like members of the same social grouping." Of course this perception of an inclusive and cohesive middle class in the United States is an illusion. Class differences do exist, and they matter. The difficulty that arises by not paying attention to them is that the influence of individuals' structural positions is often overlooked. This can, and does, lead to poor outcomes, like poverty, being blamed on the failings of individuals without consideration of the structural constraints they may have experienced.

Unfortunately this lack of appreciation for the presence and impact of class differences is not limited to public dialogue in the United States. It extends to neoliberal political discourse as well. The United States, for example, is one of the only developed Western nations that does not routinely report health statistics by class (Krieger, Chen, and Ebel 1997). Health policy in the United States also tends to neglect class disparities and instead focuses on race—a related issue as race is often an antecedent to class, but also a fundamentally different construct. Kawachi and colleagues (2005, 347) suggested that the focus on race in U.S. health policy is "the culmination of a longstanding ideological effort to suppress any consideration of class." They go on to argue that the purpose of early overt racism and later dog whistle politics in health and welfare reform was to undermine class solidarity and prevent support for redistribution policies and more generous social welfare provisions: "During the last 35 years, coded appeals to racism have been a consistent part of the strategy many conservative politicians have used to make the case for more limited government intervention on behalf of racial minorities and the economically disadvantaged more generally" (p. 349). They conclude by suggesting that both class and race must be considered in policy and assessments of health.

In relation to the ACA, Chernomas and Hudson (2013) make a similar argument. "The unique healthcare system of the United States is not the result of the will of the people, in any meaningful sense. Rather it is the result of a political battle between a relatively weak and disorganized working class, without any meaningful political representation, against a very well-funded and organized section of the corporate world, with an enormous stake in the continuation and expansion of a profit-making health care industry" (138). As the U.S. government began the process of health care reform after President Barack Obama was elected in 2008, it—for one reason or another—ended up working within this system. Thus, instead of a single-payer system, or even a public insurer option, the ACA maintained the existing for-profit, market-driven insurance system that had existed previously. While provisions like the expansion of Medicaid, the availability of subsidized insurance through the marketplace, and a mandate that insurance companies no longer deny coverage based on preexisting conditions arguably improved health care access for many, including many persons in the lower and lower middle classes, Chernomas and Hudson argue that members of the upper class—and particularly owners of pharmaceutical companies, insurance companies, HMOs, and other members of the medical industrial complex—were the true beneficiaries of the policy.

Texas and the ACA

With this background on class in the United States as a starting point, we can now turn to the particular case of Texas, and specifically how the ACA has played out in this area in relation to state culture and politics.

This in turn sets the stage for how the ACA differentially affected local residents because of their social class.

While generally considered part of the U.S. South, Texas is an entity unto itself. It is the second largest U.S. state, after Alaska, and has the second largest population, after California. Geographically, and in many ways culturally, Texas sits at multiple borders: between the U.S. South, the Great Plains, and the Southwest; and between Hispanic and Anglo America. It is also a bastion of island communities of Native Americans, Germans, Czechs, Poles, and other immigrant groups. Culturally, characteristics from all of these regions and peoples are blended to create a unique Texan worldview—and admittedly one that is ideologically "middle class," white, and Christian—which is held together by a fervent sense of devotion to the state by the majority of its citizens.

Before the Affordable Care Act went into effect, Texas boasted the highest rate of uninsured persons in the United States: 6.9 million people, or 23.7% of the state's population (U.S. Census Bureau 2011). In spite of these high numbers, most Texas politicians, including then governor Rick Perry, were strongly opposed to the implementation of the ACA. The state unsuccessfully sued the federal government to prevent the legislation from moving forward. When that was unsuccessful, the state leadership chose (1) to opt out of the Medicaid expansion portion of the program, (2) to not develop a state-based insurance exchange, and (3) to impose strict regulations on navigators—those hired to assist people in signing up for insurance through the federal marketplace—resulting in approximately 500 navigators to serve almost seven million uninsured Texans (Feibel 2014; Michels 2014).

Since then, many state leaders have continued to argue against the ACA and for the right to develop a program specific to the state. Echoing the neoliberal ideologies common in conservative political circles, Texas politicians specifically sought to develop a policy that "encourages personal responsibility, reduces dependence on the government, reins in program cost and efficiently improves coordination of care" (Rick Perry as quoted in Aaronson 2013). While not actually producing such a plan for consideration, many Texas politicians at all levels of government have continuously expressed their opposition to the ACA. Rick Perry, for example, referred to the implementation of the ACA as a "criminal act" (as quoted in Maloy 2015), and Texas senator Ted Cruz, who was responsible for a shutdown of the federal government in a failed attempt to repeal the legislation, has stated that Obamacare has "killed" millions of jobs, caused millions of people to lose their insurance, and led to an increase in medical costs (as quoted in Bash and Lee 2015).

This and similar rhetoric has been widely repeated throughout Texas, in town hall meetings, on local news programs, and in conversations around family dinner tables. Two sentiments were particularly common in the resulting discourse: The ACA takes freedom away from Texans, and the ACA provides support to groups who do not deserve it, including illegal immigrants. Of course, not all Texans viewed the ACA negatively. Some individuals advocated for the legislation, and grassroots organizations like Foundation Communities in Austin organized enrollment centers to help local residents understand the law (Jervis 2013). Overall, however, neoliberal calls for freedom and personal responsibility, as well as dog whistling, were the most prominent refrains. What was missing from the discussions was any consideration of social class.

One result of this situation was a slow decline in the number of uninsured persons in the years following the implementation of the ACA. By 2016, the percentage of uninsured Texans had decreased by 5.8 percentage points (to 17.9%), but it was still the highest percentage in the country and almost double the national average (Marks, Ho, and Sim 2016). Additional research showed that improvements in insurance coverage were directly related to income: Among Texans with incomes above 138% of the federal poverty level, uninsurance rates dropped by 42.3%, compared to only 15.0% for Texans with incomes below federal poverty level (Marks et al. 2016). While several possibilities exist for this trend, it is primarily the result of the coverage gap, which existed due to the state government's decision to not expand Medicaid. This gap made it virtually impossible for poor citizens in Texas to obtain health insurance; they were ineligible for Medicaid, often because they were adults under the age of 65, and they made too little to qualify for federal insurance subsidies through the marketplace.

Methods

The case studies examined in this chapter were collected as part of a larger ethnographic investigation into the experiences of uninsured Texans. The research took place in Hays County, a county in central Texas between the Austin and San Antonio metro areas, where demographic trends, including rates of health insurance uptake, mirrored the state averages (U.S. Census Bureau 2012). The interview portion of this project was limited to persons who were U.S. citizens and who had been uninsured for at least six months in the past year. Interview participants were recruited through a variety of methods, including fliers posted at job centers and food banks; handouts provided at health clinics and WIC offices; and messages posted to online neighborhood message boards including neighborhood Facebook pages. Interviews typically lasted between one and two hours and were conducted either in participants' homes or in public areas such as the meeting rooms at local libraries.

Thirty-one persons (18 women and 13 men) participated in interviews in the first year of the study (2013). In the following two years, a subsample of these individuals participated in follow-up interviews. The subsample was chosen based on a combination of personal characteristics and availability. Nine persons were excluded from subsequent interviews because they were insured at the time of their first interview. Seven additional persons could not be located for follow-up interviews—the phone numbers they provided were no longer in service and/or their email addresses were no longer valid. I had questionable interactions with two male informants and opted to not re-contact them, and finally, three persons chose not to be re-interviewed. This left ten people (seven women and three men) in the follow-up study.

The data presented in this chapter stem from interviews with three women who participated in the project for the duration of the research (from 2013 to 2015). Their interview data were specifically chosen for this chapter because the women were of similar ages, they were representative of different social classes, and they all lacked serious chronic medical conditions (which, among other things, directly influences social class). The fact that all three were women was not a purposeful decision but rather an artifact of the sample. Two out of the three male participants had serious chronic medical conditions—as did one of the female participants who was excluded for the same reason—and the third was a graduate student whose social class was indeterminate.

To ascertain social class, I followed the classification system described by Ortner (2006). Using a combination of the women's incomes, employment (or the employment of their husbands), and descriptions of their social support systems, I placed them into one of three categories: lower class, lower middle class, and upper middle class (no upper-class individuals were involved in any stage of the research). I also took into account how the women positioned themselves in relation to others during their interviews. These descriptions, included in the case studies below, strongly coincided with my own external assessment of their social classes. All of the women gave informed consent for each of their interviews, which were audio recorded and transcribed verbatim. Their names have been changed in this chapter to protect their identities.

Case Studies

Ana, Lower Class

Ana, who was 36 in the summer of 2013, grew up in central Texas, the only daughter of Mexican immigrants. Her family was poor and often had to scrape by to make ends meet. Growing up, Ana received periodic health care through county and state programs. As an adult, the only time she had health insurance was when she was 21 and a full-time employee at a local retail store. That job lasted just over a year. Since that time, Ana continued working at a string of different jobs—retail, seamstress, belly dance instructor, house sitter—but none offered even the option of health insurance.

When we first spoke in August 2013, Ana described herself as pre-diabetic and was experiencing pain in her right knee. Neither of these issues was being addressed. As Ana explained, she lacked the $75 needed to see her local doctor and she had little hope of ever having health insurance: "I just don't see [having insurance] as a possibility. I don't even count it as existing in my life. I just kind of deal with things and go 'Oh well, I'm sick. I'll get over it.' It's the way this country is." To address her health needs, Ana used a variety of strategies, including watching what she ate, praying, practicing Reiki, using over-the-counter medicines, and "sneaking" in questions when she accompanied her mother to appointments with health care providers. Ana had heard about "Obamacare," as she put it, from ads on the radio but did not know if or how it could help her. Her only hope for insurance, she said, was getting married to a man who had insurance through his employment.

In July 2014, Ana was not married, but she was receiving health care through Hays County Indigent Care—a county safety net program supported through property taxes that has limited funds and stringent eligibility requirements, including a condition that recipients make less than $300 per month. When Ana lost her retail job the previous May, she decided that this period of unemployment was a good time for her to enroll in this program (if she worked even part-time her income would likely exceed the $300 cutoff). While Ana was happy for an opportunity to have her health needs addressed, she was, at the same time, unhappy about the personal toll it took to apply for and be part of the county program: "I walked out of the interview feeling like life is horrible. They want you to stay down because if you advance, you're not worthy of that coverage. It's designed to keep you down." While Ana had continued to hear about the ACA from radio ads and from a few acquaintances over the past year, she emphatically stated that she did not understand it and did not know if it could help her, but she was upset about the tax penalty she heard she would need to pay.

Despite Ana predicting that she would only be able to stay with Indigent Care for six months (the time period before re-enrollment is required), when I spoke with her again in August 2015, she had been on the program for just over 14 months. The situation was a direct result of her mother's worsening condition. Ana spent the majority of her days taking care of her mother, whose dementia was quickly progressing, and was only able to work intermittently. During the past year she had gotten a suspicious mole removed, had physical therapy for her knee, received birth control, and had regular blood work to check for diabetes. She was, however, still unhappy about the toll the program took on her: "I don't pay a dime, but I do pay a price. I mean, you're constantly under the microscope. You're at the mercy of their paperwork. It's like constantly being watched by the cops. Anything you make, anything you do, something gets back to them . . . they'll drop me." Looking forward, Ana was not sure what her future would hold. Her primary concern was choosing between a job and her participation in Indigent Care, "You can't win. Be successful (which Ana later defined as being able to pay her basic utility bills without scrambling for money every month) and be up the creek with no help or stay down and miserable." Ana stated that she still did not understand Obamacare and wondered if it really worked. She was not able to get coverage from it, she did not understand how someone could, but she had not been penalized either, which confused her. In the last tax year, Ana hadn't made enough money to file income taxes, hence she did not incur a tax penalty.

Like many lower-class individuals in Texas, Ana fell into the Medicaid coverage gap. Even when she was working, she made too little to qualify for subsidized insurance through the marketplace. If the state of Texas had agreed to expand Medicaid, Ana's situation could have been quite different. She could have received the health care she needed without the constraints imposed on her by Hays County Indigent Care. Particularly, being on Medicaid would not have precluded Ana from earning more than $300 per month. In fact, as of 2016, Ana could have made $983.33 per month and still remained on Medicaid (Healthcare.gov), and if her income exceeded that she would have become eligible to receive subsidized insurance through the marketplace. The financial freedom this could offer Ana would likely be life-changing. Unfortunately, because Ana lived in Texas she did not have that option.

The other aspect of class that needs to be considered with regard to Ana's situation, and the reason why I wrote that Ana's condition *could* have been different (instead of *would* have been different), is that Ana existed so far outside of mainstream, "middle-class" Texas society that she knew almost nothing about the ACA. Like many lower-class individuals in Texas, Ana did not have a computer or Internet access in her home. Her main source of information about the ACA stemmed from radio ads that she listened to while driving her car. These ads, a minority from the federal government explaining the ACA and the majority from Texas government officials and other interested parties decrying the ACA, was the only exposure Ana had to the legislation. Her social network—her family, friends, and neighbors, who were largely in a similar social position to hers—was not well-informed about the ACA either, leading Ana to claim that not only did she not understand the ACA, but that neither did any of the people she knew. In a very real way, the legislation simply did not exist in her world. This issue, stemming from a combination of Ana's social class and a general lack of ACA promotion in both local and state arenas, would need to be addressed in order for Ana, and others like her, to be able to consider taking part in this program if it is ever made available to them.

Beth, Lower Middle Class

Beth, who was 34 in 2013, grew up in what she described as "a white, middle-class family" in Louisiana. She first moved to Texas with her husband and three children in 2008. Beth had insurance coverage as a child and in her early adult years while she worked full time. She stopped working after the birth of her first child and since then, ten years before our first interview, she had been living without health insurance. Her husband worked in construction and had intermittent personal coverage for himself through the years, but the costs to add Beth and their children to this insurance were prohibitively expensive for the family. While their children occasionally had insurance coverage through the Children's Health Insurance Program (CHIP), Beth had no coverage except Medicaid when she was pregnant.

When we first spoke in July 2013, Beth alternated between saying she was "fine" not having insurance because her children were "relatively healthy" and stating that she was afraid that one of her children would have an accident and she and her husband would not be able to pay the associated medical expenses. "We've just been lucky that we haven't had any major meningitis or broken bones or anything. So really, we live on a prayer, you know, that Bon Jovi song, 'Living on a Prayer,' I feel like we do that a lot." At this point, Beth had heard conflicting reports about the ACA, but she was not sure what to think about it herself: "It would be good to force us to get insurance, really, but at the same time, I don't know. It's going to be hard to bite that bullet and to have the extra monthly expense [of premiums]." She later explained that she was not happy about the government forcing her to do something, even if she needed to be forced. In the end, Beth planned on doing additional research on the ACA and talking with her husband to decide what they would do when the open enrollment period began the following October.

In July 2014, Beth reported that she and her family had gotten insurance coverage through the online marketplace. The deciding factor, she explained, had been the tax penalty. "We were just dragging our feet hoping that something would come through and they wouldn't require us to get insurance, but when we realized that wasn't going to happen then we figured if we were paying a fee anyway we might as well have health insurance." Beth and her family received a subsidy for half of her family's premium bill, leaving them to pay $450 per month for a mid-level (silver) plan. Her husband's employer offered to split the cost with them, but even with that help the family was struggling to make payments: "The insurance is expensive. . . . When you're living paycheck to paycheck already, that extra money is a lot." To compensate, Beth and her husband decided to have a "year of healing" where they aggressively took care of all of their health care needs, including vaccinations, wellness checks, and an overdue hernia repair for her husband. While Beth was happy to have this option, and more "relaxed" about what would happen if one of her family members had an accident, she was also very conflicted about the ACA itself. "I feel a little conscious about my insurance coming from the marketplace. Like socially. I've had people say, 'Well it's not Obamacare is it?' I really don't know how to answer them. . . . We aren't really supporters of Obamacare either." Despite these feelings, Beth stated that she was planning on continuing her insurance coverage through the marketplace the following year.

By August 2015, Beth and her family were again uninsured. In December 2014, they were informed that the cost of their premium (for the lowest priced silver plan, their only option for subsidized insurance) was going to double in the next calendar year and the family felt they could not afford the new cost. "We were barely making it as it was and we knew we wouldn't be able to afford [the cost increase] so we just let it lapse. We just let it go. Now we're uninsured again." Beth was not happy about this situation. She liked having health insurance because it allowed her family to address their health needs and because it was a "relief" to not worry about how they would pay for their medical costs if an accident occurred. Consequently, Beth wanted to get insurance coverage again "as soon as possible," but she was not sure how this could happen. In the past year her husband had started his own business, their family income varied significantly from month to month, and Beth had heard from family and friends that navigating the marketplace was doubly complicated if you were self-employed. She felt overwhelmed and wondered where she could go for help. With regard to the ACA specifically, Beth's feelings had become more negative over the past year, "So it just seems like it's a scam. 'You have to get insurance. Here's this great plan. You can afford this, right?' Well, not really, but we kind of had to make it work so we did. Then just a few months later, 'Oh, that plan is going to be double now. You can make that work now too right?' No, no we can't." She felt that the legislation should be overturned, or at a minimum drastically reconfigured, because it did not work for her family and because they were now going to be financially penalized for not being able to afford their insurance premiums.

As people living in a lower-middle-class household, which had an income of approximately $40,000–50,000 per year from 2013 to 2015, Beth and her family were eligible for subsidized insurance through the marketplace. For a time, Beth and her family were able to obtain health insurance and receive care for a number of pressing health needs, including her husband's hernia repair and surgery for Beth to treat previously undiagnosed ovarian cysts. In this way, Beth's experience highlights how the ACA benefited individuals and families.

At the same time, Beth's case also highlights a problematic aspect of the ACA that is common to many individuals in the lower middle class: confusion and concern about income-based tax credits. In Beth's case, she and her husband were completely confused about how to purchase insurance as a self-employed household. In large part because of the Texas government's decision to downplay the navigator program, Beth and her husband were unaware of where they could go for help. Even if they had accessed the navigator program, however, Beth and her husband would still have needed to guess how much income they would make in the following year. As described by Mulligan (this volume), this situation—disproportionately experienced by low-wage workers—often resulted in churning between coverage types as well as stress stemming from the uncertainty of making accurate income estimates. If a household underestimated how much they would earn, they would need to repay the subsidies. If they overestimated, however, they would end up spending more money every month for insurance and would have to wait for their tax refund to receive the offsetting credits.

Cate, Upper Middle Class

Cate, who was 35 in 2013, grew up in Texas. She met her husband while living in New York; after they were married they moved back to Texas where they had lived since. Cate and her husband had three children when we first spoke in 2013 and four, soon to be five, in 2015. Cate grew up in a white, upper-middle-class family and had insurance her entire life until she quit her job after giving birth to her first child. While Cate's husband had been employed continuously since they married, the job he had held for the past ten years, a contract position with the state government, did not offer health insurance. While Cate and her husband had considered private insurance "a few times," they had never purchased it because they felt it was cost-prohibitive. "The premiums for private insurance were around $1,200 a month, which was more than our mortgage. So we couldn't justify doing that." Instead Cate paid out of pocket, regularly negotiating prices with health care providers and, on occasion, hospitals. She felt that she and her husband were perfectly capable of meeting their family's health needs in this way and stated they did not want to have health insurance.

When I first spoke to Cate in September 2013, she was adamant that she was opposed to the ACA: "I was raised in Texas in a very conservative home where my rights and freedoms and liberties were really appreciated and so I don't appreciate being told that I have to do something. I like choice. I like being able to choose what I do for my family including making the choice to not have health insurance." At the same time, Cate and her husband had resigned themselves to the idea of getting health insurance to avoid paying the tax penalty and giving money to the government "unnecessarily." Cate did admit that having insurance would reduce her family's risk, specifically for paying high medical costs if they had an accident, and increase her own peace of mind, but she also felt it was not cost-effective nor, except in the case of medical emergencies, necessary. Citing years of experience, she felt that her family was generally healthy and that paying medical costs out of pocket, for regular checkups, prescriptions, dental and eye exams, and even occasional medical emergencies, was the most practical solution for her family.

Despite her negative feelings about the ACA, in July 2014 Cate reported that she and her family had chosen a plan from the marketplace. Because of their yearly household income, around $90,000 at that time, they did not qualify for assistance and were paying the full cost of a bronze plan premium (about $600 per month). Cate reported that the process of getting insurance through the marketplace had been problematic, even for her computer programmer husband. She couldn't understand how Healthcare.gov could be as bad of a website as she felt it was. In addition, Cate was very unsatisfied with her coverage. "The deductible is huge! We picked the plan that had the premiums we felt we could afford every month, but the deductible is like $6,000 for each individual, $12,000 for the family. It doesn't cover anything until you meet the deductible and I can tell you right now, we will never meet that deductible in a year." Part of Cate's dissatisfaction stemmed from the fact that she felt she could do better if allowed to manage on her own, negotiating prices and paying only for what was necessary instead of "$6,000 to $7,000 in premiums that isn't doing any good." Cate was still very opposed to the ACA and stated that she wasn't certain if she and her husband would keep their insurance coverage in the coming year. As alternatives, Cate was considering joining a health co-op or just paying the tax penalty, "depending on how much that really is."

Somewhat surprisingly, Cate still had the same insurance plan when we spoke again in August 2015. During the open enrollment window she became pregnant again and she and her husband became "too overwhelmed" to look into other options at that time. Instead they decided to try the coverage for another year to "see whether it was going to be worth it." By August, Cate did not think it was. While her family had used their insurance for well checks, they were left to pay for two of their children's broken bones on their own due to their plan's high deductible. Cate was certain that they were paying more for their health care now than they did before. Not only were they paying just over $700 a month in premiums at this point, Cate was also no longer able to negotiate the costs of care with her health care providers. "That negotiation process is eliminated entirely because 'Well, we billed your insurance and this is going towards your deductible. You can't negotiate a price that's going toward your deductible.' So now whatever the cost is what I'm paying." To address this issue, Cate had stopped using her health insurance for her family's sick visits. Instead, she told their health care providers that she was a cash patient and paid the cash patient rate instead. She stated that this practice saved her $25–$40 a visit. In the future, if her new baby was healthy, Cate was certain that she would cancel her insurance coverage, which she felt benefits others, particularly people with chronic conditions who need expensive care, but not her family. She questioned both the costs of health care in the United States and the way that the government was "interfering" with regard to insurance. In relation to the ACA, Cate stated, "It's a train wreck. We need to do something about it now. I think that should be, regardless of who comes into office next, one of their number one priorities to figure out how to fix this mess."

The situation described in Cate's experience, of having the ability, and particularly the income, to purchase health insurance prior to the ACA but purposefully choosing not to do so, was a phenomenon exclusive to the upper middle and upper classes. How the ACA affected these groups was also fundamentally different from how it impacted persons in the lower and lower middle classes like Ana and Beth. Instead of offering free care through Medicaid or reduced-cost insurance through tax credits, i.e., "carrots" to allow or entice individuals to enroll in insurance, the ACA only provided a "stick" to members of the upper middle and upper classes in the form of tax penalties for not being insured. Of course the tax penalties had more influence on members of the upper middle class like Cate, who had fewer assets than the truly wealthy. In Cate's case, these tax penalties directly led to her resentment of the ACA, which she saw as a form of government interference in her life that benefited others but not her family.

The other aspect of the ACA that disproportionately affected the upper middle class, and that Cate alluded to in her interviews, was the increasing cost of insurance premiums. When the ACA went into effect in 2014, many plans were priced aggressively low in order to entice healthy individuals—and particularly young, healthy individuals—to sign up for coverage. Not enough healthy individuals purchased insurance, however. Instead, people who became newly insured were often persons with chronic conditions who used a great deal of medical care. Together with ACA requirements that all insurance plans must offer a minimum level of care, this situation led to widespread, yearly increases in the cost of plans offered through the marketplace. As just one example of this, in Texas the premiums of the lowest price bronze plan increased 27% from 2015 to 2016 (Cox et al. 2016). Referred to as market stabilization, this process was ongoing and projected to continue until insurance companies could identify the price points at which they would make money based on their enrollment. Because upper-middle-class households were not eligible for subsidies, they bore the full cost of these increases. This in turn may have led to increasing numbers of upper-middle-class households, like Cate's, to decide that the threat of a tax penalty was not worth the cost of premiums.

Women and Health Care

In considering the experiences of Ana, Beth, and Cate, which portray a range of experiences with health care, health insurance, and the ACA, it becomes clear that there are points where their narratives converged and others where they were worlds apart. One important commonality that the women shared is that they were all women. This was, once again, not a purposeful methodological decision, but it provided a convenient opportunity to consider the gendered nature of care in the United States.

In every case, men who were interviewed for the larger study only reported being responsible for their own health care. Only one out of thirteen male participants was married and he had only been married for two months when we first spoke. Without exception, when people with families were interviewed, whether they had children, were living with extended family members such as parents, or a combination of these, it was the women in the family who opted to participate in the research. As described in the case studies, the health care overseen by these women was very much tied to their roles as daughters (Ana) and mothers (Beth and Cate). It involved making sure that their family members were "eating right" as they bought and prepared food, and exercising as they set family agendas and managed their family members' time. Taking care of their families' health also involved reminding family members to avoid "accidents" and when accidents did occur, or their family members became sick, proactively addressing the related health care needs through whatever means were available, including taking over-the-counter medications, seeking alternative forms of medical care, or paying to see a health care provider when necessary. In all of these efforts the women also reported taking measures to ensure they were being "responsible consumers," which for these women meant making the best, but also the most economical, decisions possible. In some cases this meant seeking alternatives to preferred medical care, especially for themselves. Beth and Cate in particular reported forgoing medical care for their own needs, but being less likely to do so for their children.

The gendered nature of care reflected in the study sample was largely representative of the gendered nature of care in Texas and to a large extent the United States as a whole. Ideologies of traditional gender roles—very prominent in Texas culture—put the onus of caring for children and other relatives disproportionately on women (Hooyman and Gonyea 1995; Sered and Fernandopulle 2005). As Hooyman and Gonyea (1995) have noted, this is generally done without recognition and at the cost of employment opportunities for the women involved. Because of the employment-based nature of the U.S. health insurance system, this meant that many women were at risk of not being able to obtain health insurance without a partner who was capable of working and providing it for them. This was the case for all of the women in this study. Each of them had forgone employment, and likely insurance opportunities, to fulfill the roles of daughter and mother. While Ana lacked a partner who could provide her with insurance or the money to purchase insurance, Beth and Cate were in better circumstances primarily because of their marital statuses. In this way, gender and expected gender roles were intimately connected with both health care and social class.

Social Class, Health Care, and the ACA

In contrast to the women's similarities in circumstances because of their gender, the great differences in these women's experiences stemmed from their structural positions, and more particularly the social classes they occupied. Incomes and social capital—including the family members, friends, and neighbors these women interacted with, as well as the degree to which they were included or marginalized in the predominantly "middle-class," white, Christian society of Hays County—had substantial impacts on how these women experienced health, health care, and the ACA. Most obviously, the women differed with regard to their knowledge of the ACA, their abilities to access Healthcare.gov, and their abilities to purchase insurance through the marketplace. Less obvious, but not less important, was how their social classes affected their perceptions and experiences of risk, health, health care, and the changes brought about by the ACA. The following sections examine these issues.

Living without Health Insurance: Risk and Embodiment

Differences based on social class did not begin or end with these women's abilities to obtain health care through the ACA. They extended to how the women lived their lives, including how they managed risks and how their abilities to do so were manifested in their own bodies.

While all of the women in the case studies sought to manage their health as well as that of their family members through diet, exercise, lifestyle choices, and even health care when they felt that was necessary, the primary concern for Ana, Beth, and Cate was "accidents." Accidents were sometimes a vague concept in the interviews, but they always implied significant, unexpected, negative health outcomes and associated high medical costs. To mitigate the risks associated with the unknowns inherent to accidents, all of the women, including a begrudging Cate, felt that some form of insurance was necessary. Without this, all of them admitted feeling vulnerable. Beth, for example, described living with the possibility of accidents without health insurance as "living on a prayer."

The specifics of how risk was articulated, and how it was lived, however, varied by social class. For Ana, life itself was risky. The choice between finding a job to make enough money to pay her bills every month and losing her health care, or keeping her health care but "remaining down" was a constant concern that filtered through all aspects of her life. She was constantly stressed about money, caring for her elderly mother, and wondering how she could best care for herself. Not only was her income limited but so were the social networks she could turn to for help. Beth, on the other hand, felt that she had few options with regard to health care because her household could not afford any of the available insurance plans even with the government subsidy. This made her constantly worried that "something bad" would happen that would "ruin" the tenuous hold she had on her life. Particularly, Beth was concerned with the possibility of losing her home if she or one of her family members had an accident. Cate was also concerned, but less so. Her family had weathered health emergencies, including multiple emergency surgeries and hospitalizations, without health insurance in the past and had the savings and social capital necessary to negotiate all of them. Whatever happened, Cate felt that "everything would ultimately be OK."

The differences in how these women were able to manage the risks in their lives were ultimately manifested in their own bodies. Ana's lack of health care over the course of her life left its mark; she was close in age to both Beth and Cate but looked almost a decade older. While Ana was able to receive care for her medical issues, particularly her pre-diabetes and injured knee, through Hays County Indigent Care, there were a number of "cosmetic" issues the program would not cover, including a significant nail fungus and advanced periodontal disease. These conditions made Ana physically different from the other women in the study, and arguably most people in the United States who can readily access health care. Beth also reported untreated ailments, including ovarian cysts which were undiagnosed and untreated until she obtained health insurance and received care in 2014. While this was an internal issue, and consequently not as noticeable as Ana's nail fungus or gum disease, it also reflects the embodied reality of living without health insurance. With regard to Cate, however, none of this was an issue. While she had occasionally put off seeking health care for herself, this only occurred when she felt the issue was minor and would resolve on its own. She did not short her children's health care under any circumstances, and she also occasionally sought care for "cosmetic" issues including braces for her children. Like all of the women in this study, Cate embodied her social class.

Perceptions of the ACA: Reproducing Local and Class Ideologies

Differences based on social class were also apparent with regard to these women's experiences with and perspectives on health insurance generally and the ACA particularly. Ana, for instance, had lived outside of the U.S. health care system for the majority of her life. She felt disadvantaged and marginalized because of this and bemoaned her current situation, which she saw as choosing between making a living, particularly eating and paying bills, and receiving health care. Beth, however, described having health insurance as the "responsible" thing to do. She felt embarrassed by not having insurance, stating that it signified she was unable to care for herself and her family the way she should. Cate, on the other hand, argued that her personal choice to forgo insurance, which was financially the most responsible in her mind, was being undermined by the ACA. Unlike Ana, she did not feel disadvantaged or marginalized by her lack of health insurance and, like many Texas politicians who also belong to the upper middle class, bemoaned the federal government's interference in her life.

Differences caused by social class were also apparent with regard to how local ideologies of the ACA were reproduced by each of these women. Ana, and by her report the members of her largely lower-class social network, were generally uninformed about the ACA. This is directly related to her lack of access to information about the legislation. In contrast, lower-middle-class Beth reproduced local and state neoliberal ideology by referring to having insurance as the responsible thing to do. She felt guilty about not being in a position to be insured because of both her income and her lack of knowledge about how to navigate the marketplace. At the same time she also felt guilty about obtaining health insurance through "Obamacare" and, once that became unaffordable for her household, for wanting it back. Cate was the most well-informed about the ACA. In addition to information she obtained from the Internet, she had read newspaper articles; listened to advertisements, news programs, and public debates on television; and discussed the legislation with those around her who were similarly informed. While Cate reported that some members of her social network expressed approval at her getting health insurance, the majority of her social network felt as she did, that government interference was inherently wrong and that the ACA should be overturned. Thus, while all of these women lived in close geographical proximity to one another, and while they each were similarly affected by local ideologies including gender role expectations, they also were very much the products of their particular social classes.

Reconciling Lived Experiences

In reconciling the neoliberal ideal prominent in Texas—one based on independence and self-reliance—with their lived experiences, it is apparent that all of the women in this study fall short. Even Cate, who is generally representative of the "middle-class" ideal in this area of Texas, was unable to obtain health care through employment-based insurance. In response, each of the women in this study sought to reconcile the disjunctions between the ideal and their own experiences, albeit, once again, in ways that reflected their particular social class.

Ana, for example, repeatedly cited the structural barriers that prevented her from getting health insurance, including being responsible for an ailing parent, the limited number of full-time jobs available to her, and the fact that she would lose the safety net medical coverage that she had if she started making more than $300 a month. Likewise, Beth explained how her best efforts at obtaining insurance through the marketplace were thwarted by a combination of a confusing and difficult to access Healthcare.gov website and insurance plans that were too costly based on her family budget. Cate meanwhile took an extreme neoliberal view by posturing that health insurance in her case was generally unnecessary because she was capable of managing her own risks. While excusing themselves in these ways, the women also occasionally questioned if others in similar or worse circumstances to their own were deserving of help or just "lazy." In this way they perpetuated state and even national stereotypes of uninsured persons as lazy, incapable, and hence undeserving of help, while at the same time recognizing that this was not true in their own lives. In other words, they questioned whether their experiences were the exception rather than the rule.

Another aspect of their experiences that the women in this study sought to reconcile was their questioning of the U.S. health care system and their role in changing that system. While their particular questions varied, all of the women wondered about the true costs of health care. They collectively felt that costs for everything, including doctor visits, hospital stays, prescriptions, and medical equipment, were inflated and argued that there was no way to know what the true cost of anything was. For Ana and Beth this was a point of irritation, for Cate it was a reason to negotiate prices. In all of the cases it went against the neoliberal ideal of a "rational consumer" who is fully informed and able to make their own health care decisions.

Coinciding with the belief that actual costs of health care were inflated and true costs were unknowable, all of the women in this study also questioned the health care system in the United States generally, including why insurance, and an insurance-driven health care system, was necessary. They further suggested that significant changes, from the government tweaking the ACA to address burgeoning health care costs to a complete overhaul of the existing system, were necessary. However, none of the women were willing to make a call to action to change the system. Instead, they argued, like Beth, that as individuals there "isn't much that [we] can do." In this way all of the women in this study, as suggested by Chernomas and Hudson (2013), lacked the class consciousness to challenge the well-funded and politically powerful health care industry that benefits the upper class in the United States at the expense of everyone else.

Conclusion

While one of the primary purposes of the ACA was to increase access to health insurance, and thus health care, the results of the legislation so far have produced mixed results that—as the research presented in this chapter has shown—were not unrelated to issues of social class that existed prior to the implementation of the legislation. In Texas, the state government opted to not expand Medicaid, which resulted in a coverage gap that prevented hundreds of thousands of lower-class individuals and families in the state, including Ana, from accessing health care coverage (Garfield and Damico 2016). And even when subsidized coverage could be obtained, affording that insurance in light of increasing costs was still an issue for some lower-middle-class households like Beth and her family. Finally, as the example of Cate and her household illustrated, even when insurance could be obtained and maintained, it did not mean that the coverage translated to health care. High deductible plans left many people underinsured, and the increasing cost of premiums might have pushed reluctant upper-middle-class households, who did not already receive health care through employment, away from purchasing health care through the marketplace.

Thus, even though the women in this study were around the same age, lived in close geographical proximity to one another, and were subject to the same legislation in the form of the ACA, they experienced strikingly different outcomes based on their social class. At the same time, their social class alone did not determine their particular outcomes. None of the women in this study were simply victims of their incomes or social capital. They made complex decisions based on their own histories and current situations. In this way, even though they were constrained by their structural positions, as well as their own and others' perceptions of these, they were doing the best they could under their specific circumstances.

So where does all of this leave us? Studies have repeatedly shown that people without health insurance, and particularly people living in poverty, are more likely to have serious health issues that lead to disability and death (CDC 2009; Kronick 2009; Wilkinson 1997). While the ACA was, at least ideally, meant to lessen differences in people's abilities to access health care, the reality of what the ACA did was more complicated. As has been reported elsewhere (see the Mulligan chapter in this volume for one example), and as I have found in my own research, the ACA did help many obtain to access to health care. The impact of the legislation, however, was mitigated by geography and, as this chapter has shown, by social class as well.

State choices in the implementation of the ACA, together with state and local discourses around health care reform, have led to an increasing bifurcation of health citizenship based on social class and geography. As the research in this chapter suggests, an alternative is needed. While popular sentiment in Texas favored the repeal of the ACA and a return to the previous system of non-subsidized market-based care, this would not fix the problem. The better option is likely the opposite—a single-payer health care system where health care is viewed as a human right and is openly available to all, regardless of social class. Without this type of system, increasing stratification in access to health care, and through this increasing inequality between social classes, is likely to occur.

For the United States to transition to a single-payer system, however, several conditions must be met, including a recognition of social class in the United States, an understanding of how dog whistling and neoliberal politics are used to obscure class differences (i.e., viewing being uninsured as a choice, like the public health official I once spoke to did), and an appreciation for how class differences lead to disparities in health. Widespread recognition of these factors could provide the impetus for members of the lower, lower middle, and even upper middle classes— the vast majority of Americans—to join together to challenge the economically and politically powerful medical industrial complex. As the women in this study described, as individuals there is not much we can do to change the U.S. health care system, but collectively there is. Class consciousness and a class-based movement for change that this would bring could provide the impetus for significant health care reform in the United States.

ACKNOWLEDGMENTS

My research into this topic would not have been possible without the participation of many Hays County residents, health care providers, and directors and administrators of county programs. I would especially like to thank the women known as Ana, Beth, and Cate in this chapter for their time and their willingness to share their stories with me. The overall project was funded by a Research Enhancement Program grant from Texas State University.

REFERENCES

Aaronson, Becca. 2013. Texas Again Has Highest Uninsured Rate in Nation. *Texas Tribune*, August 18.

Bash, Dana, and Lee, M. J. 2015. Ted Cruz Going on Obamacare. CNN, March 24.

Becker, Gay. 2004. Deadly Inequality in the Health Care "Safety Net": Uninsured Ethnic Minorities' Struggle to Live with Life-Threatening Illnesses. *Medical Anthropology Quarterly* 18(2): 258–275.

———. 2007. The Uninsured and the Politics of Containment in U.S. Health Care. *Medical Anthropology* 26(2): 299–321.

CDC. 2009. The Power of Prevention: Chronic Disease: The Public Health Challenge of the 21st Century, www.cdc.gov.

Chernomas, Robert, and Ian Hudson. 2013. *To Live and Die in America: Class, Power, Health and Healthcare.* Halifax: Fernwood Publishing.

Cox, Cynthia, Michelle Long, Ashley Semanskee, Rabah Kamal, and Gary Claxton. 2016. Analysis of 2017 Premium Changes and Insurer Participation in the Affordable Care Act's Health Insurance Marketplaces. *Kaiser Family Foundation*, kff.org.

Feibel, Carrie. 2014. Texas Issues Tough Rules for Insurance Navigators. *Houston Public Media*, January 23.

Garfield, Rachel, and Anthony Damico. 2016. The Coverage Gap: Uninsured Poor Adults in States that Do Not Expand Medicaid—An Update. *Henry J. Kaiser Family Foundation*, kff.org.

Healthcare.gov. 2016. Federal Poverty Level (FPL), www.healthcare.gov.

Hooyman, Nancy R., and Judith Gonyea. 1995. *Feminist Perspectives on Family Care: Policies for Gender Justice.* Thousand Oaks, CA: Sage.

Horton, Sarah, and Judith C. Barker. 2010. Stigmatized Biologies: Examining the Cumulative Effects of Oral Health Disparities for Mexican American Children. *Medical Anthropology Quarterly* 24(2): 199–219.

Jervis, Rick. 2013. "Obamacare" and You: Resistance in Texas, Where Many Are Uninsured. *USA Today*, September 23. www.usatoday.com.

Kawachi, Ichiro, Norman Daniels, and Dean E. Robinson. 2005. Health Disparities by Race and Class: Why Both Matter. *Health Affairs* 24(2): 343–352.

Krieger, Nancy, Jarvis T. Chen, and Gregory Ebel. 1997. Can We Monitor Socioeconomic Inequalities in Health? A Survey of U.S. Health Departments' Data Collection and Reporting Practices. *Public Health Reports* 112(6): 481–491.

Kronick, Richard. 2009. Health Insurance Coverage and Mortality Revisited. *Health Services Research* 44(4): 1211–1231.

Maloy, Simon. 2015. Obamacare Is Helping Texas, No Thanks to Rick Perry and Ted Cruz. *Salon*, www.salon.com.

Marks, Elena, Vivian Ho, and S-C Sim. 2016. Changes in Rates and Characteristics of the Uninsured among Texans Ages 18–64 from 2013 to 2016. *Rice University's Baker Institute and the Episcopal Health Foundation*, www.episcopalhealth.org.

Michels, Patrick. 2014. Texas' Health Care Navigator Rules Could Be Sweet Deal for Pearson and Other Companies. *Texas Observer*, www.texasobserver.org.

Ortner, Sherry B. 2006. *Anthropology and Social Theory: Culture, Power and the Acting Subject.* Durham, NC: Duke University Press.

Rank, Mark R. 2004. *One Nation, Underprivileged: Why American Poverty Affects Us All.* New York: Oxford University Press.

Sered, Susan S., and Rushika Fernandopulle. 2005. *Uninsured in America: Life and Death in the Land of Opportunity.* Berkeley: University of California Press.

U.S. Census Bureau. 2011. *Current Population Reports: Consumer Income. Income, Poverty, and Health Insurance Coverage in the United States*, www.census.gov.

———. 2012. *State and County Quickfacts: Hays County, Texas*, quickfacts.census.gov.

Wilkinson, Richard G. 1997. Health Inequalities: Relative or Absolute Material Standards. *British Medical Journal* 314: 592–595.

The ACA's Accountability Contradictions

The ACA created new responsibilities for the provision and financing of health insurance. Primary among these responsibilities was the individual mandate, which required most people to obtain insurance or pay a fine. The chapters collected in this third section describe the social distribution of new responsibilities under the ACA and relate how people responded to the call to get enrolled, improve their health, and pay for coverage. These chapters collectively demonstrate that the accountability, responsibility, and transparency that were demanded of patients, clients, and providers were not equally expected from lawmakers, administrators, and insurance companies.

Rather than providing the uninsured with government health care, the ACA followed a structure of *delegated governance*—namely, the public/private partnership—that had been the primary model for public policy provision in the United States since the 1990s. Under a delegated governance model, core government-financed services are administered by non-profit organizations as well as for-profit companies through contractual arrangements. In the case of the ACA, consumers were required to purchase coverage from private carriers on publicly regulated insurance exchanges. Even most of those who qualified for coverage under Medicaid received their services via private insurers because the majority of Medicaid programs in the United States follow a privatized managed-care model.

A major issue that arises when services are delegated is that of accountability and trust. How can government funders be sure that services are provided according to federal and state guidelines? How does the public know that monies have been spent responsibly? The major tool for ensuring accountability under delegated governance is the audit. Some argue that the proliferation of auditing that is common in health care settings is actually indicative of a profound lack of trust in the major institutions that govern social life (Power 1997). The rise of

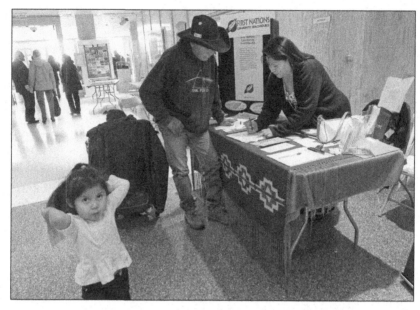

Figure S3.1. New Mexico Insurance Sign-Up. Delbert Saunders speaks with Marsha Pino of First National Community Health Service at the State Capitol on Tuesday, February 4, 2014, in Santa Fe, New Mexico. They spoke about medical enrollment and health insurance exchange. Saunders's granddaughter, Samara Garcia, age 3, waits in the foreground. (AP photo/*Santa Fe New Mexican*, Jane Phillips)

populism and social movements calling for the repeal of the ACA are also evidence that trust has waned in government institutions and in the power of government to affect positive change. Ironically, this lack of trust makes auditing even more pervasive.

The first accountability contradiction in the ACA is that it asks the most of those who are least in a position to change the system, what policy anthropologists Shore and Wright have termed "responsibility without power" (2000, 70). Susan Shaw illustrates this contradiction with her chapter on people who gained access to coverage in Massachusetts, only to then be subjected to cost accounting and audit procedures used by their new insurance companies. She shows how attempts to rein in prescription drug prices by managing drug formularies (the list of covered drugs) placed huge burdens on patients and providers, who were forced to adjust their care plans. Rather than addressing the costs of prescription drugs at a national or state level, delegating this fiduciary responsibility to insurance companies meant that they in turn passed on the cost and inconveniences to consumers.

The second core contradiction of accountability under the ACA is that audits can spiral out of control; sometimes accountability talk can be used to make accusations against one's political foes or to mask a lack of oversight. Cathleen E. Willging's and Elise M. Trott's chapter illustrates some of the cynical uses to which accountability talk can be put in their chronicle of the dismantling of New Mexico's behavioral health safety net amid false allegations of fraud. Good governance goals can produce a fear of corruption that allows accusations to be wielded against politically vulnerable or unpopular groups (Cruikshank 1999).

The final accountability contradiction is found in the chapter by Mary Alice Scott and Richard Wright, which explores ACA implementation

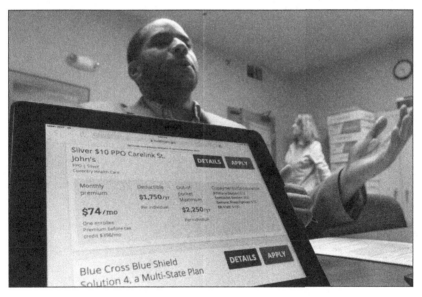

Figure S3.2. "You're Responsible to Sign Up For Coverage." In this March 31, 2014, file photo, navigator John Jones explains the many options to a client seeking help buying health insurance at the Family Guidance Center in Springfield, Illinois. According to a report published Monday, April 28, 2014, by market research firm Avalere Health, the click-by-click hunt for a health plan that would cover a particular drug or a favorite doctor proved frustrating for many consumers navigating the new insurance exchanges. It's the first systematic analysis of consumer experience on the new insurance exchanges. (AP photo/Seth Perlman, file)

in a formerly free clinic in southern New Mexico. Here, the use of terms like "patient engagement" and "co-responsibility" by health care providers obscures the structural limitations on people's ability to act in the "responsible" ways that ACA policy requires. Initiating and following through on enrollment transactions, obtaining eligibility documents, and getting to and from appointments require overcoming, often insurmountable, barriers for the homeless, marginally housed, and undocumented population served by Family Health Care Clinic. While health policymakers often assume that people are not taking enough responsibility for their lives, ethnographic attention shows that they are drowning in responsibilities.

REFERENCES

Cruikshank, Barbara. 1999. *The Will to Empower: Democratic Citizens and Other Subjects*. Ithaca, NY: Cornell University Press.

Power, Michael. 1997. *The Audit Society: Rituals of Verification*. Oxford: Oxford University Press.

Shore, Cris, and Susan Wright. 2000. Coercive Accountability: The Rise of Audit Culture in Higher Education. In *Audit Cultures: Anthropological Studies in Accountability, Ethics and the Academy*. Edited by Marilyn Strathern, 57–89. London and New York: Routledge.

8

The Responsibility to Maintain Health

Pharmaceutical Regulation of Chronic Disease among the Urban Poor

SUSAN J. SHAW

The ACA was modeled after Massachusetts's 2006 health care reform law, known as Chapter 58. Envisioned at the time as then-Governor Mitt Romney's signature legislative achievement that would undergird his eventual bid for the White House, Chapter 58 embodied the neoliberal goals of transparency and strict cost control measures to slow the state's rapidly increasing health care costs (Seifert and Cohen 2010), at the same time as it expanded access to health insurance for low- and moderate-income families. Despite the rise of Tea Party conservatism that required Romney to disavow Chapter 58 as his signature accomplishment (or to claim it as only a cost control measure), the twin demands of expanded access and controlling costs continue to guide Massachusetts's engagement with the ACA. This chapter explores the ways in which patients and health care providers at a Massachusetts community health center were made accountable to private sector rationalities of *transparency, individual responsibility*, and *cost-effectiveness* in chronic disease management under health care reform.

In many ways, Massachusetts policymakers looked to the ACA as a welcome source of new federal dollars for insurance subsidies that would "free up state dollars" for benefits not included in the ACA (Seifert and Cohen 2010, 5). In other ways, however, the federal law was less welcome: Many of its reforms and standards did not go as far as the previous Massachusetts reform: For example, the federal subsidies for insurance premiums for people with low- to moderate incomes were lower than the previous state subsidies for those groups. Furthermore,

ACA reductions in payments to safety-net hospitals could cost the state's hospitals a half-billion dollars over ten years (6–7).

The ACA replicated concerns with both expanding access and controlling costs seen in Massachusetts's 2006 health insurance reform law. Despite already high levels of insurance coverage (93% prior to 2006), Massachusetts lawmakers were able to expand access to health insurance in part by appealing to the ethical value of distributive justice. In a 2009 article in *Health Affairs*, Jon Kingsdale, director of the Massachusetts Health Insurance Connector, made the case for cost control this way:

> Massachusetts took the ethical high ground and chose to begin [its cost control battle] with near-universal coverage. To the standard arguments that we must reduce waste in order to control government spending and remain internationally competitive, we have added this imperative: only by controlling costs can Massachusetts sustain near-universal coverage. Everyone acknowledges this argument. It might not suffice to tip the balance against entrenched resistance, but it does give moral weight to the dry, abstract argument for cost containment. (Kingsdale 2009, w589)

This yoking of ethical claims to economic justifications (and vice versa) was enabled by the capacious meaning of accountability, which can encompass abstract values of good government such as transparency and cost control, as well as concrete ways of "doing business" (Harvey 2005; Shore and Wright 1999). Similar to the way ideals of "empowerment" can morph uncomfortably into "individual responsibility" (Gupta and Sharma 2006; Shaw 2012) as techniques of good governance, accountability and transparency may exacerbate inequality as much as they ameliorate it.

Anthropologies of Accountability

Anthropologists and others have adopted the rubric of "accountability" to analyze the extension of neoliberal policies into diverse sectors of social and economic life. In contrast to the norms of justice, service, or humanitarianism that previously governed the nonprofit sector (Clarke 2007; Rose 1996) and certain areas of health care (Rivkin-Fish 2011), *practices of accountability* extend private sector policies such as cost control, "outcome funding," or "return on investment" (Li 2009; Pels 2000) to new domains including safety-net health care organizations.

In studies of accountability, anthropologists and others have examined the social relations invoked by the actual technologies of accounting and audit (e.g., Strathern 2000b), as well as rhetorics of accountability in public education (Sloan 2007), higher education (Shore and Wright 1999; Strathern 2000a), international development (Clark et al. 2003; Young et al. 2007), and finance and business (e.g., contributors to Strathern 2000a). Accountability has also been understood as the ethical injunction to take responsibility or be held responsible for wrongdoing (Borneman 1997; Drexler 2006; Li 2009; Sawyer 2006). Calls for increased transparency in the nonprofit or philanthropic sector reveal the social injunction to be accountable to others (Bornstein 2009). Despite the breadth of these studies, fewer anthropologists have turned the lens of accountability to analyses of health care in the United States.[1]

Opinions remain divided as to whether Massachusetts's health care reform law and the ACA each represented neoliberal health policy; however, it is clear that the practices through which the ACA was implemented, including the guiding norms of transparency, responsibility, and cost control, reflected broader trends in social policy. Norms of transparency and cost control are key values in what Maryon McDonald calls the "new managerialism" of the nonprofit sector, where "Discipline and accountancy, financial and human accountability, were merged" (McDonald 2000, 109–110). An anthropological understanding of accountability highlights both the practices through which these policies are implemented and the ideologies that frame them. An accountability framework focuses our attention on both the organizational actors who carry out such policies (Boehm 2005; Lamphere 2005) as well as the citizens who are subject to demands for individual responsibility (e.g., López 2005). Pat O'Malley has examined the ways in which individual responsibility intertwines with practices of accountability. He terms the neoliberal injunction for rational citizens to maximize their personal resources while taking steps to minimize risk "privatized actuarialism" (O'Malley 1996, 198, cited in Raikhel and Garriott 2013). O'Malley writes,

Following privatized actuarialism, individuals reflexively apply to their own lives the same technique used to audit . . . corporations and bureaucracies. As in the spheres of insurance, finance, and global politics, the application of risk assessment techniques at the scale of individual lives is a means for controlling and even profiting from the particular contingencies of post-Fordist, finance-based capitalism. Specifically, the model actuarial self is expected to indemnify itself against the increased risks of unemployment and lack of health . . . while simultaneously reaping the economic rewards that come with exercising their own flexible and sometimes risky responses to this field of contingency. (O'Malley 1996, 198)

Analyses of accountability can help us understand the ways in which individual subjectivities are shaped through their encounters with overarching social and economic structures, while making visible ideologies of individual responsibility and risk minimization. Under the ACA, for example, individuals are expected to select the most advantageous health insurance plan with a minimum of (allowable) guidance from navigators or enrollment counselors. Health care and other service providers are also affected: as technologies of accountability reshape our encounters with each other, health care providers must enact and understand their work in new ways. Both health care providers and patients experience increased burdens of documentation and verification (López 2005; Power 1997). Part of a larger project that examines the forces and rhetorics of accountability in chronic disease management under health care reform, this chapter explores the experiences of patients and health care providers in Massachusetts who struggled to manage chronic illnesses under contradictory policies of expanded access and cost control regimes.

Methods

Caring Health Center, where I have conducted research since 1998, is a federally funded, Section 330 primary care clinic that cares for predominantly low-income and minority patients. It is located in Springfield, Massachusetts, a city with a population of 157,000 people, 29% of whom live below the poverty level. The burdens of poverty are not equally distributed, however: more than three times as many Latinos (42%) and twice as many African Americans (26.2%) as whites (13.5%) lived in poverty in 2008.[2]

This chapter presents qualitative findings from a four-year, prospective study that combined a self-report survey, medical chart abstracts, and four qualitative methods. The quantitative survey sample includes 76 African American, 97 Latino, 38 white, 56 Russian-speaking, and 100 Vietnamese immigrant patients at Caring Health Center who were diagnosed with diabetes and/or hypertension.[3] Our sample reflects the clinic's general population, which tends to be publicly insured and to have relatively low income and education levels. A subsample of 61 survey participants also completed one or more qualitative data collection activities. We conducted 50 in-depth interviews, 27 chronic disease diaries, 11 home visits, and one focus group. Interviews were audio-recorded, transcribed, translated into English if conducted in another language, and entered into the qualitative database for coding.[4] Transcripts were coded following an open-coding method and analyzed using Atlas.ti, a qualitative data management program. In addition, between 2008 and 2012 I periodically attended monthly meetings of western Massachusetts outreach workers, employed by area community health centers and hospitals, that were sponsored by a local nonprofit health care advocacy organization. Field notes were transcribed and entered into the qualitative database for analysis.

Techniques of Cost Control

After Massachusetts passed its Chapter 58 reforms in 2006, policymakers and advocates heralded the subsequent increase of the state's insured rates to 97% (Long 2008). To accomplish this, the state led the way with two innovations that were later incorporated into the ACA: state-funded outreach workers and an online health insurance exchange, both designed to help recruit and enroll uninsured people into publicly funded plans (see also Joseph, this volume). With expanded access came expanded costs, however (Blendon et al. 2008; Steinbrook 2008), and during the first few years after Chapter 58 and the ACA, the enrollment apparatus seemed designed to fail as often as it succeeded. While many residents benefited enormously from their expertise, at monthly meetings Massachusetts outreach workers detailed the multiple ways the MassHealth bureaucracy effectively deterred applicants from enrolling in state-supported health insurance. Outreach workers narrated a process of what Shari Danz (2000) calls *bureaucratic disentitlement*, in which citizens are denied their "statutory entitlements" when representatives of the state are literally unavailable or demand long wait times for access (Danz 2000, p. 1006, cited in Lopez 2005, 28).[5] Leslie Lopez provides a similar account of the frustrations encountered by both patients and outreach workers seeking to enroll clients into New Mexico's Medicaid managed care program, known as Salud!: "The complexity of Salud! enrollment, the lack of information on how to achieve it, the systemic disjunctures between Medicaid and Salud!, and the deterritorialized phone system it required added a layer of almost surreal gateways that made enrollment more difficult, especially for very vulnerable populations" (29).

Under both Chapter 58 and the ACA, the Massachusetts enrollment bureaucracy seemed to actively hinder the completion and submission of paperwork in response to eligibility verification requests. Massachusetts outreach workers cited frequent examples of such obstruction, as when the enrollment center lost a patient's application or supporting documents, or sent out multiple notification letters on a single day, each with a different response or directive.[6] In an online survey conducted in 2008 by the Boston-based Community Partners, one outreach worker wrote, "When you ask for a supervisor they disconnect you," and another, "when I request a supervisor they never come to the phone." Outreach workers described spending hours on hold waiting to speak to a customer service agent,[7] sending and re-sending requested paperwork that was never received, or submitting information online that was somehow mangled in transit. Fixing these errors frequently required access to the supervisor of the customer service representatives who staffed the phone lines, but supervisors were rarely available. Danz argues that "bureaucratic disentitlement, effectuated through such practices [as these] prevents the transformation of statutory rights into tangible benefits" (Danz 2000, 1006, cited in Lopez, 28), even as New Mexico's health insurance reform was "buttressed by discourses that emphasize competition, efficiency, and individual choice" (Lamphere 2005,19).

These measures of deferral, disinformation, and delay in enrollment served the larger goal of limiting state expenditures on health benefits by shrinking the pool of insured people and limiting the number of days per year of their publicly subsidized coverage. Other cost control measures designed to promote greater accountability, such as periodic (every year or even more frequent) eligibility recertification, also turned away current and would-be enrollees. As a result, many of the uninsured were those who fell into the gap produced by "churning the rolls"— when problems completing, submitting, or processing eligibility re-certification forms terminated coverage. If this happened, patients had to re-apply for coverage, starting the whole process over again (Seifert and Littell-Clark 2013). Since this could take months, poor people who were sick could have significant gaps in care even while theoretically "covered" by expanded access programs (see also López 2005). Eligibility re-certifications were just one of the "rituals of verification" (Power 1997) inherent in accountability measures that enacted the deterrent function of bureaucracy in Massachusetts health care reform.

Cost control efforts in Massachusetts were driven by the state's contradictory desire to expand access to health insurance coverage while balancing the budget. These contradictions and ambiguities were experienced by health care providers and patients who were subject to state health insurance and other programs that sought to implement norms of accountability, cost control, and transparency. The resulting stark contradictions were lived by low-income patients with chronic illness at a safety-net community health center. An analysis that focuses on discourses of accountability can reveal the meeting point of social structures, such as health policies and the health care organizations that enact them, and subjectivities which may be shaped by new forms of social relations invoked by specific techniques of governing. The state's effort to implement contradictory goals of expanded access and cost control produced feelings of distrust and insecurity in patients, and could lead to profound health consequences when patients were unable to access needed appointments or medications.

Findings: Experiences of Accountability in Chronic Disease Management

Patients and physicians at Caring Health Center experienced account-ability in chronic disease care in at least three ways. First, patients and their physicians were subject to MassHealth and other insurers' chang-ing formularies (the list of covered medications for a given insurance plan), a common cost-saving technique.[8] Second, patients were confronted by the costs of their care in the form of statements mailed from their insurance companies detailing the patient's share compared to the actual costs of their medications. Third, many patients we spoke with struggled to pay the out-of-pocket costs for their medications. If patients were uninsured or a medication was not covered by their insurance formulary, a patient was responsible for the drug's full cost. These challenges affected patients' overall health and their ability to stick to their medication regimens, and may even have shaped their relationships with their health care providers.

Experiences of Formulary Changes

In the absence of direct price negotiation efforts by the federal government on behalf of Medicaid (or Medicare) recipients, patients and state-subsidized plans offered by third-party payers became the locus of significant cost control efforts in Massachusetts and across the United States. While total Medicaid spending for prescription drugs has been relatively stable for some time, "government projections point to rapid escalation in Medicaid expenditures in the near future" due to Medicaid expansions under the ACA and a slowed rate of new generic drugs (Bruen and Young 2014, 3). Medicaid pharmacy benefit managers pointed to the importance of switching patients to generic drugs from brand names, since brand name drugs were only one-fifth (20%) of 520 million prescriptions reimbursed by Medicaid in 2012 but they accounted for more than three-quarters (76%) of Medicaid's total medication costs. Other cost control measures included "more stringent authorization and review strategies" (Bruen and Young 2014, 2) and better management of the "small percentage of Medicaid beneficiaries [who] are responsible for large shares of total program expenditures in each state, and the same is true for prescription drug benefits. These individuals tend to have multiple medical and/or mental health conditions" (11). It is important to examine the consequences of these policies for patients at safety-net clinics, for whom chronic disease management was an ongoing challenge. More than half (60%) of the participants in our study estimated their household income to be less than $1,000 a month.

Public, private, and publicly subsidized health insurance companies all attempt to control the costs of providing coverage by adding and subtracting brand name and generic drugs to and from their formularies (the list of covered drugs) (Goldman et al. 2007). While these practices are long-standing, insurance companies may increasingly turn to tiered formularies with higher co-pays for "non-preferred" drugs (Hodgkin et al. 2008, 67) as the pool of insured people expanded, particularly in those states that expanded Medicaid. These changes may have important effects on patients' health: tiered formularies are associated with decreased adherence among patients with chronic illness (Johnston et al. 2012; Morgan et al. 2009) and greater use of inpatient and emergency services (Goldman et al. 2007). In addition, changes in insurance coverage disrupted patients' relationships with both their medications and their health care providers. Health care providers at CHC were also subject to these new forms of accountability. As they described in a focus group, providers I interviewed were all too aware of the effects of these changes on their patients' ability to maintain their medication regimens.

PROVIDER 2: One barrier . . . is health insurance. Because, you see, insurances, some of them have specific medications they will pay for, like HMOBlue or MassHealth. MassHealth doesn't cover this particular diabetic med, so sometimes the providers have to switch around to see which medication will work for that patient because the insurance doesn't cover the one [that works best]. Sometimes this one is working for the patient, but insurance doesn't cover it, and they have to switch to something else, which doesn't work as well.

PROVIDER 3: That's why they lose control. That's when they lose track.

PROVIDER 2: And then the patients are frustrated because they think, well, that one used to work so well but they don't pay for it.

SUSAN: And that's when they lose control of their blood sugar?

PROVIDER 3: The blood sugar, everything! The tracking, everything! Because they change so much their medication so often they may be taking their meds twice a day instead of once. They lose control. They get tired. They don't want to do it anymore.

One way physicians at the clinic managed these changes, particularly when a preferred drug would be dropped from the MassHealth formulary, was by using medication samples provided by pharmaceutical companies. At the time the use of drug samples was not subject to the same kind of scrutiny it later received, and health care providers seemed to regard them as a useful but clearly stopgap measure in helping low-income patients obtain needed medications. Even this measure had its drawbacks, however, because the supplies in the "medication closet" were constantly shifting, as Provider 3 explained.

> PROVIDER 3: The other issue is that we have to treat the non–health care patients with samples because they can't afford the medications. We just had a big issue with Avandia. It had a production issue. Avandia was giving us lots of samples of Avandia and Avandamet, which was great because it had the Metformin in it, but when they had a production issue, that dried up. Now . . . you have to make sure that whatever you give them is generic and none of the TZDs are generic, like Actos and Avandia, are not generic.
>
> SUSAN: Generic for MassHealth?
>
> PROVIDER 3: Generic in general. If they have no insurance, I have several patients who are buying their Glyburide because it's generic and it's less than $12 a month. And I'm giving them samples of Actos . . . But if a person has no insurance, you're working out of the closet [referring to the cabinet where the samples are stored that have been donated to the clinic by the drug companies] which in some cases, you know, you never know what you're going to see when you go in there the next time, you may have to change their medication.
>
> PROVIDER 1: But that's another issue. If you have someone who doesn't read or write, and you put them on multiple medications, it's a potential source for confusion, errors, and I know what I'm doing in terms of trying to save the patient some money. But it could be disastrous.
>
> PROVIDER 3: Change the medicine and they didn't understand, they take it like the other medicine.

Patients had their own experiences of these formulary changes. In a single interview, Lien, a Vietnamese participant, reported no fewer than three formulary changes. After more than three years' successful use of Avalide by prescription for her hypertension, she had been relying on samples for six weeks since MassHealth removed Avalide from its formulary. She feared that she might soon lose access altogether. As we sat in her kitchen going over the pill bottles she produced when I began to ask her about her medications, she worried, "But if there's no more sample[s] the doctor could give me, then I don't know what to do. I tried many other medications, [which didn't] seem to work, so the doctor had me try this and so far it's worked." Lien reported a similar experience with a cholesterol medication, Zetia, which was also removed from the MassHealth formulary. She explained how she's been hoarding her remaining pills: "I'm saving it. MassHealth stopped covering that also, so this is left over, so I'm saving it for as needed." In fact, she read on the label of a bottle of glucosamine that it "helps reduce bad LDL cholesterol," so she took glucosamine "more regularly" than her Zetia, to make it last longer. This way, she could ration her use of Zetia, which was no longer covered by insurance but which she only took in moments when she really felt she needed it, when she felt "uncomfortable." She reported the over-the-counter cost of Zetia as beyond her means at "more than $100" for 30 pills. Finally, she had a prescription for Nexium which also went off formulary, after which she said that she would get "the purple pill" from a friend who had the same prescription: "When I'm done with mine and it's [my stomach is] hurting me, then I call my friend up. My friend will give me some." Lien's repeated experiences of formulary change created a feeling of insecurity in relation to the medications she's come to rely on. Instead of being able to simply take a Nexium pill to relieve her discomfort, Lien had to decide if she "really" needed it enough to use one of her few remaining pills. Her experience of her illness and its symptoms was shifted by formulary change to become one of more intensive self-monitoring involving repeated decisions about the necessity of each pill she takes. Cost control measures can easily produce perceived conditions of scarcity that may shape patients' medication decisions.

Other participants said that the experience of arriving at a pharmacy to pick up a prescription only to be told that a drug was not covered by their health insurance led them to doubt their physician's recommendations. Robin, an African American woman with diabetes, had this experience with a cholesterol medication.

ROBIN: I had a problem with one medication, and they said, they just wouldn't, um, they ended up stopping me taking it, the doctor she

said just forget about it. It was a cholesterol pill. 'Cause at that one
point I was taking three pills for cholesterol 'cause that's how bad
it was.

SUSAN: So what happened?

ROBIN: Yeah, I went to put in a refill and they said that the insurance
won't pay for it, something something something. And I told the
doctor and they was trying, they was battling it out [with the insurance company], and [finally] she just said not to take it no more, that
she's taking me off of it.

SUSAN: How long did that process take?

ROBIN: I'm not even sure. Maybe like a couple of months. I mean I did
have a medication still but it's just, I was on that pill for a while too.
But it kind of felt like, why am I taking all these pills for just that one
thing. But at the time, like my [cholesterol,] it was really high. So
they was trying to work whatever they could to get it level.

While Robin seemed happy enough that her insurance company's
refusal to pay for a medication led to its discontinuation, the denial
did seem to provoke questions about her doctor's judgment. Similarly,
Edward, another African American participant, experienced a crisis of
trust in his health care provider when his insurance didn't cover a medication prescribed following a hospital discharge. He explained,

When I had the colonoscopy done the doctors prescribed me that Pre-
vacid. I took it to the pharmacy, and the pharmacy says the insurance
won't cover it. I went back to Caring Health Center and spoke with the
doctor there. . . . She had to rewrite the scrip in a certain way in order for
me to get this medicine. And I said, well, you know, I had the prescription in hand but MassHealth wouldn't honor it. So she went and talked to
her, and she said "well don't worry about it." I went back to the pharmacy,
thinking that everything had been taken care of. It didn't go through.
Why would they give me a prescription if you can't honor it? Either it
costs too much or you're second-guessing the doctor and you're thinking
I don't need it. That's counterproductive to me.

Shifting costs to low-income patients such as these only exacerbated their challenges obtaining and paying for medications (Balkrish-

nan 1998), and patients we spoke with experienced these challenges as worries that compounded their existing concerns about sticking to their medication regimens. MassHealth-eligible patients, who made up the majority of patients at safety-net clinics such as Caring Health Center, experienced these reductions in coverage as part and parcel of broader state interventions in their lives, in which frequent "re-certs" (re-certifications) were required not only for health insurance but food stamps, public housing, and other forms of public assistance.

In these ways formulary changes introduced pragmatic challenges to medication adherence by making medications more expensive and difficult to access. The emotional challenge to patients' trust in their medications and their health care providers was an equally important but perhaps less recognized consequence of formulary changes as a cost control measure. Disrupting patients' relationships with medications they had come to rely on created a level of doubt as patients were forced to question the meaning and severity of their symptoms, diagnoses, and bodily experiences.

Accountability: Paying the Costs

Even for insured patients, out-of-pocket medication costs might keep participants from taking their medications as prescribed. Almost one-third (32%) of our participants reported that they were unable to afford needed medication or supplies in the past 12 months. For example, Tim, an African American participant, described receiving a prescription for antibiotics from his physician that were not included in the formulary for his Medicaid managed-care plan. When he went to pick up the medication at the pharmacy he was told his "insurance didn't cover it, you got to pay for it yourself." When asked what happened then, Tim said, "I'll put it back. I ain't got that type of money. That was like fifty-something dollars, and I had two of them. This stuff is expensive."

For some, insurance refusals kept patients from obtaining needed medicines. For example, an immigrant from the former Soviet Union described being unable to pick up a prescription following cataract surgery. She said, "I visited a nice specialist for cataracts in both eyes and he prescribed vitamins. We went to pick them up and they said that the insurance company doesn't cover them. So we just didn't take them because they were $35, and that was too much." This participant also lived with diabetes and high blood pressure and was generally able to afford her co-pays for the medications for those conditions, but found the higher medication cost insurmountable.

This sense of insecurity affected patients' feelings about their insurance coverage. Gabriela, a Latina participant, said, "Sometimes it worries me because sometimes they will pay for the pills but sometimes they'll hold them and they have to call the doctor for the medicines to be approved by Medicaid. . . . I get angry because sometimes I come home with the pills, sometimes I come home without them. And I get scared because if I don't take that one, my blood pressure will rise." Being unable to consistently afford her co-pays left her in doubt about the reliability of her insurance coverage, and she felt she was dependent on the personal indulgence of the individuals working at the pharmacy. When she did not have the money for a co-pay, she said, "sometimes they put it on a tab . . . and I [can] take the money later," but it depends on who is working at the pharmacy: If the worker knows her then it's possible he might grant her this waiver. An immigrant from the former Soviet Union had a similar sense that the standards of individual responsibility were inconsistently applied from place to place. In an in-depth interview, she asked, "why is it some people don't have to pay co-pays?" She explained that some of her friends had switched to another clinic where they were not charged co-pays for their medications. She said, "I know it's not really up to the doctor because it's from the pharmacy, so I remember when I just came here and they would [deliver] my pills, I get it that they would charge for that. Why would they charge when we alone go to the pharmacy to pick them up?" She continued, "I wonder why people at other places don't have to pay co-pays and here I do. One time I recently paid $5.70 and it's almost $6 for a bottle and that's expensive for me."

These experiences serve as but two examples of a larger sense of the fundamental arbitrariness of entitlement programs or benefits that were shared by many of our participants—exactly what transparency policies were meant to address. In the introduction to *Audit Cultures*, Marilyn Strathern points out that efforts to rationalize expenditures while rendering policies transparent can have the paradoxical effect of *reducing* trust among parties. She notes that audit practices "evoke anxiety and small resistances, are held to be deleterious to certain goals, and as overdemanding if not outright damaging" to public welfare (Strathern 2000b, 1). Eligibility verification tests and co-payments are designed to make individuals responsible for (at least some of) the costs of their care and to make clear the guidelines by which some individuals qualify for benefits and others don't, but our participants' subjective experience of these policies was of personalistic and inconsistent implementation where it all depended on who was behind the counter the day they went to pick up their prescription.

Even written statements geared at increasing transparency by making visible the costs paid by insurance companies for participants' medications (compared to the costs paid by participants) seemed to have effects greater than simple transparency. Many low-income patients I spoke with described receiving statements from their insurance providers showing the actual costs of their prescriptions, broken down into columns headed "Amount Paid by You," "Amount Paid by MassHealth," and "Total Drug Costs." Statements such as these are increasingly common accompaniments to cost-sharing arrangements that may be distributed to both publicly and privately insured patients. For publicly insured patients, these statements could also be seen as emphasizing their positions as recipients of state largesse, or as something like a talisman against what Doran and colleagues (2005) call the "moral hazard" of universal prescription drug access (see also Stone 2011).

Being unable to afford their prescribed medications could have serious effects for people with chronic conditions, especially those living with multiple illnesses. Julieta was a Latina in recovery who was living with depression, diabetes, panic disorder, high blood pressure, asthma, anxiety, and back pain, among other things. She took at least six daily oral medications, with others to be taken as needed. When, in an in-depth interview, I began with a general question about her complex medication regimen, Julieta immediately volunteered that she was often unable to cover the cost of her co-pays despite having MassHealth and disability insurance.

SUSAN: How do you manage to stay on top of all these meds?
JULIETA: I get more medication, it's that, sometimes I can't afford to take all of them out, so I take out the most important ones.

SUSAN: How do you decide what are the most important ones?

JULIETA: Well, the most important ones is the ones for my diabetes, I know that's very, because my mother had that, and she passed away, she was diabetic. She had explained a lot to me about that, cuz it runs in the family, so I know that's the major [thing] I have to take care of. And my high blood pressure. So I do try to take out the most important ones. And then sometimes when I do can, I take all of them out.

SUSAN: How much are you paying for your meds that sometimes you can't afford them?

JULIETA: Three something each.

SUSAN: How much is too much for you to afford?

JULIETA: It comes out to 20 dollars. Then I gotta take the bus too to go pick them up.

SUSAN: So to pick up 6 bottles could be like 20 dollars a month, and that would be too much for you to afford.

JULIETA: Yeah, I got like 8 [meds that I take regularly].

SUSAN: Say all 8 came due, you had to go to the drugstore for refills—

JULIETA: Sometimes I don't have it. Sometimes I tell them just give me the most important ones, I ask for it, and I would leave the other ones behind.

SUSAN: So you would choose the metformin and the high blood pressure?

JULIETA: Yeah, the Lisinopril and the metformin. And my Doxipin to sleep and my Prozac. The other ones I leave it to the side, whenever I have the money I'll get it.

SUSAN: What are the low priority drugs?

JULIETA: Well, [the one] for the worries. They gave me something for my eyes. [The strips] to check my sugar. So far I have been on top of my diet so I don't have to worry too much but it's good to check [your sugar] just to be sure. My inhaler, sometimes, I can't have it.

SUSAN: What's the longest you've gone without an inhaler because you couldn't afford it?

JULIETA: Like a month.

This was quite a burden for her, since earlier in the interview Julieta reported that she used her inhaler every day as she climbed the steps to her fourth-floor walk-up apartment. She explained that when she was without her inhaler, she was sometimes able to borrow one from her father or her brother, both of whom used the same medication. Sometimes one of them was able to get refills before his inhaler was completely empty, and he would pass the old one on to Julieta. I pictured Julieta wheezing at the top of the stairs at her apartment, gratefully drawing on her borrowed inhaler, hoping to get her breath back.

Medication costs kept some patients from picking up their prescriptions, with detrimental effects to their well-being. Insurers and publicly supported health plans viewed these cost-sharing plans as a means of fostering individual responsibility for health while they limited overall public or plan expenditures.[9] Even seemingly nominal co-pays of $1 or $3 could be prohibitive when several medications were due for refill at once. For many, these costs seemed to have direct consequences for participants' adherence.

Conclusion

Lutfey and Wishner (1999) argue for a shift in terminology from "compliance" to "adherence," suggesting that the former term overemphasizes patients' agency and under-recognizes the roles played by health care providers, structural and environmental factors in promoting or inhibiting patients' adherence to medication (see also Hunt and Arar 2001; Rouse 2010). Cost control measures such as formulary changes are an important example of the kinds of structural factors Lutfey and Wishner mean to highlight. Pressures toward medication adherence create a web of expectations for patients with chronic illness that sharpen their experiences of constraints imposed by state-sponsored cost control measures. Patients become habituated to their medications while establishing trusted relationships with both medications and health care providers. Yet when cost control measures withdraw coverage for medications or produce gaps in insurance coverage, these changes heighten patients' experience of insecurity and confirm their perceptions of a bureaucracy that is willful and arbitrary.

Techniques of accountability such as formulary changes and eligibility verification for insurance coverage alter social relations, revealing conditions of mistrust as often as they make government more transparent. Describing the LEEDS certification process for "green" buildings in the

United States, Michael Brown shows how accountability practices can themselves provoke mistrust. Brown observes, "My goal in describing the multiple dilemmas of having buildings certified as safe and sustainable is . . . to show how the certification of virtue fosters contradictions that complicate and perhaps even imperil the moralizing process that it is designed to advance" (Brown 2010, 748). The fraught relationship between trust, accountability, and verification finds emphatic expression in the moral economy of health care reform, where the vulnerability of the sick and their hope for a cure, or at least treatment, confront protocols and policies designed to hold down costs. Patients we interviewed were already dealing with limited access to those medications no longer included on the MassHealth formulary; their coping methods included hoarding pills, skipping doses, and "borrowing" medications from friends. If such measures are interpreted as non-adherence, a feedback loop is conceivable in which "noncompliance" triggers the discontinuation of expensive medications. In Australia, where universal prescription drug coverage is met with the "moral hazard" argument that low medication costs will result in "excessive" or "wasteful" drug prescriptions, cost-sharing efforts that shift costs to patients from state insurers are on the rise (Doran et al. 2005). Health care providers are not immune to the effects of such policies, as their prescribing options are narrowed by tiered formularies and formulary changes that aim to shift physician prescribing behavior in ways that support the demand for lower costs to insurers (Joyce et al. 2011).

Discussions of cost effectiveness in health care reform share much in common with recent debates over evidence-based medicine (EBM), a quality-improvement approach that requires specific kinds of evidence (ideally, randomized controlled clinical trials) demonstrating the effectiveness of every treatment used as standard of care. Helen Lambert suggests that "In requiring the production of quantified forms of evidence, EBM is clearly an example of the 'audit culture' now found throughout [the] public sector . . . associated with the decline of public trust in authority and the perceived need for increased accountability and transparency" (Lambert 2009, 17). Lambert locates the emergence of EBM in a wider context of increasing demand for evidentiary support for policy in many domains, including higher education.[10] These demands shape the work, experiences, and subjectivities of health care providers, educators, and social service providers alike. Anthropologists such as Cris Shore and Susan Wright (1999) have criticized the disciplinary dimensions of accountability, as professionals must constantly reinvent themselves under pressure of ceaseless reviews of their performance, productivity, and efficiency. Health care providers are likewise subject to accountability measures that include both cost control and transparency policies. About a year after the focus group with health care providers quoted above, the clinic stopped accepting drug samples from pharmaceutical companies in light of concerns about safety and undue influence on physicians' prescribing practices (Adair and Holmgren 2005; Chew et al. 2000). Despite the recognized limitations of relying on the "medication closet," physicians were able to provide some short-term remedies for patients' needs, especially for un- and under-insured patients, by providing free samples from the closet. Physicians' autonomy is also circumscribed by insurance formularies in ways that are still being understood (Cox et al. 2007; Joyce et al. 2011).

The Massachusetts experience of health care reform serves as a cautionary tale of the diverse costs of health care reform in neoliberal moral economies of care. Both Chapter 58 and the ACA enacted a moral economy of care, which entitled citizens to limited conceptions of health care within a larger framework of individual responsibility. When the state withdraws benefits as an accountability measure, patients experience it as yet another arbitrary subtraction of resources, which may further violate a tenuous trust between patients and health care providers. In the interests of fiscal accountability, the state's health plans for the poor disregarded patients' comfort with their medications and the burdens placed on providers. In Massachusetts, which has been held up as a model of reform for the nation, mandated health insurance coverage faces serious challenges on the ground due in part to a recalcitrant bureaucracy bent on displacing the costs of care of those deemed too expensive to cover.

ACKNOWLEDGMENTS

The project described was supported by Award Number R01HL120907 from the National Heart, Lung and Blood Institute. The content is solely the responsibility of the author and does not necessarily represent the official views of the National Heart, Lung and Blood Institute or the

National Institutes of Health. My deepest gratitude to the providers, staff, and patients at Caring Health Center for sharing their expertise. I am grateful for the diverse contributions of our entire research team, including Cristina Huebner Torres, Molly Totman, Dina Gavrilyuk, Khanh Nguyen, and Yoeli Pacheco at Caring Health Center, and Jeannie Lee, Josephine Korchmaros, William Robertson, and Amanda Hilton at the University of Arizona. I appreciate the thoughtful feedback on this chapter from editors Heide Castañeda and Jessica M. Mulligan and the participants in the 2015 School for Advanced Research Seminar on health care reform.

NOTES

1 But for exceptions, see Boehm (2005), Lamphere (2005), López (2005), and Taylor (2014).

2 Source: U.S. Census Bureau, American Community Survey Five Year Estimates, Subject Tables B17020B, B17020C, B17020D, and B17020H. Developed by Randy Albelda, Francoise Carre, Eugenia Cheah, and Lyden Marcellot for the Center for Social Policy, 2014. Downloaded from www.umb.edu.

3 Participants' mean age was 56 years old, ranging in age from 26 to 85. Our qualitative sample is nearly evenly divided between men and women, but the larger survey sample is predominantly female (147 and 215, respectively). A third of the participants in our study had less than or equal to an eighth grade education.

4 For in-depth interviews not conducted in English, on-the-spot translation was provided by bilingual interviewers. Transcripts were then transcribed and all sections in Russian, Spanish, or Vietnamese were re-translated into English to add any information not captured by the on-the-spot oral translation.

5 See also Joseph, this volume.

6 These findings echo reports from Lamphere (2005), Boehm (2005), and López (2005) on the impediments to enrollment faced by low-income New Mexicans, particularly rampant error rates in the state Medicaid system and burdens placed on safety-net health care providers.

7 Rather than arming outreach workers with direct lines to enrollment supervisors with the power to solve individual problems, these staff members, employed by area hospitals and clinics rather than state welfare agencies, were forced to dial in to the same 1–800 numbers used by the general public for help solving their insurance access problems. Understaffing and poor training meant that hold times averaged at least 30 minutes *per call*. Putting outreach workers on hold for extended periods of time had profound effects not only on their own emotional anxiety levels but on the practical help they could provide to clients, who could be sick or even hospitalized when they came up for eligibility re-review. In one notable complaint, an outreach worker wrote, "I called into Tewksbury, waited on

hold for 30 minutes to have someone pick up the phone and place it down on the desk. Then I listen to someone typing on a keyboard. The first time it happened, I waited it out for 5 minutes, only to then have the phone hung up."

8 Massachusetts has Medicaid managed care; MassHealth recipients were insured by private HMOs under contract with the state.

9 Yet cost-benefit analyses may support cost-sharing and tiered formularies only as long as the only costs considered are medication expenditures rather than overall health care expenditures. When Pitney-Bowes recently shifted all diabetes drugs and devices to its most affordable formulary tier, to "eliminate financial barriers to preventive care, . . . preliminary results in plan participants with diabetes indicate that overall direct health care costs per plan participant with diabetes decreased by 6%" (Mahoney 2005).

10 For a useful, if disturbing, analysis of the ways in which demands for, especially, quantitative evidence in support of global women's health programs has overtaken value- or ethics-based justifications, see Storeng and Behague (2014).

REFERENCES

Adair, Richard, and Leah Holmgren. 2005. Do Drug Samples Influence Resident Prescribing Behavior? A Randomized Trial. *American Journal of Medicine* 118(8): 881–884.

Balkrishnan, Rajesh. 1998. Predictors of Medication Adherence in the Elderly. *Clinical Therapeutics* 20(4): 764–771.

Blendon, Robert J., et al. 2008. Massachusetts Health Reform: A Public Perspective from Debate Through Implementation. *Health Affairs* 27(6): w556–w565.

Boehm, Deborah A. 2005. The Safety Net of the Safety Net: How Federally Qualified Health Centers "Subsidize" Medicaid Managed Care. *Medical Anthropology Quarterly* 19(1): 47–63.

Borneman, John. 1997. *Settling Accounts: Violence, Justice, and Accountability in Postsocialist Europe*. Princeton, NJ: Princeton University Press.

Bornstein, Erica. 2009. The Impulse of Philanthropy. *Cultural Anthropology* 24(4): 622–651.

Brown, Michael F. 2010. A Tale of Three Buildings: Certifying Virtue in the New Moral Economy. *American Ethnologist* 37(4): 741–752.

Bruen, Brian, and Katherine Young. 2014. *What Drives Spending and Utilization on Medicaid Drug Benefits in States?* Menlo Park, CA: Henry J. Kaiser Family Foundation.

Chew, Lisa D., et al. 2000. A Physician Survey of the Effect of Drug Sample Availability on Physicians' Behavior. *Journal of General Internal Medicine* 15(7): 478–483.

Clark, Dana, Jonathan Fox, and Kay Treakle, eds. 2003. *Demanding Accountability: Civil-Society Claims and the World Bank Inspection Panel*. Lanham, MD: Rowman and Littlefield.

Clarke, John. 2007. Subordinating the Social? Neo-liberalism and the Remaking of Welfare Capitalism. *Cultural Studies* 21(6): 974–987.

Cox, Emily, Amit Kulkarni, and Rochelle R. Henderson. 2007. Impact of Patient and Plan Design Factors on Switching to Preferred Statin Therapy. *Annals of Pharmacotherapy* 41(12): 1946–1953.

Danz, Shari M. 2000. A Nonpublic Forum or a Brutal Bureaucracy? Advocates' Claims of Access to Welfare Center Waiting Rooms. *New York University Law Review* 75(4): 1004–1044.

Doran, Evan, Jane Robertson, and David Henry. 2005. Moral Hazard and Prescription Medicine Use in Australia: The Patient Perspective. *Social Science & Medicine* 60(7): 1437–1443.

Drexler, Elizabeth. 2006. History and Liability in Aceh, Indonesia: Single Bad Guys and Convergent Narratives. *American Ethnologist* 33(3): 313–326.

Goldman, Dana, Geoffrey Joyce, and Yuhui Zheng. 2007. Prescription Drug Cost Sharing: Associations with Medication and Medical Utilization and Spending and Health. *JAMA* 298(1): 61–69.

Gupta, Akhil, and Aradhana Sharma. 2006. Globalization and Postcolonial States. *Current Anthropology* 47(2): 277–307.

Harvey, David. 2005. *A Brief History of Neoliberalism*. Oxford: Oxford University Press.

Himmelstein, David U., and Steffie Woolhandler. 2007. Massachusetts's Approach to Universal Coverage: High Hopes and Faulty Economic Logic. *International Journal of Health Services* 37(2): 251–257.

Hodgkin, Dominic, et al. 2008. The Effect of a Three-Tier Formulary on Antidepressant Utilization and Expenditures. *Journal of Mental Health Policy and Economics* 11(2): 67–77.

Hunt, Linda M., and Nedal H. Arar. 2001. An Analytical Framework for Contrasting Patient and Provider Views of the Process of Chronic Disease Management. *Medical Anthropology Quarterly* 15(3): 347–367.

Johnston, Stephen, et al. 2012. Association Between Prescription Cost Sharing and Adherence to Initial Combination Antiretroviral Therapy in Commercially Insured Antiretroviral-Naive Patients with HIV. *Journal of Managed Care Pharmacy* 18(2): 129–145.

Joyce, Geoffrey, et al. 2011. Physician Prescribing Behavior and Its Impact on Patient-Level Outcomes. *American Journal of Managed Care* 17(12): e462–471.

Kingsdale, J. 2009. Implementing Health Care Reform in Massachusetts: Strategic Lessons Learned. *Health Affairs* 28(4): w588–594.

Lambert, Helen. 2009. Evidentiary Truths? The Evidence of Anthropology Through the Anthropology of Medical Evidence. *Anthropology Today* 25(1): 16–20.

Lamphere, Louise. 2005. Providers and Staff Respond to Medicaid Managed Care: The Unintended Consequences of Reform in New Mexico. *Medical Anthropology Quarterly* 19(1): 3–25.

Li, Fabiana. 2009. Documenting Accountability: Environmental Impact Assessment in a Peruvian Mining Project. *PoLAR: Political and Legal Anthropology Review* 32(2): 218–236.

Long, Sharon K. 2008. On the Road to Universal Coverage: Impacts of Reform in Massachusetts at One Year. *Health Affairs* 27(4): 270–284.

López, Leslie. 2005. De Facto Disentitlement in an Information Economy: Enrollment Issues in Medicaid Managed Care. *Medical Anthropology Quarterly* 19(1): 26–46.

Lutfey, K. E., and W. J. Wishner. 1999. Beyond "Compliance" Is "Adherence": Improving the Prospect of Diabetes Care. *Diabetes Care* 22(4): 635–639.

Mahoney, J. J. 2005. Reducing Patient Drug Acquisition Costs Can Lower Diabetes Health Claims. *American Journal of Managed Care* 11(5 Suppl): S170–176.

McDonald, Maryon. 2000. Accountability, Anthropology and the European Commission. In *Audit Cultures: Anthropological Studies in Accountability, Ethics and the Academy*. M. Strathern, ed. Pp. 106–132. London: Routledge.

Morgan, Steve, Gillian Hanley, and Devon Greyson. 2009. Comparison of Tiered Formularies and Reference Pricing Policies: A Systematic Review. *Open Medicine* 3(3): e131–139.

O'Malley, Pat. 1996. Risk and Responsibility. In *Foucault and Political Reason*. A. Barry, T. Osborne, and N. Rose, eds. Pp. 189–208. Chicago: University of Chicago Press.

Pels, Peter. 2000. The Trickster's Dilemma: Ethics and the Technologies of the Anthropological Self. In *Audit Cultures: Anthropological Studies in Accountability, Ethics and the Academy*. M. Strathern, ed. Pp. 135–172. London: Routledge.

Power, Michael. 1997. *The Audit Society: Rituals of Verification*. Oxford: Oxford University Press.

Raikhel, Eugene and William Garriott. 2013. Introduction. Tracing New Paths in the Anthropology of Addiction. In *Addiction Trajectories*. Eugene Raikhel and William Garriott, eds. Pp. 1–35. Durham, NC: Duke University Press.

Rivkin-Fish, Michele. 2011. Learning the Moral Economy of Commodified Health Care: "Community Education," Failed Consumers, and the Shaping of Ethical Clinician-Citizens. *Culture, Medicine and Psychiatry* 35(2): 183–208.

Rose, Nikolas. 1996. The Death of the Social? Re-Figuring the Territory of Government. *Economy and Society* 25(3): 327–356.

Rouse, Carolyn. 2010. Patient and Practitioner Noncompliance: Rationing, Therapeutic Uncertainty, and the Missing Conversation. *Anthropology & Medicine* 17(2): 187–200.

Sawyer, Suzana. 2006. Disabling Corporate Sovereignty in a Transnational Lawsuit. *PoLAR: Political and Legal Anthropology Review* 29(1): 23–43.

Seifert, Robert, and Amanda Littell-Clark. 2013. *Enrollment Volatility in MassHealth: A Progress Report*. Worcester, MA: Massachusetts Medicaid Policy Institute, Center for Health Law and Economics, University of Massachusetts Medical School.

Seifert, Robert W., and Andrew P. Cohen. 2010. *Re-forming Reform (Part 1): What the Patient Protection and Affordable Care Act Means for Massachusetts*. Worcester: University of Massachusetts Medical School, Center for Health Law and Economics, and the BCBS Foundation.

Shaw, Susan J. 2012. *Governing How We Care: Contesting Community and Defining Difference in U.S. Public Health Programs*. Philadelphia: Temple University Press.

Shore, Cris, and Susan Wright. 1999. Audit Culture and Anthropology: Neo-Liberalism in British Higher Education. *Journal of the Royal Anthropological Institute* 5(4): 557–575.

Sloan, Kris. 2007. High-Stakes Accountability, Minority Youth, and Ethnography: Assessing the Multiple Effects. *Anthropology & Education Quarterly* 38(1): 24–41.

Steinbrook, Robert. 2008. Health Care Reform in Massachusetts—Expanding Coverage, Escalating Costs. *New England Journal of Medicine* 358(26): 2757–2760.

Stone, Deborah. 2011. Moral Hazard. *Journal of Health Politics, Policy and Law* 36(5): 887–896.

Storeng, Katerini T., and Dominique P. Behague. 2014. "Playing the Numbers Game": Evidence-Based Advocacy and the Technocratic Narrowing of the Safe Motherhood Initiative. *Medical Anthropology Quarterly* 28(2): 260–279.

Strathern, Marilyn, ed. 2000a. *Audit Cultures: Anthropological Studies in Accountability, Ethics and the Academy*. London: Routledge.

———. 2000b. New Accountabilities: Anthropological Studies in Audit, Ethics and the Academy. In *Audit Cultures: Anthropological Studies in Accountability, Ethics and the Academy*. M. Strathern, ed. Pp. 1–18. London: Routledge.

Taylor, Janelle S. 2014. The Demise of the Bumbler and the Crock: From Experience to Accountability in Medical Education and Ethnography. *American Anthropologist* 116(3): 523–534.

Young, John A., Susan L. Fischer, and Catherine P. Koshland. 2007. Institutional Resistance to Assessment: A Case Study of Rural Energy Development in Chinese and International Contexts. *Urban Anthropology and Studies of Cultural Systems and World Economic Development* 36(1/2): 39–72.

9

Outsourcing Responsibility

State Stewardship of Behavioral Health Care Services

CATHLEEN E. WILLGING AND ELISE M. TROTT

In February 2016, concerned citizens gathered in the rotunda of the New Mexico (NM) State Capitol in Santa Fe to demand that legislators inter- vene into what they called a statewide "behavioral health crisis." Just days before, a dozen nonprofit agencies specializing in mental health care and substance use treatment services had been cleared of fraud charges by the state's attorney general. These charges had forced the majority of the agencies to shut their doors in disgrace two years prior. The crowd within the Capitol building attested to widespread disruptions in ser- vices with profoundly injurious effects on New Mexico's most vulnerable citizens. One former patient of a shuttered agency spoke passionately of family and friends who "were completely lost" when the agencies could no longer sustain services, lamenting, "If services were still here, they might still be here (that is, alive)." For their part, current and former employees described being "confused," "devastated," and "embarrassed" by claims that their agencies had committed fraud.

As the bustling daily business of the Capitol proceeded, sometimes drowning out the voices of speakers, the crowd pointed to banners hang- ing from the second floor to the ground level of the rotunda, each de- picting patients endeavoring to "piece together services" in the wake of the fraud allegations. Paying homage to the many patients whose com- ments emblazoned the banners, one event organizer commented, "They want to be heard and live the life they deserve to live." She continued, "People are afraid to use the word 'crisis,' but we have to call it what it is." In this chapter, we illustrate how contestation over this crisis reflects a deepening pattern of systemic failure, top-down reform, and corporate profit in New Mexico's behavioral health care system, culminating in the use of federal fraud provisions within the 2010 Patient Protection and Affordable Care Act (ACA) by state officials and others to curtail availability of and access to publicly funded services. This pattern represents the "organized irresponsibility" of decision makers in "higher circles" (Gonzalez and Stryker 2014, 3; Nader 1972; Mills 1951), whose actions have adversely affected a group of citizens lacking the social capital and political clout to advance meaningful change in how their services are structured, financed, and delivered.

We contend that politically driven efforts in the past shape the contemporary context of behavioral health care delivery in New Mexico, a largely rural state that has led the nation in death related to alcohol, drugs, and suicide (NM Department of Health 2016). With a population of slightly more than 2 million people, close to 20% of adults in New Mexico likely struggle with mental health concerns (Substance Abuse and Mental Health Services Administration [SAMSHA] 2014). Yet, New Mexico is distinguished for its long-standing shortages of specialty services for people with serious mental illness and substance use problems. Importantly, the ACA has offered the state the possibility of improving access and services through Medicaid expansion, outreach to underserved populations, and new initiatives to improve quality of care and workforce locally. We illustrate how and why such desirable outcomes are likely to elude the state for the foreseeable future, as its behavioral health care system is enmeshed in a complex web of privatization, bureaucratization, and the intrigues of public stewards and corporate actors. These intrigues are influenced by neoliberal ideologies of transparency, accountability, and reliance on quantifiable (yet questionable) data, and scientific strategies "to stamp out the 'cancer' of corruption" (Anders and Nuijten 2009, 8).

Drawing on 16 years of ethnographic work with system stakeholders, we trace New Mexico's history of state-led reform. Beginning with efforts to make "greedy" service providers "accountable" for their clinical work, these reforms culminated in the use of newly instituted ACA provisions, technocratic governance mechanisms (i.e., the audit), and allegations of "egregious mismanagement," "fraud," and "corruption" to shut down decades-old nonprofit agencies that, until June 2013, had delivered 87% of all behavioral health care to low-income New Mexicans. The majority were community mental health centers that comprised the state's already beleaguered behavioral health safety net by delivering comprehensive services to individuals who otherwise lacked access to care, particularly in rural areas of the state.

Total Bureaucratization, Transparency, and "Truthiness"

We situate our analysis of reform and crisis within a broader theoretical understanding of neoliberal ideology in U.S. health care systems, its characteristic discourses of transparency, accountability, and corruption, and its specific technologies of governance, notably the audit. Anthropologists have described the ascendance of neoliberal ideology and the consequent marketization of health care (Horton et al. 2014; Rylko-Bauer and Farmer 2002). According to neoliberal logics, escalating health care costs are primarily the fault of inefficient government management. Privatization is heralded as the remedy, resulting in growing corporatization and the dismantlement of social welfare programs based on justifications of encouraging individual choice and government accountability. The marketization of health care typically involves a complex partnership of government agencies and profit-motivated private entities, such as managed care organizations (MCOs). Such partnerships are accompanied by the multiplication of new standards of management and accounting, and technologies of supervision, such as utilization review, software to detect fraud, and the audit. The anthropologist David Graeber (2015, 17) calls this phenomenon "total bureaucratization," describing it as "the gradual fusion of public and private power into a single entity, rife with rules and regulations whose ultimate purpose is to extract wealth in the form of profits."

More than an increase in bureaucracy and paperwork, the growth of total bureaucratization and "audit culture" in public systems is underpinned by the imperative to create "accountability," a concept in which "the financial and the moral meet" (Strathern 2000, 1). The rise of audit culture since the 1980s and '90s has been accompanied by calls for greater transparency and openness in the operation of public services (Anders and Nuijten 2009). In the case of behavioral health care in New Mexico, this imperative undergirds portrayals of nonprofit and community providers as both opaque and corrupt.

The ideology of transparency and accountability makes these portrayals particularly powerful, despite the presence or absence of evidence, as they become shrouded in an aura of "truthiness," a term coined by comedian Steven Colbert (cited in Wedel 2009, 41) to refer to "the truth that comes from the gut, not books." It is "the quality of seeming or being felt to be true, even if not necessarily true" (Truthiness n.d.). Truthiness is seductive, attracting the attention of both the media and the public, and bestowing upon accusations of corruption a life of their own. In this sense, calls for "transparency" are political acts that function on a symbolic level by evoking emotions such as "patriotic pride, anxieties, remembrances of past glories or humiliations, [or] promises of future greatness" (Edelman 1985, 6). As political scientist Murray Edelman (1985) describes, these symbols operate independently of evidence or outcomes because they fulfill a psychological, not an objective, need. Transparency is thus fickle (Hetherington 2012), utopian, i.e., strived for but never achieved (Graeber 2015), and available for appropriation by multiple actors and agendas (Barrera 2013; Comaroff and Comaroff 2003; Shore 2008; Zizek 1997). Scholars of transparency and audit culture have shown that proponents of transparency are as likely to hide crucial information as they are to reveal it, creating exclusions from knowledge and citizenship for select populations, such as the poor (Dotson 2014; Hetherington 2011). Transparency discourses have grown alongside the managed-care industry and the proliferation of its tools for determining and quantifying use of medically necessary services and identifying fraudulent practices. Focusing on New Mexico, we explain how public-private partnerships in the Medicaid arena, discourses of transparency, and technologies of accountability can engender truthiness claims, obscure vital information, destabilize a behavioral health care safety net, and deny low-income citizens care.

Methods

New Mexico has overhauled behavioral health care under three successive gubernatorial administrations. Since 1999, the first author has employed team-based ethnographic methods (Guest and MacQueen 2008) involving participant observation, semi-structured interviewing, and document review to describe the rise of complex bureaucratic structures within the behavioral health care system that, according to state officials, would enhance transparency, streamline service delivery, and maximize limited monetary resources. The application of these ethnographic methods, study participants, and iterative coding procedures for analyzing the resulting qualitative data are detailed in three separate publications (Willging, Wagner, and Waitzkin 2005; Willging, Waitzkin, and Nicdao 2008; Willging, Lamphere, and Rylko-Bauer 2015). We summarize findings from this work here to historicize the merging of public and private power in the policy regimes that have dominated a subpar service infrastructure.

Starting in June 2013, the first and second authors resumed pursuit of the above research trajectory, undertaking what Hugh Gusterson (1997) calls "polymorphous engagement" to understand a suddenly changing behavioral health care landscape, including participant observation at state legislative hearings, town halls, and other public events, and at professional association coalition meetings; and informal interview, phone, and email exchanges with concerned parties (e.g., patients, families, and providers). We have also turned to official government and court documents, newspaper articles, and other media coverage to construct a comprehensive understanding of the actions and possible motivations of those in power. We are not without bias, however, having organized large events and consulted with local media, legislators, and advocates to encourage public awareness, discussion, and intervention. Yet because of this involvement, we can pursue an analysis of public policy that anthropologists Janine Wedel and Gregory Feldman (2005, 2) call "studying through," defined as "following the source of a policy—its discourses, prescriptions, and programmes—through to those affected by the policies," to illuminate "the cultural and philosophical underpinnings of policy." By problematizing formal and de facto behavioral health care policy in New Mexico, we trace a pattern of organized irresponsibility and the entities and people that profit from reform and crisis.

The Past Repeats Itself: "Reform" and Public/Private Partnerships in New Mexico

In 1997, New Mexico's Human Services Department (HSD) instituted the first of three major reforms: a Medicaid managed-care program for physical and mental health care. HSD officials embraced managed care as a means to impart public-sector accountability and decrease costs. The new program aimed to control revenue through utilization review to transform mental health providers into responsible custodians of expensive services (Willging 2005). In practice, this multitier system of contractors and subcontractors diverted funds from care to corporate administration and profit, and created financial hardship for providers. More than 60 programs closed, while specialty clinicians stopped accepting Medicaid patients. The situation was so dire that the Centers for Medicare and Medicaid Services (CMS), then run by the Democratic Bill Clinton administration, mandated in October 2000 that the HSD restore the mental health portion of the Medicaid program to a traditional fee-for-service structure. However, New Mexico's Republican governor, Gary Johnson, convinced the administration of president-elect George W. Bush to overturn this unusual mandate from the CMS, thus undercutting the capacity of CMS to implement its regulatory responsibilities to hold state Medicaid programs accountable (Willging, Wagner, and Waitzkin 2005), a topic to which we will return later.

In 2005, under the next governor, Democrat Bill Richardson, the HSD led the second reform termed "Transformation," which emphasized seamless systems of care to support the "recovery" of persons with mental illness. Here, the state carved out Medicaid dollars and all other public monies for behavioral health care, and entered into a $400 million management contract with ValueOptions, the nation's largest for-profit behavioral health organization, and later its competitor, OptumHealth, an affiliate of United Healthcare and a subsidiary of the even bigger UnitedHealth Group, Inc. Economic considerations remained a driving force of the Transformation, which also facilitated increased centralization and cost containment via rigid spending and reimbursement rules, without decreasing either expense or bureaucracy, as promised by its key architects (Willging, Lamphere, and Rylko-Bauer 2015).

Controversy surfaced around both reforms, fueled by rumors of corruption, such as the state's awarding of a lucrative managed-care contract to a company headed by a former governor, or a sitting governor ensuring that another company won a contract in exchange for campaign contributions. Both reforms were also marked by top-down decision making by political appointees and corporate entities, and the wresting of traditional oversight functions from the state legislature. The HSD leadership proclaimed that each reform was crucial to ensuring transparency in the delivery of public services, but consistently ignored requests from the state legislature, healthcare researchers, and others for data to assess the reform's impacts.

When this chapter's first author began undertaking ethnographic studies of system reform in NM in 1999, the HSD lacked the technical capacity, funding, and political will to analyze and disseminate system performance information. In a 2000 interview, the director of the state Medicaid agency (part of the HSD) explained that his agency was especially reluctant to evaluate Medicaid encounter data detailing the purpose and outcome of clinical interactions, owing to fears that providers and advocates would use this evidence to criticize the Medicaid managed care program (Willging 2005). This same reluctance pervaded the HSD during the later Transformation, as state officials hesitated to release data for fear that it would reflect negatively on their system-change efforts and attempts to promote recovery-oriented services.

The first author's research into both reforms highlighted recurring implementation problems related to faulty enrollment, utilization review, and claims-processing systems. Designed and owned by state-contracted MCOs, these systems were subject to frequent change, as were service definitions and billing procedures. In navigating these complicated systems, providers incurred higher overhead and labor costs to get paid. During the later Transformation years, OptumHealth even stopped reimbursing providers for four months because of problems with its claims-processing system. Cash-strapped providers had little choice but to accept "prepayment" disbursements from OptumHealth to stay open. These monies, distributed quickly by OptumHealth without quality assurance mechanisms in place, were later subjected to an onerous accounting procedure called "reconciliation," which led to further overhead costs for providers. During both reforms, HSD officials attributed such financial woes to the failure of providers to adjust to the new private-sector logic of public-sector services.

For almost two decades, public behavioral health care in New Mexico has been influenced by the global trend toward the fusion of public and private power. As Wedel (2014, 2009) describes, this fusion involves entrenchment of state-private networks in which key players manipulate rules about governmental accountability and market competition, and strategically produce, control, and block access to information to exert influence and achieve mutual goals. All the while, the state and its corporate contractors have developed an adversarial relationship with service providers, characterizing them as "special interests" motivated by greed and disgruntled with reform because they can no longer misuse public-sector dollars due to the stringent scrutiny exercised under managed care. These characterizations endure today, as yet another governor purportedly committed to promoting transparency and rooting out corruption has set out to "modernize" behavioral health care through a new Medicaid system that is reminiscent of the earlier multitier Medicaid program. The governor's administration has referred to this new system as "Centennial Care" in recognition of New Mexico's 100th year of statehood.

The Past Repeats Itself Again: Fraud and Transparency under Centennial Care

In June 2013, five months prior to Centennial Care implementation, top HSD officials announced that 15 nonprofit agencies had bilked Medicaid for financial gain. In an unattributed memo released to the press, the HSD declared that the agencies had received $36 million in Medicaid overpayments due to unlawful billing practices, asserting "potential fraudulent activity by certain behavioral health executives" (NM HSD 2013). The HSD based its allegations on an audit undertaken at its request by the Public Consulting Group (PCG) of Massachusetts, and abruptly suspended reimbursement for services that the nonprofits had rendered. In consultation with OptumHealth, the HSD had secretively awarded the PCG a $3 million no-bid contract to audit services delivered by these specific agencies as far back as 2009, the year OptumHealth had stopped reimbursing providers statewide. The arrangement with PCG also entitled OptumHealth to a portion of any overpayments identified in the audit and returned to the state.

The HSD deemed the nonprofits ineffective, contending that OptumHealth and PCG had documented "an alarming rise in critical incidents affecting consumers' lives from injuries and the need for emergency services, to homicide, attempted suicide, and suicide" (NM HSD 2013,

3). The decontextualized examples of "mismanagement, fraud, waste, and abuse affecting real lives" cited by the HSD included "egregious lack of treatment [that] resulted in a suicide"; "disregard for follow-up care after a suicide attempt"; and "an inpatient psychiatric facility not [following] its policies of keeping all suicidal tendency consumers in the 'line of sight'" (NM HSD 2013, 3–4). Though grave, these accusations obscured the fact that not one of the nonprofits provided inpatient hospitalization. Ironically, OptumHealth had assigned these nonprofits high marks on prior audits. The chief executive officer (CEO) of one nonprofit testified before the state legislature, "[We] never scored below a 94 [of 100 points] in the last five years. . . . I've been here in New Mexico 39 years and have never had allegations or suspicions of fraud [against us]."

The HSD officials claimed that federal law, referring to Section 6402(h) (2) of the ACA, compelled them to halt payment "when there is pending an investigation of a credible allegation of fraud . . . as determined by the state," and argued that New Mexico risked losing all its federal Medicaid funding if this course of action was not followed (Heyeck 2013, 1). In 2011, Section 6402(h) (2) lowered the legal threshold for determining Medicaid fraud, changing the standard from "reliable evidence of fraud" to "credible allegation of fraud," and afforded state Medicaid agencies a wide berth of authority to cease a vendor's participation in the Medicaid program. Yet, the definition of a "credible allegation of fraud" was unusually broad: "A 'credible allegation of fraud' may be an allegation that has been verified by a State and that has indicia of reliability that comes from any source" (CMS 2011, 3). Thus, for example, it "could be a complaint made by an employee of a physician alleging that the physician is engaging in fraudulent billing practices. . . . Upon review of the physician's billings, the State may determine that the allegation has indicia of reliability and is, in fact, credible" (CMS 2011, 3). Through an overly rigid interpretation of Section 6402(h), HSD officials asserted that a state Medicaid agency "must suspend payments" based on such allegations without divulging the "particulars" of an investigation to prevent potential tampering with evidence required for a criminal trial (Heyeck 2013, 5).

The ACA empowered states to aggressively crack down on fraud and waste, but CMS noted several circumstances constituting "good cause" for a state *not* to suspend payments to providers suspected of such abuse. For example, a state could (1) implement other remedies to more effectively or quickly protect Medicaid funds; (2) allow providers to furnish "written evidence that persuades the State that a payment suspension should be terminated or imposed only in part"; (3) find "that certain specific criteria are satisfied by which recipient access to items or services would otherwise be jeopardized"; or (4) conclude "that payment suspension . . . is not in the best interests of the Medicaid program" (CMS 2011, 2). Despite these alternatives, HSD officials elected to suspend payments to the accused immediately and completely.

The HSD submitted the audit to the attorney general for a criminal investigation, and then presented the leaders of the nonprofits with the following option: either shut down their operations or allow five companies already selected from nearby Arizona to "take over" their facilities, internal operations, and clinical care functions. In a heated July 2013 exchange with state legislators who criticized the vaguely described statistical extrapolation methods used in the audit to determine fraudulent billing behavior, the HSD cabinet secretary defended concerns about possible impacts of such an abrupt transition on persons with mental illness: "They're saying that people will go without services but that is not true. It's made up by somebody." The secretary later stormed out of the hearing after refusing to answer questions from a state legislator, whom she accused of "inciting a public riot" at a previous public event regarding Centennial Care.

In the local media, possible motivations for and consequences of the crisis were disputed. Top HSD officials portrayed the MCO, OptumHealth, as a hero by alerting them in November 2012 to "aberrant billing practices" among the nonprofits; their decision to suspend payments to the providers writ large was also publicly affirmed by the CMS in the press (Terrell 2013a). Whereas the coverage by the state's largest newspaper—the *Albuquerque Journal*—tended to support HSD's actions, the *Santa Fe Reporter*, *Santa Fe New Mexican*, *New Mexico In Depth*, and local public radio stations were far more critical. Several journalists from these outlets began documenting what appeared to represent backdoor dealings on the part of current Republican governor Susana Martinez's administration, OptumHealth, and the out-of-state companies brought in to deliver services. While OptumHealth executives were warning state officials of fraud in the Medicaid system, the company was also attempting to sell the HSD new fraud detection products. Lobbyists from its parent company hosted political appointees of the Martinez administration, including the HSD secretary and the governor's chief of staff, at expensive restaurants and resorts (Horwath 2015). Journalists also published government records and emails showing that in January 2013 (months before the audit was made public), representatives of HSD, OptumHealth, and PCG, a contributor to the Republican Governors Association that donated $1.3 million to elect Martinez, had traveled to Arizona to initiate negotiations with the companies later contracted to assume management of the accused nonprofits. Finally, local political reporters also alleged that individuals with links to the Arizona companies held a $100-per person fund-raising dinner for the governor (Monahan 2013).

Because of "pay holds" that surpassed $13.5 million in November 2013, dwindling cash reserves, and no new state financing on the horizon, the majority of the accused nonprofits submitted to what many referred to as a "hostile" takeover by the Arizona companies. After refusing to allow a nonprofit network of federally qualified health centers that served 4,000–5,000 mental health patients statewide per quarter to rebut audit findings, HSD officials, in apparent violation of the federal Worker Adjustment and Retraining Notification (WARN) Act, pressured its leaders to swiftly fire 300 of the agency's service providers, so they could then be rehired by an Arizona company. While this network admitted to no wrongdoing, its administrators disclosed at a state legislative hearing that they had no recourse but to begrudgingly pay the state $4 million in restitution, while accruing $1.3 million in legal and administrative fees, to stay in business. During this period, the people who ran or worked for the nonprofits were not allowed to see the evidence against them while they felt that HSD officials were sullying their reputations with titillating allegations of bloated CEO salaries, suspicious business maneuverings, and undisclosed whistleblower complaints in the local press. However, without access to the audit results, the nonprofits were unsuccessful in seeking redress through state courts.

Meanwhile, the Arizona companies were paid $24 million from state general funds to participate in the changeover and promised future payments exceeding the going Medicaid rate. As the Arizona companies took over the operations of the nonprofits, a K-Street lobbying group blanketed the radio and television waves with ads praising the crackdown on Medicaid fraud (Terrell 2013b), while the governor was celebrated in *People Magazine* for caring for a sister with a developmental disability (Clark 2013, 80). Still, the hurried process of transitioning staff to the new employers was erratic and not without adverse consequences. A September 2013 statewide canvass of five of the 15 nonprofits by the advocacy group, *New Mexicans Fighting to Save Behavioral Health*, suggested that the rehire rate of the Arizona companies was closer to 60% than the 85% proclaimed by HSD officials. By October, one of the companies had laid off three counselors, leaving two to see 380 patients. During this period, an administrative executive from an accused nonprofit weepily shared with us how former staff were rehired by another Arizona company, then let go months later, and were now turning to public assistance to make ends meet. Because the Arizona companies were not paid for outreach to former patients of the nonprofits, it was unclear how many people stopped receiving services.

Inundated with complaints from patients, families, and caregivers, federal and state legislators placed pressure on the CMS to examine access and quality of care problems in September 2013. Although largely based on a small number of visits to clinical sites, the resulting report confirmed that the Arizona companies were operating with far fewer staff than the New Mexico nonprofits had previously. Clinicians also had to revamp clinical activities for bureaucratic reasons, such as patient assessment and treatment planning, thus delaying care for persons in need (CMS and SAMHSA 2013). These concerns were reiterated through data from a July 2014 online survey developed and administered by the advocacy group, *New Mexico Rising Up for Community Mental Health*, which we were later asked to analyze and present at a town hall organized by congressional delegation staff and attended by CMS staff. Of the 115 participants who had used mental health services in the past year, 52% had to change providers in the same time period. In open-ended comments, participants expressed frustration that they could no longer access trusted clinicians with whom they had long-established relationships when their care was transitioned to the Arizona companies without their consent. They also complained of long wait times for services, inconsistency and insecurity of their care, and premature discharge. Several participants reported that they did not just change providers but stopped accessing care altogether.

Nevertheless, HSD officials publicly contended that the transition had worked out well, claiming their data revealed that more patients were actually being served than when the 15 nonprofits were in existence (Boyd 2014), in contrast to what they characterized as "anecdotal" information mustered by local advocacy groups. At a state legislative hearing, the HSD presented a utilization report that credited Centennial Care (rather than Medicaid expansion under the ACA) with increasing the total number of [Medicaid] recipients who received behavioral health care in 2014 by 30.8% over 2013. This statistic, however, was derived from an unspecified "alternative method" for tracking data rather than a conventional analysis of claims records, which had fallen into further disarray as the Arizona companies gained their footholds in New Mexico. Despite their questionable veracity, such assertions from HSD constituted a justification for these companies to cut salaries and terminate the staff inherited from the accused nonprofits. Notably, no one—not even state and federal legislators—was privy to the actual data fueling these truthiness claims.

Conclusion

While complaints of fraudulent provider activity are a mainstay in critiques of Medicaid and other social programs (Smith 2002), the use of new ACA provisions and technocratic governance mechanisms (i.e., the audit) in New Mexico sheds light on how the actions and behaviors of public stewards and corporate actors can give way to abuses of authority in public systems. In particular, we must problematize the audit as a political symbol of our neoliberal orientation toward public systems. On the one hand, the audit evokes the moral and emotional qualities of efficiency, accountability, and transparency of those in power, while on the other, it foments distrust and suspicion toward those who rely on public assistance (i.e., those with mental illness and their providers). Authorities can put this process in motion by cultivating the impression that data exist and by circulating truthiness claims, regardless of their basis in fact. Indeed, in a separate investigation, the state auditor, a Democrat later elected to the post of attorney general, chastised the HSD for "poor oversight" and "mismanagement of federal funds," and identified a litany of improprieties related to HSD's spending on behalf of the PCG audit. His investigation revealed that the audit subpoenaed by his office was altered by HSD staff to eliminate language that PCG "did not uncover what it would consider to be credible allegations of fraud" (Office of the State Auditor 2014, 3). His investigation also found that HSD violated established requirements for assessing and referring credible allegations of fraud when bypassing its own Program Integrity Unit, which should have conducted the first inquiry into the overbilling problems, and by entering into a contract with the PCG that contravened state procurement codes.

Importantly, audits beget audits and intensify distrust (Power, 1994). Mirroring findings from its earlier audit of the 1997 Medicaid managed-care program (State of New Mexico Legislative Finance Committee 2000), results of a 2015 audit commissioned by the state legislature questioned the capacity of Centennial Care to contain rising Medicaid costs, as promised, and the poor reporting of utilization data by HSD and the participating MCOs. Even more disconcerting were findings regarding the "deteriorated" quality of these data, begging the question of whether Medicaid enrollees were receiving more or less behavioral health care. The report concluded that "it is unknown if the current system under Centennial Care is adequate or cost-effective compared to previous years" (State of NM Legislative Finance Committee 2015, 5).

Despite the growing concern over the PCG audit and Centennial Care, the CMS has declined to intervene in the HSD, even at the repeated request of the New Mexico congressional delegation. Both state and federal legislators, let alone the public, still cannot access reliable information about the Medicaid system. At the urging of the largely Democratic delegation, the CMS undertook a second site visit in the summer of 2014 followed by a series of closed conference calls with select patient and provider constituents in March 2015, but did not share its findings or implement any formal administrative action against the HSD. At a July 2015 congressional hearing in Washington, DC, a New Mexico delegation member pressed a high-ranking CMS official to explain why the state and the CMS were slow to release reliable information regarding the audit and its fallout, but received no satisfactory response (Medicaid at 50, 2015).

All of the accused nonprofits were exonerated of wrongdoing by the attorney general between February and March 2016 (at a minimum cost of $1.9 million to New Mexico taxpayers), prompting Democratic members of the congressional delegation to write a letter to the U.S. Department of Health and Human Services requesting "oversight and assistance" from CMS "to ensure that this vulnerable population in New Mexico is able to access the care they need." An HSD spokesperson referred to the letter as "a partisan stunt" in the media (Horwath 2016). Silence from the CMS and the dearth of data with which to critique the knowledge claims of the HSD, OptumHealth, and PCG, however, further fomented distrust and cynicism. Many in the state legislature and advocacy community suspect that the CMS refrained from intervening at the request of the Obama administration to appease Governor Martinez, one of the few Republican governors to move forward with major components of the ACA, including Medicaid expansion and establishment of a health insurance exchange partly managed by the PCG via another sizeable contract.

Epilogue: The ACA and Accountability

The pronouncement of innocence by the attorney general received a bittersweet reception among providers and patients. Of the cleared nonprofits, most were out of business. At a March 2016 town hall, one CEO reflected on the pain of "attacks on our personal integrity or our personal financial losses and the indescribable unnecessary upheaval in our lives," concluding that "what is truly the injustice is the damage to the many consumers across the state." A second CEO tearfully recounted a phone conversation with a third CEO who had recently passed away, quoting him as hoping that "before I die, that it be found out that I'm not a criminal." Nonetheless, the HSD maintains that the investigation was warranted, telling the *Albuquerque Journal* that "We respect but disagree with" the Attorney General's findings and insisting that "the undeniable facts are that a significant amount of public money was misspent" (Baker 2016).

Health reform advocates should stand forewarned by recent events in New Mexico. With loose definitions for what is a "credible allegation of fraud" and without due process protections under the law, the same ACA provision invoked in New Mexico can justify the deliberate outsourcing of health care in other states. We should also not count on states to apply this provision equally to their managed-care contractors. In 2011, when OptumHealth was but two years into its multimillion-dollar contract with New Mexico and involved in "reconciling" the prepayments that were hastily dispersed to providers in 2009, its upper-level management instructed employees to destroy and falsify records to obtain a higher audit score for appeals and grievance processing. A three-year grand jury investigation—knowledge of which was not made public until October 2014—verified that these acts constituted actual fraud, during which the state continued to pay OptumHealth to run the behavioral health care system (Heild 2014).

Public contestations over the origins, perpetrators, and very existence of the crisis are ongoing. The executives of the Arizona companies complained to the media that once the financial incentives ran out, low reimbursement rates left them essentially subsidizing services that they could not afford to provide (Baumgartel 2015). Four of the companies have pulled out of New Mexico, rendering large swaths of the state and thousands of New Mexicans without services entirely. In a shocking turn of events, one Arizona company, La Frontera, also filed a lawsuit against United Healthcare alleging that the original fraud accusations were invented by OptumHealth in an attempt to conceal its own defective claims-processing system, and that its contract with La Frontera was intended as an "exit strategy" for the company to avoid losing money once its contract with New Mexico expired and Centennial Care was fully implemented. Furthermore, court documents allege that OptumHealth did not pay La Frontera for the first six months of services provided by the agency, instead keeping the money from the state government for itself (*La Frontera Center, Inc. v. United Behavioral Health, Inc.* 2016). An ongoing April 2013 whistleblower suit of a former OptumHealth employee hired to investigate fraud also criticized the claims-processing system, and alleged that OptumHealth had covered up false Medicaid claims to retain a percentage of the provider reimbursements for its coffers (*Clark v. UnitedHealthGroup, Inc.* 2013). These proliferating accusations of fraud point in manifold directions, making it increasingly difficult to disentangle the decisions and actions that have compromised behavioral health care under the ACA.

Anthropologists are only now beginning to document the complexities of ACA implementation and its outcomes. Like other reforms before it, the ACA is subject to various forms of misuse and appropriation. For example, Jessica M. Mulligan (2014) has described how insurance companies game key provisions of the ACA, such as the requirement that no less than 85% of insurance costs must go toward medical care, by reclassifying administrative tasks as medical services. Similarly, she describes an insurance company that offered welcome physicals to new enrollees to record as many diagnoses as possible and thus report "having the sickest beneficiaries in the country (and, by extension, the highest risk-adjusted premium rates)" (13). In New Mexico, a public-private partnership has undercut expanded Medicaid services for persons with mental illness by using fraud provisions under the ACA to advance unsubstantiated claims of corruption. By then depriving nonprofits of due process, this partnership reduced direct service delivery dollars by denying payments to the discredited nonprofits, liquidating their staff, and denying access to their patients.

Anthropologists studying ACA implementation have the responsibility to attend to the "total bureaucratization" of government-funded health care systems that allow the kinds of abuse of authority by public stewards and their corporate partners described here. These systems are simultaneously the main source of care for the most politically disenfranchised segment of our population and an attractive source of revenue for corporate interests. In this way, they embody the core problem of market-based health care identified by Barbara Rylko-Bauer and Paul Farmer (2002, 476): "the fundamental conflict between what is *just* and what is *profitable.*"

This example of politicking in the behavioral health care arena illustrates how the "clamorous rhetoric of transparency" (Anders and Nuijten 2009, 3) can be deployed by a "new breed of players, who operate at the nexus of official and private power," "test the time-honored . . . cannons of accountability of the modern state and the codes of competition of the free market," manipulate the media and the law, and "reorganize relations to bureaucracy and business to their advantage" (Wedel 2009, 7). Within this nexus, political symbols of transparency, such as the audit, mask rather than engender "openness in the exercise of power" (Anders and Nuijten 2009, 3), demonizing and excluding certain classes of citizens (e.g., persons with mental illness) from critical public services that may be essential to their well-being. Encountering relatively little resistance from what remains of New Mexico's diminished and thoroughly frightened provider workforce, the MCOs contracted under Centennial Care (including United Healthcare) echo neoliberal calls for greater patient responsibility rather than admitting to any corporate obligation in addressing the unmet behavioral health care needs of state residents.

The events, media coverage, lawsuits, and outcomes described in this chapter underscore the need for an ACA research agenda that focuses on what anthropologist Colin Hoag (2011, 786) describes as "the sometimes secretive realm of powerful bureaucracies," to elucidate the beliefs, motivations, and practices of privileged decision makers who shape our structures of service delivery. This is no easy task, given that the work and the worldviews of these decision makers are likely influenced by tacit imperatives to protect state interests, or rather, the interests of the administration under which they serve, in addition to corporate interests, as in the case of OptumHealth/United Healthcare. Because public stewards are today powerful players within the behavioral health care marketplace, we must expend greater effort to dissect their relationships with various corporate stakeholders and to reveal the role of vendor influence in our systems of governance. One way to do this is through detailed examinations of political campaign contributions and government contracting (Bromberg 2014). We must also attend to "revolving-door relationships between government and industry officials," a trend that took root during the Medicaid managed-care years, continued in the Transformation, and was most recently epitomized by the state Medicaid agency director—an instrumental player in leveling the accusations of fraud—terminating her HSD employment to take on a position at OptumHealth.

In the midst of the ongoing contestation in New Mexico, testimonies from individuals with mental illness and their families indicate that they are suffering the consequences of this conflict between state agents, corporate actors, and providers. In 2014—the year after fraud allegations shut down the nonprofits statewide—the suicide rate in New Mexico was higher than it had been in the previous two decades; already alarming alcohol- and drug-induced death rates also increased (NM Department of Health 2016). At the March 2016 town hall meeting, a patient recounted his confusing transfer of services to an Arizona company: "I felt like I was slipping through the cracks. If I died, who would care?" In an April 2016 commemoration of "Behavioral Health Day" at the state capital, the mother of a young boy with suicidal ideation, who also happened to be a seasoned child and adolescent therapist, recounted to us how her son's MCO (United Healthcare) repeatedly denied the family access to services locally, placing him instead in a less costly inpatient facility in Texas, where he repeatedly suffered from bullying, violence, and death threats at the hands of other patients. After filing a report with state authorities in Texas, she later learned that her son was the victim of neglect due to lack of supervision on five occasions. Navigating bureaucratic and legal channels to advocate on behalf of her son for in-state care had become her full-time occupation. Troubled that his condition would soon decompensate to the point at which he was likely to become a danger to himself and to others, her family was planning to relocate to another state with a more robust service infrastructure.

Over the last three years, videos produced by local advocates and young journalists (Generation Justice 2016; Jim Cooney Productions 2014; New Mexicans Fighting to Save Behavioral Health 2013) have detailed the experiences of New Mexicans whose access to services has been compromised. These videos offer nuanced perspectives of the crisis and its aftermath, which are not captured in the incomplete utilization data shared by the HSD. One such video tells the story of a 16-year-old with mental health concerns from the rural town of Española who died shortly after being shot by a police officer responding to his 911 call. Both his parents and local advocates attribute his death to the lack of a behavioral health safety net. Incidents like these just scratch the surface of the multiplying stories of negligence and despair from patients and former patients. Such incidents also recall Graeber's cautionary point that while institutional injustices against marginalized citizens, like those described here, take place in the realm of financial accounting, bureaucratic paperwork, and fraud-detection software, they are in fact never very far from real, physical violence. For this reason, we must continue to interrogate "how all these threads— financialization, violence, technology, the fusion of public and private—knit together into a single, self-sustaining web" (Graeber 2015, 42). We must ask: How might the lives of New Mexicans be improved today if ideologies of social justice and equity had shaped public behavioral health care, rather than decades of non-stop reform fueled by privatization, profiteering, and political maneuvering? In the era of the ACA, the crisis in New Mexico exemplified the urgent need to question the organized irresponsibility that was concealed by the circulation of discourses of transparency and the production of accountability while having such deleterious downstream effects on some of our most vulnerable citizens.

ACKNOWLEDGMENTS

The authors wish to thank Louise Lamphere, Sarah Horton, and Patricia S. Hokanson.

REFERENCES

Anders, Gerhard, and Monique Nuijten. 2009. Corruption and the Secret of Law: An Introduction. In *Corruption and the Secret of Law: A Legal Anthropological Perspective*, edited by Gerhard Anders and Monique Nuijten, 1–24. Burlington, VT: Ashgate Publishing.

Baker, Deborah. 2016. AG Clears 10 More Behavioral Health Providers of Fraud. *Albuquerque Journal*, February 8. www.abqjournal.com.

Barrera, Leticia. 2013. Performing the Court: Public Hearings and the Politics of Judicial Transparency in Argentina. *Political and Legal Anthropology Review* 36(2): 326–340.

Baumgartel, Elaine. 2015. Nonprofits Cut Services in Arizona While Expanding into New Mexico. *KUNM*, February 28. kunm.org.

Boyd, Dan. 2014. Behavioral Health Service Rolls Up 30%, State Says. *Albuquerque Journal*, September 24. www.abqjournal.com.

Bromberg, Daniel. 2014. Can Vendors Buy Influence? The Relationship Between Campaign Contributions and Government Contracts. *International Journal of Public Administration* 37(9): 556–567.

Centers for Medicare and Medicaid Services. 2011. *Affordable Care Act Program Integrity Provisions—Guidance to States—Section 6402(h)(2)—Suspension of Medicaid Payments Based upon Pending Investigations of Credible Allegations of Fraud (CPI-B 11–04)*. Baltimore, MD: U.S. Department of Health and Human Services. oig.hhs.gov.

Centers for Medicare and Medicaid Services, and Substance Abuse and Mental Health Services Administration. 2013. *Site Review Report: New Mexico Behavioral Health 9/16/13–9/18/13*. Dallas, TX: Centers for Medicare and Medicaid Services Dallas Regional Office.

Clark, Champ. 2013. Gov. Susana Martinez: Caring for Her Sister. *People*, August 5. www.people.com.

Clark v. UnitedHealthGroup, Inc. 2013. No. 13-CV-372. U.S. District Court for the District of New Mexico.

Comaroff, Jean, and John Comaroff. 2003. Transparent Fictions; or the Conspiracies of a Liberal Imagination: An Afterword. In *Transparency and Conspiracy: Ethnographics of Suspicion in the New World Order*, edited by Harry G. West and Todd Sanders, 287–299. Durham, NC: Duke University Press.

Dotson, Rachel. 2014. Citizen-Auditors and Visible Subjects: Mi Familia Progresa and Transparency Politics in Guatemala. *Political and Legal Anthropology Review* 37(2): 350–370.

Edelman, Murray. 1985. *The Symbolic Uses of Politics*. Chicago: University of Illinois Press.

Generation Justice. 2016. New Mexico Speaks. www.generationjustice.org.

Gonzalez, Roberto J., and Rachael Stryker. 2014. Introduction: On Studying Up, Down, and Sideways: What's at Stake? In *Up, Down, and Sideways: Anthropologists Trace the Pathways of Power*, edited by Rachael Stryker and Roberto J. Gonzalez, 1–24. New York: Berghahn Books.

Graeber, David. 2015. *The Utopia of Rules: On Technology, Stupidity, and the Secret Joys of Bureacracy*. Brooklyn, NY: Melville House.

Guest, Greg, and Kathleen M. MacQueen, eds. 2008. *Handbook for Team-Based Qualitative Research*. Lanham, MD: Altamira Press.

Gusterson, Hugh. 1997. Studying Up Revisited. *Political and Legal Anthropology Review* 20(1): 114–119.

Heild, Colleen. 2014. AG: Behavioral Health Boss Falsified Records." *Albuquerque Journal*, October 10. www.abqjournal.com

Hetherington, Kregg. 2011. *Guerilla Auditors: The Politics of Transparency in Neoliberal Paraguay*. Durham, NC: Duke University Press.

———. 2012. Commentary: Agency, Scale, and the Ethnography of Transparency. *Political and Legal Anthropology Review* 35(2): 242–247.

Heyeck, Larry. 2013. *Medicaid Payment Holds Due to Credible Allegations of Fraud*. Santa Fe: New Mexico Legislature Health and Human Services Committee.

Hoag, Colin. 2011. Assembling Partial Perspectives: Thoughts on the Anthropology of Bureaucracy. *Political and Legal Anthropology Review* 34(1): 81–94.

Horton, Sarah, Cesar Abadia, Jessica Mulligan, and Jennifer Jo Thompson. 2014. Critical Anthropology of Global Health "Takes a Stand" Statement: A Critical Medical Anthropological Approach to the U.S.'s Affordable Care Act. *Medical Anthropology Quarterly* 28(1): 1–22.

Horwath, Justin. 2015. Access Peak. *Santa Fe Reporter*, March 18. www.sfreporter.com.

———. 2016. Calls Grow for Federal Probe into Provider Shake-Up. *Santa Fe New Mexican*, February 14. www.santafenewmexican.com.

Jim Cooney Productions. 2014. New Mexico's Behavioral Health Crisis. www.youtube.com.

La Frontera Center, Inc. v. United Behavioral Health, Inc. 2016. No. D-202-CV-2016-00857. County of Bernalillo Second Judicial Court.

Medicaid at 50: Strengthening and Sustaining the Program. 2015. Hearing Before the Energy and Commerce Subcommittee on Health, Representatives, 114th Congress. www.youtube.com.

Mills, C. Wright. 1951. *White Collar: The American Middle Classes.* New York: Oxford University Press.

Monahan, Joe. 2013. Exploring the Political Connections of Arizona Firms Called in to Take Over Health Care. *New Mexico Politics with Joe Monahan.* joemonahansnewmexico.blogspot.com.

Mulligan, Jessica. 2014. Insurance Accounts: The Cultural Logics of Health Care Financing. *Medical Anthropology Quarterly* 30(1): 37–61.

Nader, Laura. 1972. Up the Anthropologist: Perspectives Gained from Studying Up. In *Reinventing Anthropology*, edited by Dell H. Hymes, 284–311. New York: Pantheon Books.

New Mexicans Fighting to Save Behavioral Health. 2013. The Shutdown of New Mexico's Behavioral Health Providers. www.youtube.com.

New Mexico Department of Health. 2016. *New Mexico Health Indicator Reports.* ibis.health.state.nm.us.

New Mexico Human Services Department. 2013. *Behavioral Health Provider Audit Results.* Santa Fe: State of New Mexico.

Office of the State Auditor. 2014. State Auditor Balderas Releases Financial Audit that Finds Poor Oversight and Mismanagement of Federal Funds by the Human Services Department [Press Release]. www.saonm.org.

Power, Michael. 1994. *The Audit Explosion. No. 7.* London: Demos.

Rylko-Bauer, Barbara, and Paul Farmer. 2002. Managed Care or Managed Inequality? A Call for Critiques of Market-based Medicine. *Medical Anthropology Quarterly* 16(4): 476–502.

Shore, Cris. 2008. Audit Culture and Illiberal Governance: Universities and the Politics of Accountability. *Anthropological Theory* 8(3): 278–298.

Smith, David G. 2002. *Entitlement Politics: Medicare and Medicaid, 1995–2001.* New Brunswick, NJ: Transaction Publishers.

State of New Mexico Legislative Finance Committee. 2000. *Audit of Medicaid Managed Care Program (SALUD!) Cost Effectiveness and Monitoring.* Santa Fe, NM.

———. 2013. *LFC Program Evaluation Progress Report: Human Services Department Costs and Outcomes of Selected Behavioral Health Grants and Spending (#13–04).* Santa Fe, NM. www.nmlegis.gov.

Strathern, Marilyn. 2000. *Audit Cultures: Anthropological Studies in Accountability, Ethics and the Academy.* New York: Routledge.

Substance Abuse and Mental Health Services Administration. 2014. *The NSDUH Report: State Estimates of Adult Mental Illness from the 2001 and 2012 National Surveys on Drug Use and Health.* Rockville, MD: Substance Abuse and Mental Health Services Administration.

Terrell, Steve. 2013a. Behavioral-Health Probe: A Primer. *Santa Fe New Mexican*, July 27. www.santafenewmexican.com.

———. 2013b. Radio Spot Touts Martinez's Tough Stance on Medicaid Fraud. *Santa Fe New Mexican*, September 10. www.santafenewmexican.com.

Truthiness. n.d. *Oxford Dictionaries Online Dictionary.* www.oxforddictionaries.com.

Wedel, Janine R. 2009. *Shadow Elite: How the World's New Power Brokers Undermine Democracy, Government, and the Free Market.* New York: Basic Books.

———. 2014. *Unaccountable: How Elite Power Brokers Corrupt our Finances, Freedom, and Security.* New York: Pegasus Books.

Wedel, Janine R., and Gregory Feldman. 2005. Why an Anthropology of Public Policy? *Anthropology Today* 21(1): 1–2.

Willging, Cathleen E. 2005. Power, Blame, and Accountability: Medicaid Managed Care for Mental Health Services in New Mexico. *Medical Anthropology Quarterly* 19(1): 84–102.

Willging, Cathleen E., Louise Lamphere, and Barbara Rylko-Bauer. 2015. The Transformation of Behavioral Healthcare in New Mexico. *Administration and Policy in Mental Health and Mental Health Services Research* 42(3): 343–355.

Willging, Cathleen E., William Wagner, and Howard Waitzkin. 2005. Medicaid Managed Care for Mental Health Services in a Rural State. *Journal of Healthcare for the Poor and Underserved* 16(3): 497–514.

Willging, Cathleen E., Howard Waitzkin, and Ethel Nicdao. 2008. Medicaid Managed Care for Mental Health Services: The Survival of Safety Net Institutions in Rural Settings. *Qualitative Health Research* 18 (9): 1231–1246.

Zizek, Slavoj. 1997. *The Plague of Fantasies.* New York: Verso.

10

Increasing Access, Increasing Responsibility

Activating the Newly Insured

MARY ALICE SCOTT AND RICHARD WRIGHT

"The Affordable Care Act is making sure that we do our jobs," said Cheryl,[1] the clinical coordinator at a formerly free clinic in southern New Mexico. We were sitting with her in an office that barely fit her desk and our three chairs. Her office was situated in an equally cramped facility that frequently provided the only medical care for the area's large homeless and undocumented immigrant population. We came to the clinic to understand the changes that were happening in the provision of health care under the Affordable Care Act. The clinic was in the process of becoming Medicaid eligible, which required new credentialing for its health care professionals and conversion to an electronic medical record, among other major changes. In a sometimes chaotic environment in which patients frequently arrived with no records and serious complications due to long-standing untreated mental and physical health issues, Cheryl described her changing role in light of the new health policy. Before the ACA, her job was to shepherd patients through a complex process of piecing together resources to increase the possibility that patients could obtain medications and see specialists. With the implementation of the ACA, she argued, patients could better engage in and take charge of their own health care because clinic staff had to be "a little more accountable" for educating patients.

This idea of "co-responsibility"—health care professionals do their part, but patients are ultimately responsible for their own health and health care—permeated the clinic site where we conducted ethnographic research. We borrow the term "co-responsibility" from the language of international development and poverty alleviation programs, but it also reflects an emerging moral discourse of patient engagement and accountability in the United States. On the surface, it is easy to see the practicality of patient responsibility—medicine only works if it is actually taken. However, the staff member quoted above also identified her patients as marginalized through homelessness, irregular immigration status, and mental illness. She saw herself as an advocate for patients without access to health care. In both identifying "co-responsibility" and recognizing the need for structural change, she and her colleagues demonstrated a complex but common discourse among health care professionals in our research. This chapter explores the intersections of seemingly opposing understandings of health—a "right" or a "responsibility"–in health care professionals' commentaries on ACA implementation in a formerly free clinic in southern New Mexico. In doing so, we challenge a moral framework that obscures structural barriers to achieving health and defines health solely according to biomedical parameters.

Discourses of Co-Responsibility and Patient Engagement

In our analysis of clinic staff discourse, we see the concepts of co-responsibility and of patient engagement reflected in staff framing of health care problems, clinic activities, and conceptualizations of patients. These concepts are increasingly central to health care and other social programs globally. In this section, we explain each of the concepts as they are defined by researchers and program administrators who actively study and participate in social programs and health care reform throughout the United States and Latin America. We begin with a discussion of co-responsibility as it is used in Latin American poverty alleviation programs and then move to more recent discussions of patient engagement within U.S. health care reform processes. Although the concepts are similar, the frameworks that emerge contribute to our analysis in different ways. Additionally, these concepts support neoliberal understandings of health and health care that continue to undergird the ACA, although perhaps more subtly than in former health care models. This is not to say that the ACA has not been beneficial to patients. In a recent focus group we conducted with patients of the clinic, patients universally expressed gratitude for their new health insurance, particularly considering the complex health issues all had been struggling to manage, understand, and keep from overpowering their daily lived experiences. We will return to this point in the conclusion following detailed analysis of the way that co-responsibility played out in this particular clinic setting.

Co-responsibility, as it has been established in international development programs, refers to the idea that recipients of assistance and providers of that assistance each have responsibilities to ensure that program goals are met. Often, recipients are required to engage in practices aimed at improving health, educational, or economic status, while providers are required to focus assistance (usually monetary, but sometimes informational or instrumental) in areas of greatest potential benefit. The concept of co-responsibility in health care has worldwide currency. The World Bank and the World Health Organization have advocated for co-responsibility in health care through supporting conditional cash transfers (CCTs) as part of an approach to poverty alleviation (Fiszbein and Schady 2009; Huntington 2010). For example, Mexico's *Oportunidades* program, which is the second largest in Latin America and widely considered to be the most successful of such programs, focuses on alleviating poverty by reducing the "risk" of becoming or remaining poor. The program focuses in particular on increasing educational attainment and improving health outcomes for children by entering into a contractual arrangement with mothers. Mothers have the responsibility to use the financial and informational resources provided through *Oportunidades* to achieve these goals in their own households. *Oportunidades* fulfills its responsibility through disbursing funds and presenting workshops and other educational activities. As Maxine Molyneux (2006, 433) argues, the program is premised on the idea that "poor households do not invest enough in their human capital, and are thus caught in a vicious cycle of intergenerational transmission of poverty, with children dropping out of school and destined to suffer the long-term effects of deprivation." *Oportunidades* gives people the "opportunity" to actively engage in their own poverty alleviation, thereby reducing the paternalism that is sometimes associated with welfare programs. Rather than being "clients of the state," those participating in *Oportunidades* are cast as "empowered, active citizens capable of formulating their own needs" (Molyneux 2006, 429).

This conceptualization of client (or patient) participation in achieving the goals of state-funded programs is in many ways similar to ideas of patient engagement that have recently gained significant traction in the United States, particularly in connection to the Affordable Care Act. Although there are several definitions of patient engagement in the literature, one of the most widely used is that developed by Angela Coulter: "the relationship between patients and health care providers as they work together to 'promote and support active patient and public involvement in health and healthcare and to strengthen their influence on healthcare decisions, at both the individual and collective levels'" (Coulter cited in Carman et al. 2013). Patient engagement relies on "shared responsibility"[2] and *collaboration* among patients, providers, health care administrators, and communities (Danis and Solomon 2013; Robert Wood Johnson Foundation 2014). It requires *motivating* patients to increase their participation in their own health care (Carman et al. 2013; Hibbard and Greene 2013) and to become more *proactive* in managing health and health care issues (Natale and Gross 2013). This definition of patient engagement involves supporting patients' increased *responsibility* for their own health (Carman et al. 2013), *empowering* patients to develop *self-efficacy* (Danis and Solomon 2013), and improving health literacy so that patients can be more fully *informed* in making health care decisions (Koh et al. 2013). These and other similar processes aim to increase patient accountability.

Patient engagement has become imagined as one of the primary tools for achieving the "Triple Aim" in health care—reduced health care costs, improved patient experience, and improved health outcomes (Dentzer 2013; Institute for Healthcare Improvement, n.d.). Patient-centered care, which was central to the ACA's provisions, did not necessarily require patient engagement. However, the ACA did mandate measurement of the quality of health care (Millenson and Macri 2012). This mandate created a framework for new metrics such as the Physician Quality Reporting System (Centers for Medicare and Medicaid Services, n.d.) and meaningful use of electronic health records (HealthIT.gov, n.d.). Clinics funded through some federal grants, like FHCC (Family Health Care Clinic), were required to report through the Uniform Data System on nearly 70 metrics, including measures of cost and quality of care, effective use of electronic health records, health outcomes, and health disparities (Health Resources and Services Administration 2015). Many of these metrics were added through the ACA.

Numerous commentaries across health professions proclaim the power of patient engagement to transform health care (cf. Mayer 2014; Schiavo 2014) and improve the results of measurements such as those mentioned above. The research literature on patient engagement connects it to several outcomes including higher quality patient experience (Carman et al. 2013; Hibbard and Greene 2013), higher self-reported quality of life (Danis and Solomon 2013), and lower rates of high-cost health care usage (Hibbard and Greene 2013). While there is often a nod to vulnerable populations, who may not be able to engage at the same level as non-vulnerable populations, usually the answer is not to engage the health care system or its authoritative actors to refocus on structural inequalities, but instead to suggest modified interventions that recognize the diminished capacity of vulnerable populations to fully engage (see Carman et al. 2013) and "help patients begin to manage these vulnerabilities" (Koh et al. 2013, 361).

Those individuals and organizations who adopt the concepts of co-responsibility and patient engagement often claim that these frameworks reduce or eliminate the paternalism associated with older programs that sought to alleviate poverty. For example, in establishing co-responsibility, patients become *empowered* with increased information offered through workshops. Through patient engagement, doctors *share* health care decision making with patients, thereby giving patients *control* over their own health and health care.

While the concepts of co-responsibility and patient engagement are similar, they highlight different aspects of neoliberal thinking about the relationships between the state and its citizens as well as health care organizations and patients. Co-responsibility implies that patients and health care professionals are on equal footing, each able to support equivalent responsibilities for achieving health. Patient engagement perhaps opens slightly more space for recognizing the inequities in social position and the effects of structural inequalities on patients' health and health care, but it remains focused on the individual patient as the source of potential responsibility (or "activation," to use the language of patient engagement). Bringing together these ideas of co-responsibility and patient engagement allows for a complex analysis of FHCC's process of becoming Medicaid eligible following the implementation of the Affordable Care Act.

In many ways, patient engagement and co-responsibility were taken for granted as foundations of patient health care in this clinical setting. This is not surprising, as individual responsibility, autonomy, and choice are frequently cited as core values in the United States, and these values are embedded in health policy. As noted in the introduction to this book, notions of personal responsibility codified in federal policy certainly pre-date the ACA, notably through PRWORA. It continued in the language of the ACA: "This Act puts individuals, families, and small business owners *in control of their health care* . . . Americans without insurance coverage will be able to *choose the insurance coverage that works best for them* in a new open, competitive insurance market" (U.S. Department of Health and Human Services, n.d., emphasis added). The ACA, then, guaranteed access to insurance[3] by giving people choices that put them in control. As our research participants pointed out, access to insurance is only one of many barriers to health care and is limited in its ability to put patients in control. However, health care professionals in our research understood patients to retain a significant responsibility for their own health care, a responsibility that became more explicit with the implementation of the ACA. At that point, clinic staff began drawing on the ACA as a symbolic support for their already existing beliefs that patients needed to have some responsibility for their health.

Their perceptions of health care and the ACA assumed in some ways the inevitability of neoliberal models of health care that have been critiqued by health scholars. These critiques challenge the idea that market-based models of care that hold individual responsibility, autonomy, and choice (or freedom) as core values are the best way to address health, health care, and health inequalities. While the ACA did expand access to health care, it still operated within this market model. Moving health care to the "marketplace" supports the notion of health as a commodity rather than a human right, a private rather than a public good (Iriart et al. 2001; Maskovsky 2000). When health is viewed as a commodity, it becomes the individual responsibility of the consumer to maintain (Maskovsky 2000). This process increases health inequalities (Maskovsky 2000; Rylko-Bauer and Farmer 2002; Waitzkin and Iriart 2000). The ACA focused on improving the quality of health care through expanded access and fiscal management. However, there was relative inattention placed on disparities in health care related to factors such as sex, race/ethnicity, social class, insurance status, and language, which often limit how much overall health quality can improve (Davis and Walter 2011). If an effective model of co-responsibility is to be implemented in U.S. health care, then these disparities need to be more thoroughly addressed. Individual choice and autonomy in the health care marketplace become constrained as long as these issues of health inequality remain unaddressed.

The Affordable Care Act, as well as Medicaid and Medicare more broadly, are balanced somewhat between health as a commodity and health as a right. In her review of recent health care reforms in the United States, legal scholar Erika Blacksher (2010, 42) notes that those at the highest levels of government, including the president of the United States and the secretary of Health and Human Services, have "declared health a collaborative enterprise." In other words, patients, legislators, health care professionals, and others share co-responsibility for health—both the patient and the system must do their parts.

One of the most frequent challenges for patients in our research was to fulfill their responsibility for obtaining a Medicaid card indicating their eligibility for the insurance as well as their new accountability for accessing care. While the Affordable Care Act expanded access to Medicaid in the state of New Mexico, the process for obtaining a Medicaid card was confusing to patients. Additionally, health care professionals sometimes equated the Medicaid card with actual access to health services and therefore believed that patients could shoulder more of the responsibility for their own health care. Both staff and patients at FHCC also narrated another story—one that offers a more complex understanding of the challenges to accessing health care and achieving health. The dominant narrative of responsibility, choice, and autonomy often obscured this more subtle story.

Methods

The setting of this research is Family Health Care Clinic (FHCC). FHCC began in the mid-1980s as a first aid table in a soup kitchen at a local church. A nurse who was volunteering at the soup kitchen saw that people were coming in with injuries, and she wanted to help. Other health professionals began to get involved, and the first aid table eventually grew into a community health care clinic over the next five years. At the time of our research, the clinic still served the same population as it did at the soup kitchen, mostly homeless and immigrant patients.

That continues to be the case. In 2015, approximately 90% of patients were homeless.[4] Fifty-five percent of patients attending the clinic were male, and 45% were female; 2.5% of patients were veterans; approximately 63% of FHCC's patients identified as Hispanic/Latino. It was difficult for the clinic to determine how many patients were undocumented. In 2015, 50% of patients were uninsured and 46% received Medicaid; 4% of patients were on Medicare; and 90% of patients were between the ages of 18 and 64.

This clinic was located on a campus that also included many other services: a soup kitchen, a food pantry, a supportive housing agency, a place to shower and wash clothes, a tent city, and a day care center. The clinic operated within a large county in southern New Mexico where approximately two-thirds of the population identified as Hispanic/Latino, and just under one-third identified as non-Hispanic White. Twenty-seven percent of the population lived below the poverty line. A number of *colonias* were present within the county's borders. A colonia is a community in the U.S.-Mexico border region "with marginal conditions related to housing and infrastructure" (U.S. Department of Housing and Urban Development, n.d.). Many of the clinic's patients lived in these colonias and struggled not only with access to basic services like water and sewage, but also with transportation. Bus service was limited, and a border checkpoint in the middle of the county prevented some from traveling due to fears of harassment or deportation.

Our research team conducted two interviews with each of the staff members in the clinic, including a clinical coordinator, two front office staff, the case manager, and the clinic director. We also sat in the waiting room of the clinic on different days of the week and times of the day to complete surveys and conduct short interviews with patients. This sample was a convenience sample of the patients in the waiting room on the days that we were present. The clinic served homeless and indigent patients, the majority of whom spoke Spanish as their primary language. We asked all patients in the waiting room if they would be willing to participate and completed interviews and/or surveys with those who consented. We completed 12 interviews with English-speaking patients and nine interviews with Spanish-speaking patients. We also completed 33 surveys with English-speaking patients and 25 surveys with Spanish-speaking patients.[5] Due to the difficulty in following up with patients, our interviews had to take place in the clinic itself. The interviews lasted an average of five minutes because patients had other, more pressing concerns than talking with us. Sometimes they were called back for their appointment and did not return to complete the interview. Sometimes they had buses to catch or needed to get in line for lunch at the soup kitchen. We shortened our interviews to a few basic questions to accommodate each situation. We also included surveys as a way to capture some data more quickly. Many patients were not willing to be interviewed, but they would complete a survey. In this chapter, we focus on the interviews with clinic staff, using data from patients as a counterpoint where appropriate.

Getting Patients Engaged in Their Own Health Care: The Hope of the Affordable Care Act to Increase Individual Responsibility

FHCC's director, Angela, became involved with the organization because she had experienced homelessness herself. In an interview with her, she recognized the difference between her situation and that of many of the clinic's patients.

> I was homeless myself for just a month when I was 18, and I could see that if my life were different I could very well still be homeless. If I didn't have a family who loved me, you know, they kicked me out at the time, but I had a sibling that got me a job in Boston when I was sleeping in the back seat of my car. So I think that I had a lot of benefits that a lot of people who are homeless don't, particularly family support. So I had a good education, a middle-class background, family that finally came around, and I had siblings to offer me support.

Her experience with homelessness supported her commitment to establishing quality health care for marginalized patients.

Angela frequently commented that her staff was similarly committed to the patients who came to their clinic for their health care. Cheryl, the clinical coordinator mentioned at the beginning of this chapter, came out of retirement as a nurse to work part-time in the clinic. When we asked her why, she said, "I believe in the mission that they have here, which is to help everyone to be able to have access to medical care. And if they have no other means of obtaining it, I mean, that's just the bottom line is that I believe that everyone has equal opportunity to have medical care whether they have insurance or not." Cheryl's vision was that all people have a right to *equal opportunity* for health care. The interview data presented in this section are from interviews conducted with staff members prior to the Medicaid expansion. While staff members were nervous about the transition to accepting Medicaid and the accompanying changes to the clinic, they were hopeful that the provisions of the Affordable Care Act would improve the health of their patient population. They moved from envisioning the Affordable Care Act as a policy that would at least partially address the structural barriers to health that their patients faced to seeing the ACA as a way to increase patient responsibility.

The staff recognized the marginality of their patient population and identified specific structural barriers to health care that were clearly outside an individual patient's control. These barriers included transportation, lack of both medical and behavioral health clinicians, low incomes, and lack of social support. "Transportation is a big barrier," said Cheryl. "There's a lot of people that we see that come here that are from outlying areas . . . and, you know, they'll say, 'Well you know I couldn't come because I didn't have a ride and my neighbor didn't come.'" Public transportation was very limited in the more rural areas of the county, and many residents relied on family members and neighbors for rides into town. When transportation limited the days and times that a patient could attend the clinic, the lack of physician coverage became a greater issue. The doctors who practiced at FHCC were volunteers and only worked about one day per month each.

Claudia, a front office staff member, was particularly concerned that many patients needed both medical treatment and psychological counseling, but it took two to three months to get an appointment with a counselor because of the lack of mental health professionals practicing in the area. In addition, Angela pointed to lack of steady income, mental health issues, and difficult family backgrounds. The staff articulated multiple ways that they worked against these barriers to help their patients get the treatment that they need. They pitched in money to pay for patients' medications or their bus fare to the Wal-Mart pharmacy. They pleaded with pharmaceutical companies to obtain free medicines through assistance programs. They applied for grants in order to have a paid medical provider and a behavioral health provider. In other words, they recognized and worked to address the structural barriers that patients confronted as they attempted to obtain health care.

On the other hand, they emphasized co-responsibility for health. For example, Cheryl implicitly argued that some patients clearly do not take responsibility for their own health when she discussed some of the challenges she faced in her work at the clinic.

> One of the other challenges is just getting people to—the people who come in and see the doctor, getting them to come in on a regular basis to manage their chronic illnesses. A lot of people that come here have chronic illness. In other words, they're gonna live with this illness for the rest of their life, and *they need to manage it*. But they think that one visit to the doctor and one prescription or a bottle of medicine is gonna be the cure-all. But it isn't because sometimes they have to have education on nutrition—on better nutrition. *They have to be educated* on what type of exercise they need to keep their blood pressure stable. And you try to provide these resources and services and they're not interested. They just want to see what kind of free stuff they can get . . . That's my biggest challenge . . . trying to get people to understand that if you *participate in your own health care* you're gonna have better outcomes . . . I mean it is your own health care. *You own your own health.* (Authors' emphasis)

Cheryl here focused on the patient's role in chronic disease management and the need for education. She claimed that patients *own* their health. At other times, she also called the patient a *partner* in health care. Although the health care professional can offer support, it is the patient who has to take responsibility and not just "see what kind of free stuff they can get."

Similarly, Angela said that the hardest part of working at the clinic was seeing

> *people making bad decisions* and suffering the consequences of them like giving up their housing for something else like partying; people not

growing up and *not taking responsibility for themselves*, like people doing stuff that I was doing in high school like sneaking around the corner and smoking pot behind the tree on the property. Out here they're doing it, and they're 65 and that's part of the frustration. But they're still a really small population.

Cheryl and Angela expressed frustration with their work. They saw many patients every day with uncontrolled diabetes, hypertension, obesity, and other chronic illnesses. In our interviews with them, their sincere desire to see their patients become healthier was clearly evident. Their exasperation at what at least at times seemed to be a lack of individual responsibility was understandable. They fell back on a discourse of patient responsibility perhaps without realizing that in the moment they had forgotten the structural barriers that they articulated in other moments of the interviews.

Claudia relied on a similar discourse, but articulated it differently. She said that much of her job was education. For example, when they needed to have blood work or other labs that were not available at the clinic, Claudia explained that patients often needed direction. She role-played speaking with a patient: "OK, you need to go do this first, then go do this, then go back and do this, then they'll help you at the hospital." She said that she had to write it down for some people. Others were not capable of proceeding on their own, as Claudia asserted, "Some of them need to get it by hand and say, 'OK, I need to make an appointment for this person; they're standing right here. Can I set a date?' It has nothing to do with our clinic, but we're helping them make an appointment somewhere else. We do a lot of that here . . . you gotta hold it by hand, *do it for them*" (authors' emphasis). The implication here is that patients should be able to do it themselves. As Claudia said, "This has nothing to do with our clinic," nothing to do with health care. But for *their* patients, they needed to do it anyway.

Both Cheryl and Claudia emphasized education as a central component of patient responsibility even as they described other structural barriers. If patients are educated, they argued, then they can take charge of their health even though other issues loom in the background. For example, Claudia responded to a question about the reasons people come into the clinic already very ill: "Not having a stable life is one, and two, I believe that not having someone educate them on how important it is to take care of themselves. Some of them come in, didn't even know they had diabetes and, 'Oh, I didn't know I wasn't supposed to eat that' or 'I never knew I couldn't have it' . . . 'Well, what do I do to avoid it?' A lot of them don't know." She listed language barriers for Spanish-speaking patients and cultural differences between patients and the health care system model in the United States, moving back and forth between broad structural barriers and patients' individual knowledge, as barriers to health care. She assumed that once patients *know*, they will act differently.

Angela similarly argued that if patients had options, they would become more responsible. In discussing her vision for the future of the clinic she said, "The other things I think would be great would be to have continuous outreach staff that could bring alternatives to interest people in their own health through non-traditional medical means" like yoga, tai chi, and massage. Angela also articulated a difference between the clinic's patients and herself and her friends.

> I think we had a really good training program for chronic disease management. It was a six-week program . . . We had 14 people sign up for the Spanish version and 10 people for the English and we had almost zero attendance. The two people that attended regularly was myself and another staff member, not clients. They were all enthusiastic, but life happens—my car broke down, my boyfriend left me. It happens. So I think there's an interest, it's just how to truly engage them. You know a lot of my friends, we go to things. We pay to learn about things or to get massage or acupuncture and here we can't always get them to come for free.

The staff often relied on individual stories of success—for example one patient who came to the clinic with uncontrolled diabetes and was able to change his diet and lifestyle to the point that he no longer needed medication—to underscore this belief.

Prior to the implementation of Medicaid expansion through the Affordable Care Act in New Mexico, the staff at the clinic expressed hope that when their patients were able to obtain health insurance, they would begin to care about themselves and change their perspectives so that they would take responsibility for their health and health care. At least in part, the staff recognized that having insurance could increase access to care so that people would have the ability to "participate" in their health care in a way that they did not before. Access to insurance, however, did not directly address the other barriers that staff identified. The problem for clinic patients was that increased responsibility did not come with increased resources beyond insurance.

In many ways, the staff at the clinic drew on the language of health care reform in their discussions of patient responsibility. Their reflections on their patients often mirrored the literature advocating for increased patient engagement or activation in order to improve health care quality and the patient experience. Whether they realized it or not, they echoed the language of co-responsibility in health care reform policy globally in their understanding that patients must "do their part" because staff are certainly doing theirs. Staff focused on motivating and educating patients to become partners in their own health care, ultimately determining that a patient's health will not improve unless that individual responsibility takes shape in the form of compliance with treatments and attendance in health care programs, such as those for chronic illness. Although the patient engagement literature distinguishes between engagement and compliance, the workings of engagement on the ground in this case demonstrate their continued interconnectedness.

The staff believed that access to insurance through the Affordable Care Act was the gateway to responsibility and engagement even as they continued to recognize the structural barriers that were present. Like Koh and colleagues (2013), clinic staff focused on managing vulnerabilities for individual patients. In doing so, they supported broader ideas of individual responsibility rooted in neoliberal discourses that are present even in health care policy that purports to move in a different direction.

Still Struggling: The Affordable Care Act in Action

Our research team returned to interview staff after the implementation of the Medicaid expansion in New Mexico to document the changes that had been made in the clinic and with staff experiences. The staff remained hopeful that the Affordable Care Act would indeed improve their patients' health, and they were beginning to see some benefits. For example, the clinic was able to hire a behavioral health specialist, made possible because the clinic could now bill Medicaid for patients that had enrolled in the expansion. Having an in-house counselor improved follow-up with patient referrals and made it more likely that patients would obtain behavioral health services. Just before writing this chapter, Angela informed us that the clinic had received a large "Affordable Care Act New Access Points" grant through the Health Resources and Services Administration. This grant supported behavioral health staff and a paid medical provider. However, the staff also continued to identify ongoing barriers to access. These barriers included lack of documentation, being just over the financial limit to qualify for Medicaid, challenges with the different requirements of the four managed-care organizations participating in the expansion, and a lack of awareness among patients that they even need to apply for Medicaid.

As in the first interviews, staff highlighted patients' lack of knowledge, awareness, and education as key obstacles to increasing access to insurance through the Affordable Care Act. Minerva, the case manager, said, "A lot of people don't know that they have to apply for Medicaid. And some of these people from the rural areas, or other people that are not informed of what Medicaid consists of, they're the ones who are gonna fall through the cracks." In order to address this issue, she pointed to patient education. "We put out flyers, we tell all our patients or people that come in, and then they spread the word. So we constantly educate them on how important it is and why you have to apply."

Some saw the new access to insurance as a confidence builder for patients that led them to take more responsibility for their care. Claudia felt that the Medicaid expansion had improved the quality of health care because it makes patients "more confident." She role-played a patient: "Now I can go see a doctor. Now I can follow up with this person, this doctor, this specialty doctor. It's gotten better for patients that have Medicaid." Similarly, Cheryl saw the Affordable Care Act as helping her

> to become a little more accountable to help teach patients about managing their own health care. The focus needs to change from just coming in, picking up your medicines and then leaving, to "OK, you have high blood pressure. These are the things that you can do to manage your blood pressure," and helping patients with goal setting and buying into the whole thing that they have control over their health care. The health care facility,

the clinic, the doctors, the nurses, we're not in charge of their health care. They are ... Because ultimately each individual has that responsibility to take care of themselves.

However, they also recognized the significant structural barriers that played a role as well. Staff was already aware that undocumented immigrants would not have access to health insurance through the Medicaid expansion, but they also learned that documentation was difficult for their transient population to produce in general, even if such documentation existed. Minerva mentioned, "we just find it hard that some of our people that walk in don't have money to get IDs or get their birth certificates. So that's a big challenge for us, and not just for us, but for the whole community." Cheryl echoed this concern, adding that if patients have partial documentation it is not worth it for the case manager to upload it to the system because it will be deleted after a short period of time. It can take a month or more for patients to gather all the necessary documentation. Therefore, clinic staff only process enrollments when the patient has all the necessary documentation with them that day. Minerva said that the lack of funding to support patients in getting appropriate documentation was an issue.

In our surveys, nine English-speaking patients and four Spanish-speaking patients said that they had used the Medicaid enrollment services offered at the clinic. Eight English-speaking and 13 Spanish-speaking patients said that they thought they would use that service in the future. Nine English-speaking and one Spanish-speaking patient said that they were not likely to use Medicaid enrollment services at all. These data did not tell us much about why people would or would not enroll in Medicaid, but did indicate that few patients had, in fact, enrolled. Our interviews revealed slightly more detail about what was happening with Medicaid enrollment. Only two of the Spanish-speaking patients that we interviewed clearly stated that they had enrolled in Medicaid. One patient said that she thought the clinic staff had tried to enroll her, but she wasn't sure. When asked whether she had enrolled, she said, "I don't think so. They signed us up here, but then I never learned anything more." Another patient was unsure whether he was receiving services through Medicaid or through the county's indigent funds. When asked if he was enrolled, he replied, "No, I don't know. Documents come telling me to enroll in this program—what's it called . . . I don't know if it's indigent. I think it is indigent." Other patients had not enrolled because of lack of residency in the United States, because they did not know about the Medicaid expansion, because they were unsure which programs they qualified for, and because they confused it with Medicare and thought they could not get it until they turned 65 years of age.

Of the 12 English-speaking patients, seven had enrolled in Medicaid and one was unsure whether he was enrolled or not. Those who had not enrolled thought they were not eligible (some were likely not because of new jobs), needed additional documentation such as a birth certificate, or were new to the area and currently homeless. For example, a member of our research team asked a patient whether he had enrolled in Medicaid through the expansion:

> PATIENT: Not yet. I just found out I can.
> INTERVIEWER: OK, so that information wasn't really–
> PATIENT: I was under the impression, based on my exposure to mass media, that I wasn't eligible.
> INTERVIEWER: Did the clinic let you know you were eligible?
> PATIENT: Yeah, the Medicaid representative said I might be eligible.
> INTERVIEWER: OK, so you still have to kind of see.
> PATIENT: Well, there's a document that I still have to get. When I was born I didn't get a birth certificate from the state. So I have to get a state-issued birth certificate.

The patient went on to indicate that the cost of the birth certificate was not an issue, only ten dollars, but getting there to get it was taking some time. Another patient also indicated his own responsibility in getting enrolled in Medicaid: "I need to get enrolled . . . I guess I should have taken care of this earlier, but I've been chronically homeless so . . ."

Even when patients have the appropriate documentation, Claudia expressed concern for those who are "a dollar over." They have jobs that pay just enough for them to move into the marketplace rather than qualify for Medicaid. At that point, the issue is that they "give up," according to Claudia. They have gone through a burdensome process to apply for Medicaid. "It's supposed to be transferred over to the exchange, well guess what, they already gave up because they don't have Medicaid. Well guess what, they still don't have insurance."

Cheryl echoed these thoughts in her conclusion that the Affordable Care Act had caused "a lot of confusion about who qualifies and the income requirements, who qualifies for Medicaid expansion through the state, who doesn't and who needs to go through the exchanges." Patients also experienced this confusion according to Cheryl. She explained a specific situation:

> The other day this gentleman came in, and he's had his Medicaid card for three months, since March. But he failed to tell us. And so all this time he's coming here 'cause he was our patient. But he had Medicaid, and so I went up front and I said, "Did you all know this guy had Medicaid now?" "Oh, no, we thought it was pending." So not even the patients are connecting to—"OK this card came in the mail so now what do I do with it. I should ask at the clinic what I should do with this card." Right?

With the Medicaid card, she said, patients can go get an MRI, receive foot care, or get an eye exam. "But they just, I don't know, I mean, are we so failing these people that we're not educating them?" In some sense, Cheryl equated access to insurance with access to care. The issue, she believed, was lack of knowledge, and again patient education was the solution.

The clinic staff still moved back and forth between recognizing structural barriers and focusing on patient responsibility for their own care. They still felt hopeful about the possibilities of the Affordable Care Act to make a difference in patient responsibility, but they felt doubtful about how much access to insurance would affect the structural barriers to health that their patients experienced. According to Cheryl,

> Now that they have their Medicaid, then we can say, "OK, you have your Medicaid now, so now you can go and get your eye exam, so let us make your appointment for that, and let us make your appointment for your dental exam." But the issue is still if they don't have transportation to get to that medical appointment, or they don't have bus fare to get on the bus, they're still gonna miss their appointment. So it's not the answer to everything because there's other barriers to getting health care. Some people

live out in the colonias, they live out in the rural communities . . . what do those people do? What do those people do when they have to go to the doctor and they don't have a car? They depend on their neighbor or their aunt or their sister or whatever. So transportation's still a big issue. And the Affordable Care Act doesn't cover that.

Conclusion

There is a tension in the comments made by clinic staff both before and after the implementation of the Affordable Care Act. Staff moved between an unquestioned use of the language of co-responsibility and patient engagement and a recognition that individual patients at their clinic could only shoulder so much responsibility for their own health. While some health policy researchers have documented benefits to this kind of shared responsibility for health care as we noted above, we argue that the foundations of this language prevent a complete reframing of health as a "right" and instead continue an arguably more subtle paternalistic approach. Clinic staff did continue to label patients as "good" or "difficult" depending on their level of engagement and acceptance of responsibility.

In some positive ways, the Affordable Care Act became a symbol for the professionals discussed here as for others, standing in for a broad range of changes in health systems. Its language opened up a space for challenging standard practice in health care among our collaborators that led to innovative models to address social determinants of health in clinical settings. Patient-centered care is becoming more prominent as a tool to develop patient engagement and co-responsibility—the shift in values will include patient safety, quality of care, re-centering care in the patient's community, improving the patient experience of care, and addressing the social determinants of health that patients must navigate. These ideals exemplify the social mission in medicine as well as the discursive changes in the language of health policy. The health care professionals at the Family Health Care Center, in fact, saw their work as a mission of sorts. Their commitment to caring for their patients, particularly those who were working to fulfill their responsibilities for their own health, went far beyond what might typically be expected of a health care provider.

On the other hand, the patient had become the "customer," and health care professionals must provide good customer service. The patient also had responsibilities in this new regime of care. The patient must be part of the team. They must take responsibility for their own health care even as the physician increasingly recognizes that there are limits to what patients can do. The focus remains on individual patients rather than the structural barriers that limited the possibilities for fostering health and well-being among marginalized populations. However, this analysis of how FHCC clinic staff understood their patients and enacted the requirements and opportunities of the ACA is not meant to undermine the commitments of either the staff or of emerging health policy that does move toward broader inclusion and access to humane and respectful health care. The critique articulated in this chapter is offered in the spirit of collaboration with hard-working, committed health care providers and health policy makers who constantly work to improve community health and well-being through direct care and policy development. In this complex and challenging world, the health care professionals at Family Health Care Clinic in many ways did the best that they could do—offering the resources made available through the Affordable Care Act, caring deeply for their patients, and working outside the normal bounds of their jobs to improve health in their community.

ACKNOWLEDGMENTS

The authors thank Alicia Cruz and Devin Grider for assisting with data collection, Aracely Pedraza for assisting with transcription of Spanish-language interviews, and the staff and patients at Family Health Care Clinic for sharing their time and insights with us. We also thank the School for Advanced Research for providing the opportunity to develop this manuscript during a short seminar and the participants of the seminar who provided feedback that greatly improved the manuscript. The College of Arts and Sciences at New Mexico State University generously provided funding for this project.

NOTES
1 All names are pseudonyms.
2 We understand this concept of shared responsibility to be different than that of co-responsibility in large part because it expands responsibility beyond a

relationship between citizen and state (or patient and health care system actors) to include organizational responsibility.

3 As stated in the Introduction and other chapters in this book, the guarantee of access did not extend to all populations living within the United States, including undocumented immigrants.

4 A year earlier the rate of homeless patients was approximately 60%. Before 2016, the clinic kept manual documentation. The switch to Electronic Health Records may have skewed the data.

5 Our sample was skewed toward English-speaking patients. While we did not directly ask anyone why they chose not to participate, we do know that a greater proportion of Spanish-speaking patients were undocumented. It is possible that more Spanish-speaking patients chose not to participate in our study for that reason.

REFERENCES

Blacksher, Erika. 2010. Health Reform and Health Equity: Sharing Responsibility for Health in the United States. *Hofstra Law Review* 39(1): 41–58.

Carman, Kristin L., Pam Dardess, Maureen Maurer, Shoshanna Sofaer, Karen Adams, Christine Bechtel, and Jennifer Sweeney. 2013. Patient and Family Engagement: A Framework for Understanding the Elements and Developing Interventions and Policies. *Health Affairs* 32(2): 223–231.

Centers for Medicare & Medicaid Services. n.d. Physician Quality Reporting System, www.cms.gov.

Coulter, Angela 2011. *Engaging Patients in Healthcare.* New York: McGraw-Hill Education.

Danis, Marion, and Mildred Solomon. 2013. Providers, Payers, the Community, and Patients Are All Obliged to Get Patient Activation and Engagement Ethically Right. *Health Affairs* 32(2): 401–407.

Davis, Matthew, and Jennifer Walter. 2011. Equality-in-Quality in the Era of the Affordable Care Act. *Journal of the American Medical Association* 306(8): 872–873.

Dentzer, Susan. 2013. Rx For the "Blockbuster Drug" of Patient Engagement. *Health Affairs* 2(2): 202.

Fiszbein, Ariel, and Norbert Schady. 2009. *Conditional Cash Transfers: Reducing Present and Future Poverty.* Washington, DC: World Bank.

HealthIT.gov, n.d. Meaningful Use Definition & Objectives, www.healthit.gov.

Health Resources and Services Administration. 2015. Reporting Instructions for Health Centers. Uniform Data System Manual. www.bphc.hrsa.gov.

Hibbard, Judith H., and Jessica Greene. 2013. What the Evidence Shows About Patient Activation: Better Health Outcomes and Care Experiences; Fewer Data on Costs. *Health Affairs* 32(2): 207–214.

Huntington, D. 2010. *The Impact of Conditional Cash Transfers on Health Outcomes and the Use of Health Services in Low- and Middle-Income Countries: RHL Commentary.* Geneva: World Health Organization, WHO Reproductive Health Library.

Institute for Healthcare Improvement. n.d. IHI Triple Aim Initiative, www.ihi.org.

Iriart, Celia, Emerson Elias Merhy, and Howard Waitzkin. 2001. Managed Care in Latin America: The New Common Sense in Health Policy Reform. *Social Science and Medicine* 52(8): 1243–1253.

Koh, Howard K., Cindy Brach, Linda M. Harris, and Michael L. Parchman. 2013. A Proposed "Health Literate Care Model" Would Constitute a Systems Approach to Improving Patients' Engagement in Care. *Health Affairs* 32(2): 357–367.

Maskovsky, Jeff. 2000. "Managing" the Poor: Neoliberalism, Medicaid HMOs and the Triumph of Consumerism Among the Poor. *Medical Anthropology* 19(2): 121–146.

Mayer, Deborah K. 2014. How Do We Encourage Patient Engagement? *Clinical Journal of Oncology Nursing* 18(5): 487–488.

Millenson, Michael L., and Juliana Macri. 2012. Will the Affordable Care Act Move Patient-Centeredness to Center Stage? Timely Analysis of Immediate Health Policy Issues. Princeton, NJ: Robert Wood Johnson Foundation, www.rwjf.org.

Molyneux, Maxine. 2006. Mothers at the Service of the New Poverty Agenda: Progresa/Oportunidades, Mexico's Conditional Transfer Programme. *Social Policy and Administration* 40(4): 425–449.

Natale, Carmen V., and Devin Gross. 2013. The ROI of Engaged Patients. *Healthcare Financial Management* (March): 90–97.

Robert Wood Johnson Foundation. 2014. What We're Learning: Engaging Patients Improves Health and Health Care. Quality Field Notes Issue Brief No. 3, March 2014. Princeton, NJ: Robert Wood Johnson Foundation.

Rylko-Bauer, Barbara, and Paul Farmer. 2002. Managed Care or Managed Inequality? A Call for Critiques of Market-Based Medicine. *Medical Anthropology Quarterly* 16(4): 476–502.

Schiavo, Renata. 2014. Reflecting on Community and Patient Engagement and Other Health Communication Topics. *Journal of Communication in Healthcare* 7(3): 149–151.

U.S. Department of Health and Human Services. n.d. The Affordable Care Act, Section by Section. www.hhs.gov.

U.S. Department of Housing and Urban Development. n.d. Community Development Block Grant: COLONIAS. portal.hud.gov.

Waitzkin, Howard, and Celia Iriart. 2000. How the United States Exports Managed Care to Developing Countries. *International Journal of Health Services* 31(3): 495–505.

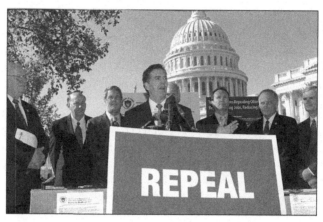

Figure C.1. Repeal. Senator Jim DeMint (R-SC), center, joins other conservative lawmakers to criticize President Obama's national health care plan, often called "Obamacare," Wednesday, October 5, 2011, during a news conference on Capitol Hill in Washington. The event was organized by the Repeal It Now.org campaign, which says the boxes are packed with petitions from American citizens asking Congress to repeal the Patient Protection and Affordable Care Act. (AP photo/J. Scott Applewhite)

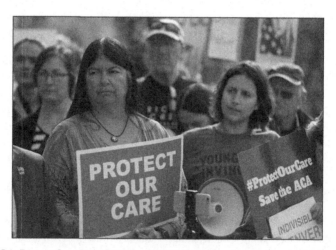

Figure C.2. Protect Our Care. State Senator Dr. Irene Aguilar (D-Denver), left, stands with activist Christina Postolowski, of the group Young Invincibles, as supporters of the Affordable Care Act who are also opponents of Colorado's GOP-led plan to undo Colorado's state-run insurance exchange hold a rally on the state capitol steps in Denver, Tuesday, January 31, 2017. The state GOP measure, a bill that would dismantle Connect For Health Colorado within a year, is an indication of how Republicans plan to chip away at Obamacare. If the federal health care law remains unchanged, it would force Coloradans shopping for private insurance to use the federal exchange. (AP photo/Brennan Linsley)

Conclusion

JESSICA M. MULLIGAN AND HEIDE CASTAÑEDA

Post Mortem: Resentment Trumped the Technocrats

When we started organizing this project in 2011, we could not anticipate how much we were studying a particular moment in time—a political, social, and historical convergence that made it possible for Barack Obama to win the presidency and then to push through health reform legislation. Nor did we anticipate how quickly that convergence would dissipate. In retrospect, we have new appreciation for how vulnerable and temporary policy programs can be, especially when promulgated by charismatic politicians instead of as the product of broader, bipartisan consensus. This ethnography of a major health policy, then, is an "anthropology of the present," where contestation was unremitting and the future always uncertain amid the unfolding of events (Wright and Reinhold 2011, 91–93).

We thought the Affordable Care Act reflected the "new normal," as a pro-market, managerial, and technocratic reform committed to for-profit insurance that also aimed to make the system a little more fair through consumer protections and funding to extend coverage. We assumed that after a period of dispute and controversy—and even a rocky rollout—the law would fade into the background and become taken for granted, following the well-worn pattern of other health overhauls.[1] This didn't happen.

Instead, riding a wave of anger largely fueled by discontented white supporters, we saw the rise of the Tea Party, major Democratic losses in the midterm elections, and then Donald Trump was elected president. In the very close 2016 election, Hillary Clinton promised to keep and fix the ACA through a series of technocratic adjustments, while Donald Trump tweeted incessantly that Obamacare was a "disaster" and the premiums were going through the roof (Diamond 2016). At the time, leading health policy scholars, however, were optimistic about the fate of the ACA and claimed that it was in fact working to expand coverage, despite small setbacks like rising premiums and insurers exiting the market (Altman 2016; Jost 2016). Trump both tapped into and fueled revulsion toward the ACA. Teasing out what this revulsion meant, however, is difficult because, when people criticized Obamacare, they did it for many different reasons that did not share one ideological viewpoint. Poll data show that major reasons for disliking the ACA included increased health costs, that it created too big a role for government, that it took the country in the "wrong direction" under President Obama, and that it did not go far enough in expanding coverage (KFF 2016c). In addition to these reasons, our ethnographic research has shown that people were dissatisfied because they felt that "others" (besides themselves) were benefiting more from the law; deductibles were too high; they experienced bureaucratic hurdles to enrollment; not all doctors would accept the coverage; they disagreed with the tax implications of the law; and the website was too difficult to navigate. While some of these reasons are ideological, many of them are related to price, the design of the law, and the growing pains of implementation. Furthermore, only a small minority of people in the United States (6%) ever actually got their health coverage through the ACA (20 million in 2016 out of a population of roughly 325 million). As we argue in this book, the law became a flashpoint for battles over inequality, fairness, and the role of government. It also became a vehicle for generating hostility toward women, immigrants, the poor, and racialized minorities. Politicians skillfully used these endless reserves of resentment to attack the law.

The ACA was also hampered by its own very complicated and multifaceted construction. It became a receptacle for all kinds of critiques, whether they were items contained in the law or not (definitely no "death panels"!) A public incident involving one of the law's architects, MIT economist Jonathan Gruber, is illustrative. A video of Gruber surfaced, in which he thanked "the stupidity of the American voter" for leading to the passage of the ACA and credited the law's lack of transparency for getting it passed (for example, the legislation painstakingly avoids calling the penalty for not enrolling in insurance a "tax") (Stoll 2016). This was a tone-deaf move, but also highlighted a tension between the policy elite and people who were experiencing the law on the ground.

Donald J. Trump @realDonaldTrump. October 25, 2013
First Titantic sunk on its maiden voyage. Next the Hindenburg explodes on its first flight to America. Now we suffer the ObamaCare rollout!

Donald J. Trump @realDonaldTrump. October 20, 2016
In addition to those without health coverage- those that have disastrous #Obamacare are seeing MASSIVE PREMIUM INCREASES. Repeal & replace.

Official Team Trump @TeamTrump, October 20, 2016
Thanks to Obama, 29 million people in America are still without health coverage

Donald J. Trump @realDonaldTrump. November 3, 2016
ObamaCare is a total disaster. Hillary Clinton wants to save it by making it even more expensive. Doesn't work, I will REPEAL AND REPLACE!

Figure C.3. Donald J. Trump tweets on Obamacare from 2013 and right before the 2016 election.

The law's architects—immersed as they were in health policy networks at elite foundations and Ivy League universities—devised many clever methods to bring people into coverage and to shepherd the law through development and passage. However, the result was so complicated and difficult to navigate that it became a stunning example of the distance between policy elites and the people for whom they supposedly design policies. While anthropologists have long been interested in the social production of expertise and experts (Carr 2010), it seems we must now look just as closely at the cracks in expertise and the ways in which people distrust and denigrate experts, often asserting the primacy of other forms of knowledge such as rumors, hoax news sources, and personal experience. The widespread discrediting of experts—from the pollsters who got the 2016 election wrong to the architects of the ACA—revealed cracks in the foundation of the technocratic project of state-making characteristic of neoliberalism. This signaled another move toward the policing and security state (Hyatt 2011) that Trump celebrated with his campaign promises to restore the honor of policing, build a wall between the United States and Mexico, and impede freedom of the press.[2]

Though some have decried that the election of Trump signified the end of truth and the beginning of a new "post-fact" era (Cohen 2016), we think it makes more sense to examine how the rules for making something true became a site of contestation. During the election, Trump's bombastic tone and demeanor evoked authenticity and spoke to a truth beyond the experts. But we should not have been surprised. In the chapter in this volume by Willging and Trott, the authors discuss how discourses of "truthiness" were widespread; they pervaded anti-fraud and audit efforts in New Mexico so that making a vague accusation, regardless of any evidence or specifics, was enough to shutter safety-net mental health institutions in the name of accountability. Rather than reviving a naïve positivism that holds that if we all just knew the facts, sound policy would prevail, we remain committed to an intersectional and post-positivist orientation to truth that recognizes that truths are social, constructed, and vary by one's subject position and perspective (Crenshaw 1991; Haraway 1999). More facts and even big data are not the antidote to new practices of truth-making. What we do need is theory, interpretive prowess, and an appreciation for the multiplicity of conflicting perspectives engendered by this novel political conjuncture. What does this all mean for the future of health reform in the United States? What does it mean for planning and evaluating health care policy? Contestation over facts and the fanning of resentment are likely to continue; as we have shown in this volume, the ACA entered into a landscape that was already highly stratified and historically volatile. A straightforward repeal of the law, however, does not appear likely, and repealing and replacing it is not supported by the majority of the American people (KFF 2016). As Republican health proposals were introduced into Congress in 2017, support for the ACA reached record levels (Pew Research Center 2017). Trump's offhanded comment that "nobody knew that health care could be so complicated" revealed how unprepared he was for the task at hand (Pear and Kelly 2017). Repealing the ACA turned into a conflict between those who wanted to maintain the ACA's coverage expansions and consumer protections and those who favored entitlement rollbacks and additional tax cuts for the wealthy.

Learning from Experiences with the ACA

Though the ACA's future remains uncertain, its tumultuous implementation offers lessons to students of policy. We turn now to synthesizing the insights and findings presented in this book. The ethnographic interventions in each of the chapters offer nuanced assessments of the ACA grounded in uninsured and newly insured people's experiences. In this final section, our frame is cross-cutting and draws together what the

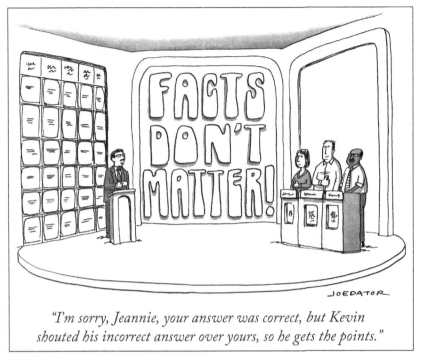

"I'm sorry, Jeannie, your answer was correct, but Kevin shouted his incorrect answer over yours, so he gets the points."

Figure C.4. *New Yorker* cartoon. Facts Don't Matter.

chapter authors learned in the nine states and from the hundreds of people they spoke to over the course of five years about the ACA. The following pages elaborate on lessons learned, and at the end of each we relate our findings to policy proposals that are on the table for the post-Obama era. Our analysis of the law is offered in the spirit of upholding its aspirations of making coverage affordable and accessible to all. To get to that place, it is important to better understand where the law succeeded, where it failed, and how it was able to generate such intense reactions from its detractors.

People Need and Want Affordable Coverage

Insurance matters, and there remains a profound unmet need for coverage and access to care in the United States. For the 20 million people who did gain access to coverage, it had profound impacts on their lives, when financial barriers like high deductibles, copays, and premiums could be overcome. For those who were able to gain access either through the expanded Medicaid program or through an affordable Marketplace plan, their lives were transformed for the better. In this book, we have recounted the stories of a person with Type 1 diabetes who could for the first time in a decade manage this chronic condition with insulin (Introduction); former cancer patients who were able to get the medication and ongoing follow-up care that they needed (Mulligan); young families able to procure health insurance for the first time in generations (Castañeda); low-income pregnant women who gained access to prenatal care (Andaya); immigrants of various statuses who were able to access primary and hospital care (Joseph); and families who got their vaccinations and attended to multiple health issues (Brunson). Without the law, these people and the millions of others who gained insurance through the ACA may again go without coverage.

But for many, financial barriers to coverage remained. Those in the coverage gap—below 100% of the federal poverty level in non-Medicaid expanding states—had no realistic options for getting covered, and their situations were made even worse as funds for safety-net and charity care dissipated. Those who were ineligible for cost-sharing reductions (above 250% of the poverty level) may have had coverage, but were priced out of all but routine, preventative care. High individual deductibles—ranging from $1,000-$6,000—proved an insurmountable barrier for many (Castañeda). Even for those on Medicaid, what might seem to policymakers like small fees—such as a few dollars for a prescription copay—prevented people with chronic disease from adhering to their medication regimens (Shaw). In these cases, people chose the medicines they thought were most important, skipped doses, or borrowed medication from family members when copays proved too high.

In addition to affordable coverage, people need comprehensive, integrated health services. The ACA went a long way toward attaining this goal by defining a package of basic required services that included things like prescription drug coverage, mental health parity, and maternity health services (which were too often left out of insurance packages prior to the ACA). The ACA improved access to behavioral health and addiction treatment for many, and these gains should be protected and extended (Frank, Beronio, and Glied 2014). Oral health, however, was not included among the Essential Health Benefits package and this continues to be a major problem. Oral diseases are among the most common and preventable health conditions in the United States (Mertz 2016). Though people could purchase dental coverage separately on ACA exchanges, it was not required. The human consequences of this policy decision are quite clear. We observed many people with unmet oral health needs attempting to access coverage, rubbing their mouths as they talked, and treating severe dental disease with over-the-counter pain medications like Advil.

In 2016, there were still more than 27 million people without coverage in the United States (KFF 2016a). Even this reduced number is unacceptable for a rich country. Every other economically advanced country provides universal access to health care (OECD 2014). But currently, the United States is poised to backslide. Without the ACA, the federal deficit will increase and the number of uninsured will skyrocket, according to CBO estimates (CBO 2015). The insured rate for non-elderly adults would drop almost immediately from its 2016 all-time high of 90% to an all-time low of 82% (CBO 2015, 8; KFF 2016a).

Though insurance certainly matters, a healthy nation is not determined only by the presence, absence, or type of health insurance. As research on the social determinants of health has shown us, stratification isn't just bad for policy, it also leads directly to poor health outcomes (Braveman et al. 2011). Social determinants of health include factors, aside from access to health care, that are determined by social and economic structures, policies, and inequalities, including the availability of healthy food, safe housing and working conditions, as well as freedom from the stressful effects of racism, sexism, and xenophobia. This too must be addressed. Massive tax cuts, downsizing the social safety net, and doubling down on aggressive and prejudicial policing would exacerbate inequality and further erode the social environment that creates the conditions for health. Instead, we desperately need health policies that expand coverage *and* reduce social inequalities.

Stratified Approaches to Expanding Access Generate Resentment

As the chapters in this book have shown, the Affordable Care Act expanded access through multiple levers: allowing young adults to remain on their parents' coverage until age 26; expanding Medicaid to poor adults up to 138% of the federal poverty level; and providing access to marketplace plans with income-based tax credits and cost-sharing reductions to help make coverage affordable. The most popular aspects of the law—outlawing limits on preexisting conditions and allowing young adults to stay on their parents' coverage—opened up access to coverage to more people. However, these popular provisions were paired with less popular ones, like the individual mandate in order to ensure that both the healthy and those with preexisting medical conditions got insured. The result was a policy compromise that balanced coverage expansions with financial guarantees for insurers.

One of the strongest lessons to be learned from this book is that when highly stratified approaches to expanding coverage are employed, it generates resentment. Means testing and the complicated formulas for calculating how much people would actually pay created multiple issues. Some people owed the IRS money at tax time, which did not create goodwill toward the law. People with seasonal, temporary, informal, or part-time work found it very difficult to navigate the income-calculating sections of the application. They were also informed—assuming that they had help with their application—that they needed to report any income changes to the exchange so that the amount of their subsidy could be recalculated each time. This burdened low-income workers with additional administrative tasks and put them at financial risk if they received too much in subsidies. As Andaya discussed with reference to the perceived disposability of poor people's time, and Joseph documented regarding intensive surveillance of poor women using public services, the poor have long been subjected to differential and more invasive and disrespectful treatment by public bureaucracies. Ongoing financial verifications, like those created by the ACA for monitoring insurance subsidies, have become common in post-welfare reform (PRWORA) social service provision (Morgen et al. 2010). However, middle-income people were not accustomed to and did not appreciate this degree of surveillance and monitoring.

Significant variations have always existed in the U.S. health care system where states are responsible for regulating insurance and setting Medicaid eligibility and coverage rules within federal guidelines. But in 2012, with the U.S. Supreme Court's decision to make Medicaid expansion optional, geography truly became destiny. Sered's research into un-insured people's experiences in five states made it abundantly clear that where one lived—in a Medicaid expanding or non-expanding state—inordinately shaped one's likelihood of obtaining affordable coverage. This in turn, impacted people's abilities to treat chronic health issues, recover from injuries, and stay in the workforce.

Another major finding related to stratification is that people did not understand how their subsidies were calculated or the other variables that affected the price of their coverage (Mulligan). They also talked to each other and compared outcomes, which were often wildly divergent in ways that did not make intuitive sense. The upshot? Obamacare seemed utterly unfair.

Though the individual mandate received a lot of attention and was the focus of challenges in the Supreme Court, it was not usually the main reason people were disgruntled. It is our belief that if people had gained access to truly affordable coverage that allowed them to meet their medical needs, the mandate would not have been such a huge issue. For many, though, the mandate stung because they felt that they were forced to buy useless insurance.

Virtually all of the major proposals for modifying the ACA will lead to erosions in coverage and will deteriorate the consumer protections created by the law, including the definition of comprehensive benefits and the law's existing (though insufficient) consumer and financial pro-tections. The proposals, if implemented, will also increase stratification, primarily by state of residence, income, gender, and race. Prohibitions on gender rating could disappear as well as protections for gender non-conforming individuals and same-sex partners. Individual states could still keep parts of the ACA if it is repealed; again, like the uneven imple-mentation we describe in this book, *where* one lives will make all the difference. Ironically, states that fully implemented the law may feel the difference most acutely if Medicaid expansion to poor adults is reversed and insurance subsidies on the exchanges eliminated.

Giving states more flexibility in designing their Medicaid programs—such as through block grants—could exacerbate existing disparities, es-pecially in terms of eligibility and ease of access to care (Rosenbaum et al. 2016). We saw in this volume how radically different Medicaid services and eligibility levels were for residents of Massachusetts, New

York, and Rhode Island compared to Texas, Mississippi, and Florida. In states that opted not to expand Medicaid, median eligibility thresholds for parents and childless adults were 45% and 0% of the federal poverty line respectively in 2015, while in states that opted to expand, both parents and childless adults were covered up to 138% (KFF 2015). States that are already among the stingiest with low eligibility thresholds and no coverage for childless adults are likely to remain that way, while more generous states will likely opt to continue providing a more robust safety net despite eroding federal support. For decades, we have seen a narrowing in health disparities by race for major outcomes such as life expectancy, infant mortality, and access to care (National Center for Health Statistics 2016). Given the racial disparities inherent in current Medicaid programs (many of the most restrictive programs serve states with large minority populations), the effects on raced-based health disparities could be catastrophic. The spillover effect on other Medicaid-eligible populations, like the elderly, children, and the disabled, is also a concern, especially if per capita spending limits are imposed on these populations (KFF 2016d). In the rush to take apart the ACA, other health programs are also vulnerable, even popular ones like Medicare, which are now being targeted for cost-cutting and additional benefit cuts, but not for supplier-side price controls like lower provider and prescription drug payments.

Enrollment and Accessing Coverage Shouldn't Be So Hard

Many chapters in this book detail how difficult it was for individuals and families to get enrolled, use their coverage, and keep up with their cost-sharing obligations. Though policymakers usually see these as distinct health policy issues, for people trying to navigate the system, they are deeply linked and experienced together.

Joseph described multiple forms of disentitlement experienced by immigrants in Massachusetts who were eligible for coverage, but not able to use it. Brunson showed how uninsured people in Texas were misinformed about the law and were excluded from coverage when they missed a deadline. Scott and Wright showed that enrolling people who are homeless requires multiple forms of ID and follow-through that might not be appropriate for this population. Shaw showed that for covered populations, changes to their drug formularies made in the name of cost-effectiveness created barriers to accessing needed care. Andaya showed that pregnant women had to navigate a complex mix of coverage options and that pregnancy afforded them temporary inclusion into the public Medicaid system which made care affordable, but also came with extra surveillance and being made to wait.

Taken together, we learn from these stories that poor and near-poor individuals are already overburdened with administrative tasks that compete with the daily struggles of getting to work, managing their chronic conditions, caring for children, and maintaining their households. Having to re-enroll annually, provide income updates, and navigate confusing plan structures and pricing is a big ask. Instead of generating increasingly clever plan designs and devising schemes to nudge poor people to behave like middle-class health care consumers, policymakers could devote their energies to simplifying the system and removing some of the burdens and responsibilities that have been hoisted onto low-income people.

Unfortunately, we are poised to move in the opposite direction. Proposed reforms to add work requirements, premiums, and other forms of cost-sharing for the poor will only exacerbate barriers to enrollment, inhibit continuity of coverage and care, and create additional administrative expense. Stringent enrollment policies join a long list of ideologically motivated efforts to limit the Medicaid rolls and reduce fraud. Ironically, these efforts can be counterproductive and far from cost-effective. A recent report from North Carolina documents that the state spent seven times more on Medicaid auditing than it recovered (North Carolina General Assembly 2016). The chapter in this volume by Willging and Trott vividly recounts the dangerous uses to which accountability talk can be put when false accusations of fraud were used to dismantle the behavioral health care safety net in New Mexico. Expanding access through insurance exchanges—which was an ideological concession to those who think that market-based private insurance is the only moral way to expand coverage in the United States—is more expensive than expanding through Medicaid. The Congressional Budget Office estimated that it cost the federal government $3,000 more for every individual who enrolled in private coverage via the Marketplace, and thus received tax credits and cost-sharing reductions, as opposed to Medicaid (CBO 2012, 4).

If our goal is to increase access to coverage and care, then enrollment and financing should be as simple and automatic as possible.

Anti-Immigrant Policies Are Anti-Health

The United States has a long history of distinguishing the "deserving" from the "non-deserving" in the design of social welfare programs. Since 1996, immigration status has become the major criterion for excluding people from health coverage and other social programs. The consequences of this policy decision are macabre and deadly, as demonstrated by Melo's research on kidney failure. Barred from insurance exchanges and Medicaid coverage, undocumented workers turned to hospitals for intermittent care, where the only requirement was that they be stabilized. Without access to the usual sources of primary and specialty care, those with chronic health conditions like diabetes and renal failure learned that the only path to treatment was to become sick enough to be admitted, over and over again, to an emergency department.

Joseph and Castañeda show how stratified forms of inclusion impacted immigrants in lawfully present statuses and in states that tried to provide universal access to coverage irrespective of immigration status. In both of their chapters, we saw how anti-immigrant policies spilled over and created downstream consequences, such as fear of driving to health facilities because of a possible traffic violation and fear of enrolling eligible family members in coverage when some members of the household were undocumented. Despite these barriers and the discrimination they faced, Castañeda found that many immigrants desired health insurance and would have liked the opportunity to purchase it on the exchange.

Thus, we see that anti-immigrant policies are anti-health. Beyond the exclusion created in the ACA, in recent years, immigration enforcement laws have aggravated undocumented immigrants' health-related vulnerabilities and threatened the health and well-being of their entire families, including U.S.-born citizen children. Enforcement efforts affect individual health behaviors and interpersonal relationships. And promote bias that can translate to poor care or experiences of discrimination in health service settings and result in people's inability or unwillingness to utilize health services for which they are eligible (Alexander and Fernandez 2014; Rhodes et al. 2015). The detrimental impact of deportation and detention on individual, family, and community health cannot be overstated (Allen et al. 2015). Immigration policy is not just a single policy issue among many, but rather part of a system of multiple components impacting health in the United States and producing structural vulnerability (Quesada, Hart, and Bourgois 2011).

Finale

The Affordable Care Act remains an important part of Barack Obama's legacy as a popular, though polemical, two-term president. The law was inherently hopeful: Its premise was that government could affect positive change, reduce inequality, and bring much-needed health care to those who were unable to access public programs or afford private insurance coverage. While the law was not perfect, it did expand coverage to 20 million people and provide new social protections through political and health inclusion.

The ACA built upon a long history of piecemeal changes to the U.S. health care system. Despite claims to the contrary, the ACA was not a radical reform—it left the entire health care system intact and simply expanded Medicaid for the poor and created new insurance marketplaces, known as exchanges, to sell private coverage. It provided new economic supports to make coverage more affordable for individuals, families, and small businesses. It did not, however, change the for-profit nature of the U.S. health care system, nor did it "socialize" medicine. In fact, in the end, it impacted only a small percentage of Americans. However, the discourse around it was radicalizing, tapping into and fueling resentments. What the law did and did not do was never well understood by the public, and this ambiguity was skillfully exploited by the law's foes, who blamed it for everything from rising prescription drug prices to factory closures.

Born of compromise, the ACA's ultimate downfall may have been that it was too modest. Its piecemeal and partial reforms left very few people satisfied—those on the left wanted more profound systemic reform and universal coverage, while those on the right decried government overreach and pointed to the law's failures (KFF 2016c). Many ordinary people, who did not identify strongly with either ideological pole, did understand that the law was not working well for them or the people they knew. The law also lacked a shared social purpose. When explaining the law and promoting it to the American people, President Obama often said, "If you like your coverage, you can keep it." In other words, for the 80% of people who were already insured, the ACA was not for them. As a strategy to build political support and institutionalize the law into a taken-for-granted entitlement, this was not an effective tactic. Future health reformers would do well to pay attention to how and why the ACA failed to garner widespread support. Perhaps in order to fully address the inequities and problems in the health care system, something much more profound is needed: attending first to widespread existing stratification in U.S. society. However, any effort in this direction must emerge from a shared social purpose and understanding of insurance rooted in mutual solidarity rather than consumer individualism.

This book illustrates four lessons. First, we learned that people in the United States want and need affordable health insurance coverage. However, stratified approaches to expanding access have the result of generating resentment. Coupled with difficult enrollment processes and barriers to accessing coverage, the law became unpopular and unusable for many. Finally, the outright exclusion of groups such as immigrants—to appeal to nationalists—had direct impacts on the law's success. These lessons are best understood through the frameworks of stratified citizenship (how different groups are viewed as deserving based on a gradation of rights and opportunities), notions of risk (since people assess and experience these as deeply connected to their class positions, sense of vulnerability, and social resources), and the devolution of responsibility onto individuals. As this book demonstrates, scholars and students of health policy need a nuanced conceptual toolkit that attends to more than just statistics, one that also examines the on-the-ground human experience of policy implementation and contextualizes experience within existing structures of inequality, modes of governance, and politics of resentment. It is our hope that future health reforms will build on these lessons rather than pursue health policies that increase inequality and stratification.

NOTES

1 The passage and implementation of Medicare and Medicaid in 1965 provides a telling counter-example for the ACA. Medicare and Medicaid represented an even more fundamental reform than the ACA, as they guaranteed a new federal role in health care financing and created a health care entitlement for the elderly (Cohen et al. 2015) Medicaid began as a welfare program, a federal-state partnership that provided care for some eligible poor people. Medicare was also responsible for legal desegregation in U.S. hospitals, since Medicare funds could not be assigned to segregated facilities. Together, these programs brought about a massive shift in the role of government, hospital financing, and the social distribution of medical care. Nonetheless, Medicare became popular very quickly, a fate the ACA never experienced.

2 Trump tweeted repeatedly during the Democratic Convention regarding law and order and restoring honor to the police. Some representative examples from the Twitter handle @realDonaldTrump include: "The Democratic Convention has paid ZERO respect to the great police and law enforcement professionals of our country. No recognition—SAD!" from July 27; "Why aren't the Democrats speaking about ISIS, bad trade deals, broken borders, police and law and order. The Republican Convention was great" from July 26; and "Shooting deaths of police officers up 78% this year. We must restore law and order and protect our great law enforcement officers!" from July 27.

REFERENCES

Alexander, William L., and Magdalena Fernandez. 2014. Immigration Policing and Medical Care for Farmworkers: Uncertainties and Anxieties in the East Coast Migrant Stream. *North American Dialogue* 17 (1): 13–30.

Allen, Brian, Erica M. Cisneros, and Alexandra Tellez. 2015. The Children Left Behind: The Impact of Parental Deportation on Mental Health. *Journal of Child and Family Studies* 24 (2): 386–392.

Altman, Drew. 2016. The ACA Marketplace Problems in Context (and Why They Don't Mean Obamacare Is 'Failing'). *Wall Street Journal*, August 29. blogs.wsj.com.

Braveman, Paula, Susan Egerter, and David R. Williams. 2011. The Social Determinants of Health: Coming of Age. *Annual Reviews of Public Health* 32: 381–398.

Carr, E. Summerson. 2010. Enactments of Expertise. *Annual Review of Anthropology* 39: 17–32.

Cohen, Alan B., David C. Colby, Keith A. Wailoo, and Julian E. Zelizer. 2015. Introduction: Medicare, Medicaid, and the Moral Test of Government. In *Medicare and Medicaid at Fifty: America's Entitlement Programs in the Age of Affordable Care*. Julian E. Zelizer, Keith Wailoo, and David C. Colby, eds. Pp. xi–xx. New York: Oxford University Press.

Cohen, Roger. 2016. Trump and the End of Truth. *New York Times*, July 25.

Congressional Budget Office (CBO). 2015. Budgetary and Economic Effects of Repealing the Affordable Care Act. www.cbo.gov.

———. 2012. Estimates for the Insurance Coverage Provisions of the Affordable Care Act Updated for the Recent Supreme Court Decision, 4, (July 2012). www.cbo.gov.

Crenshaw, Kimberle. 1991. Mapping the Margins: Intersectionality, Identity Politics, and Violence against Women of Color. *Stanford Law Review* 43(6): 1241–1299.

Diamond, Dan. 2016. How Trump Tweets about Obamacare. Politico.com. www.politico.com.

Frank, Richard G., Kirsten Beronio, and Sherry A. Glied. 2014. Behavioral Health Parity and the Affordable Care Act. *Journal of Social Work in Disability and Rehabilitation* 13(0): 31–43.

Haraway, Donna. 1999. Situated Knowledges: The Science Question in Feminism and the Privilege of Partial Perspective. In *The Science Studies Reader.* Mario Biagiolo, ed. Pp. 172–188. New York: Routledge.

Hyatt, Susan Brin. 2011. What Was Neoliberalism and What Comes Next? The Transformation of Citizenship in the Law-and-Order State. In *Policy Worlds: Anthropology and the Analysis of Contemporary Power.* Cris Shore, Susan Wright, and Davide Però, eds. Pp. 105–123. New York: Berghahn Books.

Jost, Timothy. 2016. Health Care Reform and a Failed Vision of Bipartisanship. *Health Affairs* 35(10): 1748–1752.

Kaiser Family Foundation (KFF). 2016a. The Affordable Care Act's Little-Noticed Success: Cutting the Uninsured Rate. kff.org.

———. 2016b. After the Election, the Public Remains Sharply Divided on Future of the Affordable Care Act. Kaiser Family Foundation. kff.org.

———. 2016c. Data Note: Americans' Opinions of the Affordable Care Act. Kaiser Family Foundation. kff.org.

———. 2016d. Key Medicaid Questions Post-Election. Kaiser Family Foundation. kff.org.

———. 2015. Modern Era Medicaid: Findings from a 50-State Survey of Eligibility, Enrollment, Renewal, and Cost-Sharing Policies in Medicaid and CHIP as of January 2015. Kaiser Family Foundation. kff.org.

Mertz, Elizabeth. 2016. The Dental-Medical Divide. *Health Affairs* 35(12): 2168–2175.

Morgen, Sandra, Joan Acker, and Jill Weigt. 2010. *Stretched Thin: Poor Families, Welfare Work, and Welfare Reform.* Ithaca, NY: Cornell University Press.

Mosse, David. 2006. Anti-social Anthropology? Objectivity, Objection, and the Ethnography of Public Policy and Professional Communities. *Journal of the Royal Anthropological Institute* 12(4): 935–956.

National Center for Health Statistics. 2016. *Health, United States, 2015: In Brief.* Hyattsville, MD.

North Carolina General Assembly. 2016. Medicaid Program Integrity Section Is Not Cost-Effectively Identifying and Preventing Fraud, Waste, and Abuse. Final Report to the Joint Legislative Program Evaluation Oversight Committee. Report Number 2016-10 November 14, 2016. www.ncga.state.nc.us.

Organization of Economic Cooperation and Development (OECD). 2014. OECD Health Statistics 2014. How Does the United States Compare? www.oecd.org.

Pear, Robert and Kate Kelly. 2017. Trump Concedes Health Law Overhaul Is "Unbelievably Complex." *New York Times*, February 27. www.nytimes.com.

Pew Research Center. 2017. Support for 2010 Health Care Law Reaches New High. www.pewresearch.org.

Quesada, James, Laurie Kain Hart, and Philippe Bourgois. 2011. Structural Vulnerability and Health: Latino Migrant Laborers in the United States. *Medical Anthropology* 30 (4): 339–362.

Rhodes, Scott D., Lilli Mann, Florence M. Simán, Eunyoung Song, Jorge Alonzo, Mario Downs, Emma Lawlor, Omar Martinez, Christina J. Sun, and Mary Claire O'Brien. 2015. The Impact of Local Immigration Enforcement Policies on the Health of Immigrant Hispanics/Latinos in the United States. *American Journal of Public Health* 105 (2): 329–337.

Rosenbaum, Sara, Sara Schmucker, Sara Rothenberg, and Rachel Gunsalus. 2016. What Would Block Grants or Limits on Per Capita Spending Mean for Medicaid? The Commonwealth Fund, November 2016. www.commonwealthfund.org.

Stoll, Ira. 2016. Call It the Jonathan Gruber Election. *New Boston Post*. newbostonpost .com.

Wright, Susan, and Sue Reinhold. 2011. "Studying Through": A Strategy for Studying Political Transformation. Or Sex, Lies and British Politics. In *Policy Worlds: Anthropology and the Analysis of Contemporary Power*. Cris Shore, Susan Wright, and Davide Però, eds. Pp. 86–104. New York: Berghahn Books.

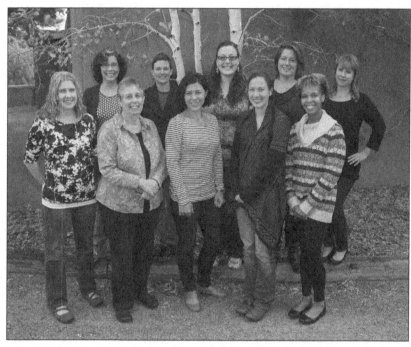

Figure AA.1. Photo of authors, School for Advanced Research, Santa Fe, New Mexico.

ABOUT THE EDITORS

Jessica M. Mulligan is Associate Professor of Health Policy and Management at Providence College. Her current research explores insurance, financial security, and health reform from the perspective of the newly insured and those who continue to lack coverage. She is the author of *Unmanageable Care: An Ethnography of Health Care Privatization in Puerto Rico* (NYU Press, 2014) as well as multiple journal articles.

Heide Castañeda is Associate Professor of Anthropology at the University of South Florida and is the author of dozens of articles on health care access for immigrant and minority populations. Her research on health care policy has been funded by the National Science Foundation, Fulbright Program, and the Wenner-Gren Foundation for Anthropological Research.

Elise Andaya is Associate Professor of Anthropology at the University at Albany (SUNY) and the author of *Conceiving Cuba: Reproduction, Women, and the State in the Post-Soviet Era* (2014), which won the 2015 Adele Clarke Book Award for Best Book on Reproduction and was awarded Honorable Mention for the 2015 Michelle Rosaldo Book Award for Best First Book in Feminist Anthropology. She has also written a number of articles and book chapters on gender and reproduction in Cuba and in the United States. Her research has been funded by the Wenner-Gren Foundation and by Fulbright-Hays, as well as by institutional faculty grants.

Emily K. Brunson is Assistant Professor of Anthropology at Texas State University and the author of several articles on topics related to health care access and decision-making.

Tiffany D. Joseph is Assistant Professor of Sociology at Stony Brook University and author of *Race on the Move: Brazilian Migrants and the Global Reconstruction of Race* (2015).

Milena Andrea Melo is Assistant Professor of Anthropology at Mississippi State University. She is the 2017–2018 Andrew W. Mellon Fellow in Latino Studies at the School for Advanced Research. Melo's research has been funded by the Ford Foundation, the National Science Foundation, and the American Anthropological Association.

Mary Alice Scott is Assistant Professor of Anthropology and affiliated faculty in Public Health Sciences at New Mexico State University. She is also adjunct research faculty at the Southern New Mexico Family Medicine Residency Program.

Susan Sered is Professor of Sociology at Suffolk University and author of *Uninsured in America: Life and Death in the Land of Opportunity* (2005) and *Can't Catch a Break: Gender, Drugs, Jail, and the Limits of Personal Responsibility* (2015).

Susan J. Shaw is Associate Professor in the Department of Health Promotion and Policy, University of Massachusetts School of Public Health and Health Sciences. She is the author of *Governing How We Care: Contesting Community and Defining Difference in U.S. Public Health Programs* (2012).

Elise M. Trott earned a PhD in Anthropology at the University of New Mexico. She researches communal water management in New Mexico in relation to social justice, environmental health, and community well-being. She is the recipient of a Mellon doctoral dissertation completion fellowship and graduated in 2017.

Cathleen E. Willging is Director of the Behavioral Health Research Center of the Pacific Institute of Research and Evaluation and is the author of numerous publications.

Richard Wright holds an MA in Anthropology. He works as a manager for a Behavioral Health Program at a Federally Qualified Health Center in Southern New Mexico.

INDEX

Printed in the United States
By Bookmasters